Men's Health

Vasan S S • Fahim L. H. Rajiwate
Peter H. C. Lim
Editors

Men's Health

Second Edition

Springer

Editors
Vasan S S
Ankur Healthcare
Bangalore, Karnataka, India

Fahim L. H. Rajiwate
Ankur Healthcare / Raja Rajeswari Medical College and Hospital
Bengarluru, Karnataka, India

Peter H. C. Lim
Department of Andrology, Urology and Continence Centre
Gleneagles Hospital
Singapore, Singapore

ISBN 978-3-031-76897-2 ISBN 978-3-031-76898-9 (eBook)
https://doi.org/10.1007/978-3-031-76898-9

This Springer imprint is published by the registered company Springer Nature Switzerland AG
The registered company address is: Gewerbestrasse 11, 6330 Cham, Switzerland

Foreword

I am delighted to writing the foreword for the second edition of Professor Peter Lim's *Men's Health*. This was long overdue, following the success of the first edition, and now with his dynamic co-editors. Dr. Fahim Rajiwate and Dr. Vasan SS, the content has been expanded with beautiful figures, diagrams, and tables.

The content has been divided into four parts: Hypogonadism, ejaculatory dysfunction, sexually transmitted diseases, and men's health. All the contents are highly informative for international specialists, while also including specific chapters that are more relevant to the local region, specifically Singapore.

The first part on hypogonadism teaches us the basic science behind testosterone pathologies and treatments, including up to date discussions on all the controversial topics, particularly when to treat and when not to. I enjoyed the chapter on traditional Asian herbs, which is new to me.

The second part on ejaculatory dysfunction mainly focuses on premature ejaculation, which is sensible, considering its prevalence. The journey starts again with basic science, classification, and etiologies, before delving into the clinical aspects. Additionally, delayed, retrograde, and anejaculation are also covered.

The next part on sexually transmitted diseases is straight to the point and covers what is relevant for the specialist in men's health. Finally, the last part focuses on men's health, which deals with areas not related to sexual function, such as cardiac protection and prevention, which, as physicians, we are obligated to promote.

Overall this is a comprehensive and easy to read book, which is a must for doctors dealing with men's health.

Prof. David Ralph

Professor of Urology
University College London,
St Peter's Andrology
London, UK

Chairman, EAU Section of Genito-Urinary
Reconstructive Surgeons
King Edward VII Hospital
London, UK

Foreword

The update of this book, first published in 2013, is long overdue. Notably, in the field of hypogonadism, remarkable progress has been made. It has become clear that optimal effects of testosterone therapy can only be achieved through long-term treatment. Consequently, hypogonadism should be considered a chronic disease, necessitating lifelong treatment. Unfortunately, it is impossible to conduct randomized, placebo-controlled studies (RCTs) over a sufficiently long period of time. Throughout the history of clinical experience with testosterone therapy spanning approximately 80 years, only four RCTs with a duration of 3 years were performed, and not all of them strictly adhered to the definition of hypogonadism as per today's guidelines. Hence, we have to rely on the second best approach to gather information about long-term testosterone therapy. This would be real-world evidence, and we are fortunate to have several registry studies which are based on very precise data collections and the highest possible level of medication adherence. From such studies, treatment data up to 11 years of follow-up have been published. The lessons learned from these studies, go far beyond the original understanding of testosterone, i.e. that it regulates reproductive and sexual functions. The most powerful findings of the observational registry studies suggest that

1. Long-term testosterone therapy is associated with substantial and sustained weight loss.
2. Long-term testosterone therapy can prevent the progression from prediabetes to type 2 diabetes.
3. Long-term testosterone therapy may result in remission of type 2 diabetes.
4. Long-term testosterone therapy is associated with a reduced incidence of prostate cancer.
5. Long-term testosterone therapy is associated with reduced cardiovascular events and mortality.

Since 2016, the three largest randomized, placebo-controlled studies in the history of testosterone therapy have been conducted. The "T4DM" study confirmed that the rate of progression from prediabetes to type 2 diabetes was indeed significantly lower in the testosterone-treated patients. It also showed that a certain proportion of men who had been newly diagnosed with type 2 diabetes at baseline no longer had type 2 diabetes after 2 years of intervention, this proportion being higher in the testosterone-treated group. The "T-Trials" demonstrated that in a population of men aged 65 years and older, there was no increased risk of prostate cancer or cardiovascular events. This was consistent with "T4DM" results. Finally, the "TRAVERSE" study was performed upon request by the FDA. The study population consisted of men at a high risk of cardiovascular events. Testosterone therapy led to neither increased cardiovascular nor prostate cancer risk.

The fact that the three largest RCTs were consistent regarding potential risks of testosterone therapy is gradually integrated into clinical guidelines, such as the guidelines of the British Society of Sexual Medicine (BSSM) and the European Association of Urology (EAU). Let us hope that in the future, testosterone therapy will be recognized for its positive effects, rather than being viewed with great caution due to its perceived risks. In the experience of many clinicians, testosterone therapy—where indicated—is one of the most beneficial and indeed life-changing treatments available to men.

This new edition covers many other aspects relating to men's health somewhat in great detail and depth to enable the clinician to treat comprehensively the disorders using the practical pearls of wisdom imparted by the respective authors not usually found in texts on *Men's Health*.

Heartfelt congratulations to the editors Professor Peter Lim, Dr. Fahim Rajiwate, Dr. Vasan SS and authors on this excellent contribution to this important new field of clinical medicine.

Hamburg, Germany Farid Saad

References

1. Saad F, Doros G, Haider KS, Haider H. Differential effects of 11 years of long-term injectable testosterone undecanoate therapy on anthropometric and metabolic parameters in hypogonadal men with normal weight, overweight and obesity in comparison with untreated controls: real-world data from a controlled registry study. Int J Obes (Lond). 2020;44(6):1264–78.
2. Yassin A, Haider A, Haider KS, Caliber M, Doros G, Saad F, Garvey WT. Testosterone therapy in men with hypogonadism prevents progression from prediabetes to type 2 diabetes: Eight-year data from a registry study. Diabetes Care. 2019;42(6):1104–11.
3. Haider KS, Haider A, Saad F, Doros G, Hanefeld M, Dhindsa S, Dandona P, Traish A. Remission of type 2 diabetes following long-term treatment with injectable testosterone undecanoate in patients with hypogonadism and type 2 diabetes: 11-year data from a real-world registry study. Diabetes Obes Metab. 2020;22(11):2055–68.

4. Yassin A, Salman M, Talib RA, Yassin D-J. Is there a protective role of testosterone against high-grade prostate cancer? Incidence and severity of prostate cancer in 553 patients who underwent prostate biopsy: a prospective data register. Aging Male. 2017;20(2):125–33.
5. Zhang X, Zhong Y, Saad F, Haider KS, Haider A, Clendenin AG, Xu X. Testosterone therapy may reduce prostate cancer risk due to testosterone deficiency at a young age via stabilizing serum testosterone levels. Aging Male. 2020;23(2):112–8.
6. Traish AM, Haider A, Haider KS, Doros G, Saad F. Long-term testosterone therapy improves cardiometabolic function and reduces risk of cardiovascular disease in men with hypogonadism: a real-life observational registry study setting comparing treated and untreated (control) groups. J Cardiovasc Pharmacol Ther. 2017;22(5):414–33.
7. Zhang X, Huang K, Saad F, Haider KS, Haider A, Xu X. Testosterone therapy reduces cardiovascular risk among hypogonadal men: a prospective cohort study in Germany. Androg Clin Res Ther. 2020;2(1):64–72.
8. Wittert G, Bracken K, Robledo KP, Grossmann M, Yeap BB, Handelsman DJ, Stuckey B, Conway A, Inder W, McLachlan R, Allan C, Jesudason D, Fui MNT, Hague W, Jenkins A, Daniel M, Gebski V, Keech A. Testosterone treatment to prevent or revert type 2 diabetes in men enrolled in a lifestyle programme (T4DM): a randomised, double-blind, placebo-controlled, 2-year, phase 3b trial. Lancet Diabetes Endocrinol. 2021;9(1):32–45.
9. Snyder PJ, Bhasin S, Cunningham GR, Matsumoto AM, Stephens-Shields AJ, Cauley JA, Gill TM, Barrett-Connor E, Swerdloff RS, Wang C, Ensrud KE, Lewis CE, Farrar JT, Cella D, Rosen RC, Pahor M, Crandall JP, Molitch ME, Cifelli D, Dougar D, Fluharty L, Resnick SM, Storer TW, Anton S, Basaria S, Diem SJ, Hou X, Mohler ER 3rd, Parsons JK, Wenger NK, Zeldow B, Landis JR, Ellenberg SS; Testosterone Trials Investigators. Effects of testosterone treatment in older men. N Engl J Med. 2016;374(7):611–24.
10. Lincoff AM, Bhasin S, Flevaris P, Mitchell LM, Basaria S, Boden WE, Cunningham GR, Granger CB, Khera M, Thompson IM Jr, Wang Q, Wolski K, Davey D, Kalahasti V, Khan N, Miller MG, Snabes MC, Chan A, Dubcenco E, Li X, Yi T, Huang B, Pencina KM, Travison TG, Nissen SE; TRAVERSE Study Investigators. Cardiovascular safety of testosterone-replacement therapy. N Engl J Med. 2023;389(2):107–17.

Contents

Part I
Hypogonadism

Chapter 1
Epidemiology: Late-Onset Hypogonadism in Singapore

Peter Huat Chye Lim

Situation in Singapore Survey on Andropause/ Late-Onset Hypogonadism

Singapore's population is aging rapidly with concurrent increase in life expectancy (74 years). Increased life expectancy and aging inflict social, health, and economic problems. A nationwide, prospective, cross-sectional, validated questionnaire-based survey was conducted in 2001 to assess andropausal symptoms and their potential implications in 228 subjects (between 45 and 70 years) of Chinese (60%), Malay (20%), and Indian (20%) races. In total, 39.5% of Singaporean males were aware of the term male menopause or andropause and 35% signified it as normal sign of aging, requiring medical treatment (12%). Physical- or vasomotor-associated problems were found to be more predominant (32%) than psychological (28.9%) and sexual (12.3%) problems. Lack of physical energy (73.7%) and pains in bones and joints (53.1%) were the most commonly felt physical problems, whereas memory impairment (47.4%) and irritability (41.7%) constituted the psychological symptoms. Absence of nocturnal erection, lack of sexual excitement, loss of interest in sex, failures in sexual act, and poor erections dominated the sexual problems in

---

P. H. C. Lim (✉)
Department of Andrology, Urology Continence Centre, Gleneagles Hospital, Singapore, Singapore

H.T. Naval Medical School, Surabaya, Indonesia

Edith Cowan University, Joondalup, WA, Australia

Society for Men's Health Singapore, Midview City, Singapore

Singapore Gleneagles Medical Centre, Singapore, Singapore

Department of Urology, Changi General Hospital, Singapore, Singapore
e-mail: tphphcl@pacific.net.sg

Vasan S S et al. (eds.), *Men's Health*,
https://doi.org/10.1007/978-3-031-76898-9_1

50.9, 42.1, 41.7, 41.2, and 38.2% of subjects, respectively. A significant proportion of population (81.2%) reported that treatment is necessary for andropause and 45.6% preferred treatment with a general practitioner. In Singaporean aging men, *diminishing sexual function (75%) including ED (51.5%) and lack of physical energy (73.7%) were the predominant andropausal symptoms* requiring treatment. Singaporeans preferred natural approaches for andropausal symptoms (84.2%), and 39.9% cited treatment is not necessary. Among the andropausal symptoms in Singaporean men, lowered sexual function figured the highest and most important symptom. As the proportion of aging men is likely to increase in the near future, providing better quality of life has become a necessity in these populations with the potential assessment of male menopause.

Singapore Survey on Perception of Male Hormone Replacement Therapy (HRT) in Singaporean Males

Hormone replacement therapy (HRT) has been accepted as a regular clinical practice in the Western world. However, the prevailing scenario with respect to HRT in Asia is still largely controversial and generally not fully accepted by the public and medical practitioners. In 2001, a nationwide, prospective, cross-sectional, validated, questionnaire-based study evaluated the perception of aging males (45–70 years) in the multiracial population of Singapore for HRT. In Singapore, only 36.8% of aging men knew about hormone replacement and its different modalities, and 63.2% were unaware of the same. Nearly 46% indicated that the risk of taking hormones outweighs its potential benefits, and 46.5% believe that hormones may lead to cancer (in particular prostate cancer). Although media (TV, radio) (26.8%) and newspapers (30.2%) were the main source of information on HRT, 41.7% did not bother to get any information on HRT. Interestingly, only 10.5% of the subjects received information from medical professionals. With respect to treatment, never, previous, and current users of HRT were 98.7, 0.4, and 0.9%, respectively. *Lack of awareness (56.3%) and preference for herbal treatment (23.9%) were the main reasons for higher proportion of nonusers of HRT*. Thus, the medical and social taboo about HRT in Singaporean males is high, suggesting the need for orientation and education to get men to achieve a better quality of life despite aging and late-onset hypogonadism.

Incidence of Hypogonadism in Primary Care

Incidence of hypogonadism in the population of primary care practices was assessed by a health screening. A primary care clinic-based health screening ($n = 1000$) was performed in Singapore. The screening assessed androgen deficiency/hypogonadism by applying the aging male symptoms (AMS) rating scale and biochemical

Demographic variable – age:

Age Group	Total	Percentage(%)
Below 45	128	12.79
45–49	127	12.69
50–54	195	19.48
55–59	212	21.18
60–64	141	14.09
65–69	77	7.69
Above 69	51	5.09
NA (age not available)	70	6.99
Mean		54.70

Fig. 1.1 Age distribution of hypogonadism patients

quantification of testosterone level. In addition, the sexual health function was also further elucidated by the International Index of Erectile Dysfunction (IIEF) scores.

Of the 1000 patients screened between 17 Oct 2007 and 30 Sept 2009, the mean age of the population was 54.7 years (Fig. 1.1), and nearly *26.37% were noted to have some form (mild, moderate, and severe) of androgen deficiency* according to the AMS rating scale (Fig. 1.2). Of this, 19.08% had mild deficiency, 3.2% had moderate deficiency, while severe deficiency was identified in 4.10% of respondents. With respect to age, higher incidence was determined in men above 69 years of age (43.4%, odds ratio 3.44), whereas men between the age of 45 and 69 had an average incidence of 17.9%, odds ratio 0.91. The primary medical conditions among the survey population were diabetes, hyper-cholesterol, hypertension, obesity, and prostate problems, respectively, in 17, 33, 35, 26, and 5%, while *androgen deficiency was 38, 25, 24, 28, and 30% in people with diabetes, hyper-cholesterol, hypertension, obesity, and prostate problems, respectively* (Fig. 1.3). The survey highlighted that our Singapore population had more physiological (97%) and sexual problems (95%) compared to psychological (91%). Sexual function as assessed by AMS rating scale showed that only 6.3% had a normal function and 90.2% had below- average function. Of this, 20 and 11.4% were androgen deficient at below-average and normal sexual function, respectively. Sexual function was further analyzed by IIEF scores and severe, moderate, mild to moderate, and mild ED were 36.1, 31.4, 22.8, and 6.3%, respectively, and in this population the presence of androgen deficiency was 37.2, 35.1, 24.9, and 30% at these grades of ED (Fig. 1.4).

These results highlight that diabetes and prostate disorders have greater influence on the status of androgen deficiency and its associated disorders compared to other medical conditions. Androgen deficiency impacts significantly on physiological and sexual function. Hence, a greater awareness of the condition and a crying need for remedial measures for androgen deficiency or hypogonadism is warranted as it has significant effect on overall health and well-being in Singaporean men in view of the aging population in Singapore.

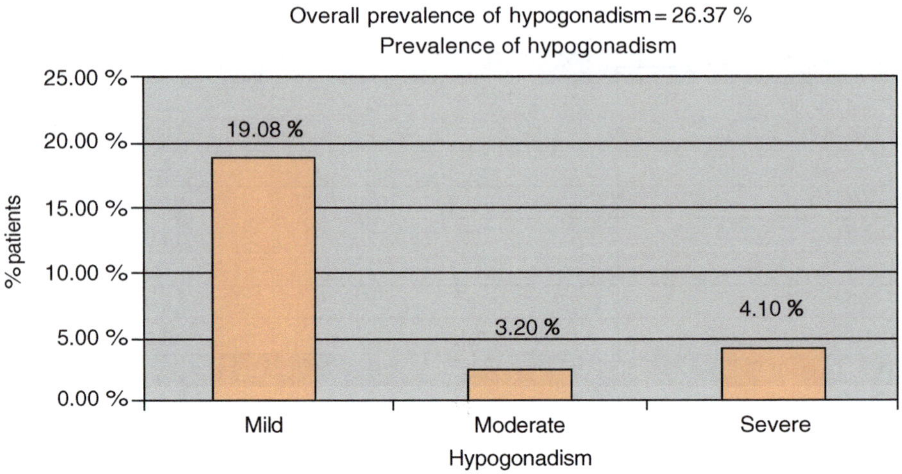

Fig. 1.2 Prevalence of hypogonadism in Singapore

Medical conditions and odds ratio of developing hypogonadism

	YES		NO	
	Odds ratio	*p*-value	Odds ratio	*p*-value
Cigarette smoking	0.163	<0.001	6.143	<0.001
Exercise	65.000	<0.001	184.000	<0.001
Overweight	6.267	<0.001	9.333	<0.001
High cholesterol	5.368	<0.00	16.842	<0.001
Drug allergy	3.857	<0.001	31.286	<0.001
Hypertension	18.000	<0.001	23.333	<0.001
Diabetes	9.429	<0.001	25.857	<0.001
Prostate problem	0.680	0.220	8.360	<0.001
Erectile dysfunction	12.824	<0.001	0.078	<0.001

odds ratio reveal that medical factors such as smoking, exercise, overweight, high cholesterol, hypertension, diabetes and ED have higher odds of developing hypogonadism

Fig. 1.3 Medical conditions and risk of hypogonadism

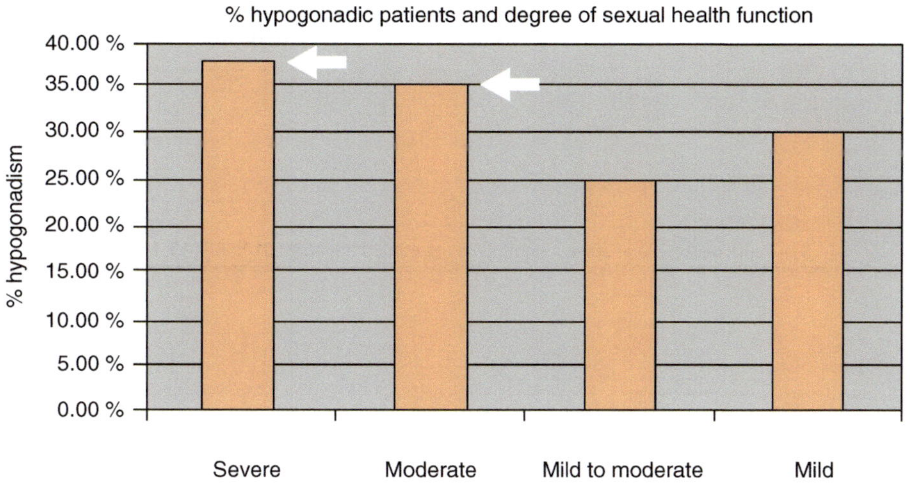

Fig. 1.4 Hypogonadism patients and degree of sexual health function

Bibliography

1. Lim PHC. Results from a men's health screening for hypogonadism in primary health care—1000 men with clinical & biochemical diagnostic confirmation. Project of the Society for Men's health Singapore, Singapore. 2007–2009.
2. Quek P, Khin LW, Lim PHC. National survey on knowledge, attitudes and practices relating to "Andropause" in Singapore. Joint project of MRC, Clinical Trials & Epidemiology Research Unit, Min of Health & the Society for Men's Health, Singapore. 2001.

Chapter 2
Physiology of Aging and Pathophysiology of Late/Adult-Onset Hypogonadism (LOH/AOH)

Fahim L. H. Rajiwate

Male "andropause" is similar to female "menopause" in terminological sense but is not functionally equivalent. In females, menopause represents the cessation of reproductive potential by near-total stoppage of gonadal sex steroid production. On the contrary, in a healthy male, androgen production as well as fertility are largely preserved, until very old age. To understand the pathophysiology of aging male, we need to have a brief about the functional physiology of male, which is discussed below.

The hypothalamic-pituitary-gonadal (HPG) axis forms the backbone of the endocrine regulation of gonadal function of a male. The key players in this regulatory circuit are the two anterior pituitary gonadotropins, namely the luteinizing hormone (LH) and follicle-stimulating hormone (FSH) and their specific receptors expressed in gonadal target cells.

(HPG) axis undergoes changes during the intrauterine, prenatal, pubertal, and adult stages of life. The HPG axis begins development in utero with the hypothalamic gonadotropin-releasing hormone (GnRH) at around 10 weeks and the pituitary luteinizing hormone (LH) and follicle-stimulating hormone (FSH) by 10–15 weeks gestation (Kaplan et al. 1976). These are responsible for the development of Wolffian duct structures, formation and descend of testis, and inhibition of Mullerian duct in an XY male fetus. At birth, in the immediate postnatal period, there is a brief surge of gonadotropins due to withdrawal of maternal hormones, called as "Mini Puberty" priming the gonads for puberty and brain for further physio-psycho-social development as an adult male.

F. L. H. Rajiwate (✉)
Ankur Healthcare / Raja Rajeswari Medical College and Hospital,
Bengarluru, Karnataka, India

Vasan S S et al. (eds.), *Men's Health*,
https://doi.org/10.1007/978-3-031-76898-9_2

The HPG Axis in Male

The cells of arcuate nuclei of hypothalamus secrete gonadotropin-releasing hormone (10 amino acid peptide). Endings of these neurons terminate in median eminence of hypothalamus. From here, gonadotropin-releasing hormone passes through hypothalamo-hypophysial portal system to anterior pituitary where it stimulates secretion of luteinizing hormone (LH) and follicle-stimulating hormone (FSH) (Fig. 2.1). Gonadotropin-releasing hormone (GnRH) is secreted intermittently a few minutes at a time once every 1–3 h. GnRH mainly controls LH secretion. LH and FSH are glycoproteins and the differences are depicted in Table 2.1.

Both these hormones affect target cells by activating cyclic AMP second messenger system, which in turn activates specific enzyme system in respective target cells (Fig. 2.2). Luteinizing hormone stimulates interstitial cells of Leydig in testes to secrete testosterone, which has a reciprocal effect on pituitary to inhibit LH secretion in two ways (Fig. 2.3):

(a) Greater part of inhibition of LH secretion results from direct effect of testosterone on decreasing GnRH secretion (negative feedback effect).
(b) Testosterone also has a weak negative feedback effect on anterior pituitary to inhibit secretion of LH. There is also a negative feedback control of seminiferous tubule activity (rate of spermatogenesis) through hormone inhibin on release of FSH and to a certain extent on release of GnRH.

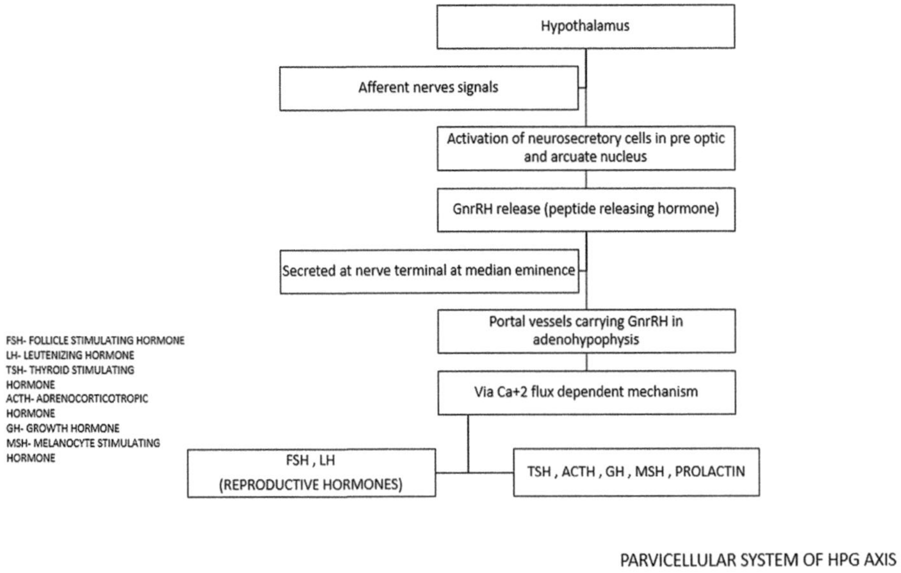

Fig. 2.1 The HPG axis in male

Table 2.1 The difference between the LH and FSH are enumerated below

	FSH	LH
Molecule	β- Polypeptide	β - Polypeptide
Alpha subunit	92 amino acid	92 amino acid
Alpha gene chromosome	6q 14.3	6q 12.21
Beta subunit	111 amino acid	120 amino acid
Beta gene chromosome	11p 13	19q 13.32
Biological half life	3–4 h	20 min
Secretory pulse	Every 1.5 h	8–10 pulse/day
Pulse amplitude	Variable and small, with fluctuations of up to 25%	Variable by one to three-fold
GnRH response	Difficult to assess Activin and inhibin affect secretion (relative secretory independence)	Easier to assess

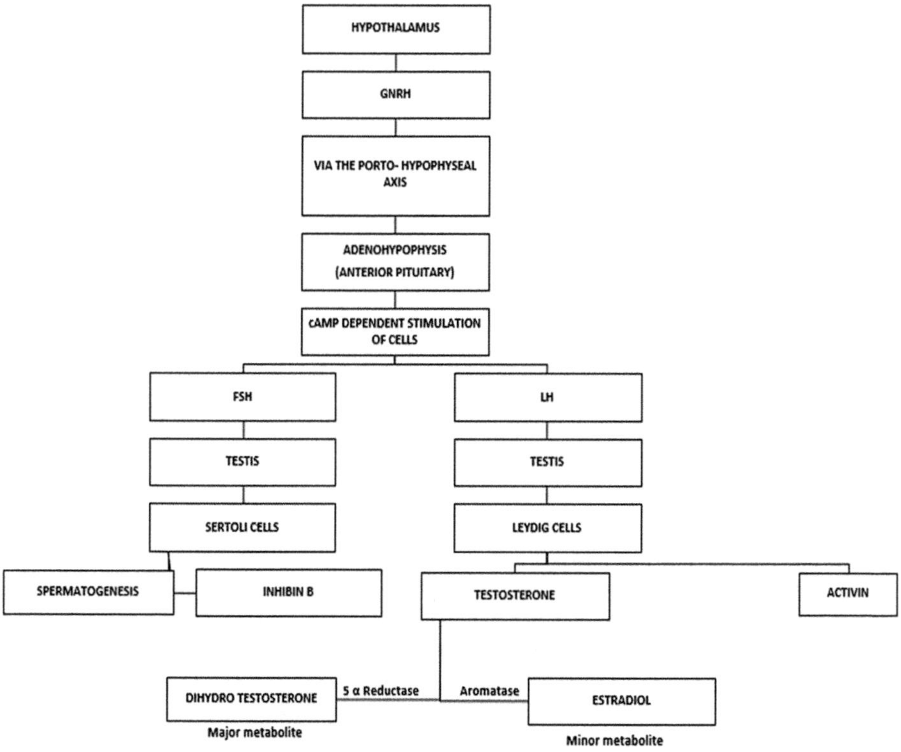

Fig. 2.2 Physiological role of male reproductive hormones

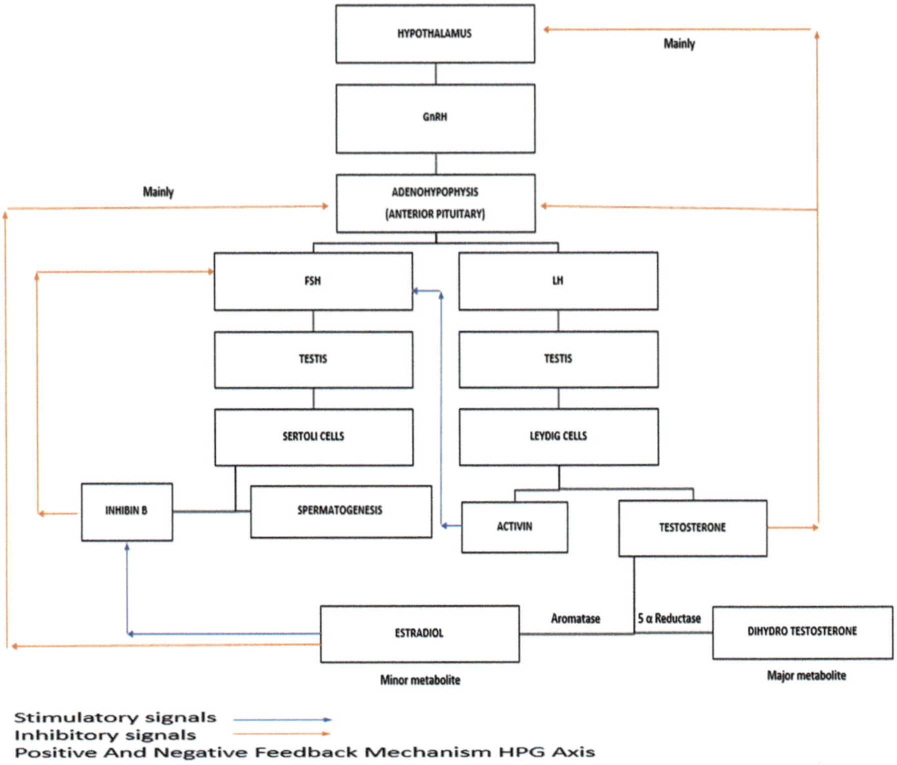

Fig. 2.3 HPG feedback mechanism

Functions of Testosterone

In utero: Fig. 2.4 depicts the intrauterine role of testosterone for development of Wolffian duct and inhibition of Mullerian duct to form the internal and external male genitalia.

Puberty

At puberty, it has the following functions:

The physiological onset and sequence of physical maturation vary greatly based on sex, race and ethnicity, and environmental factors. Tanner Stages (Fig. 2.5), rather than chronological age, are being used clinically in pediatric and adolescent stages to counsel parents about the timing of anticipated body changes, to perform appropriate medical screenings, and monitor for deviations in normal timing and sequence of physical signs of puberty that may represent physiologic problems.

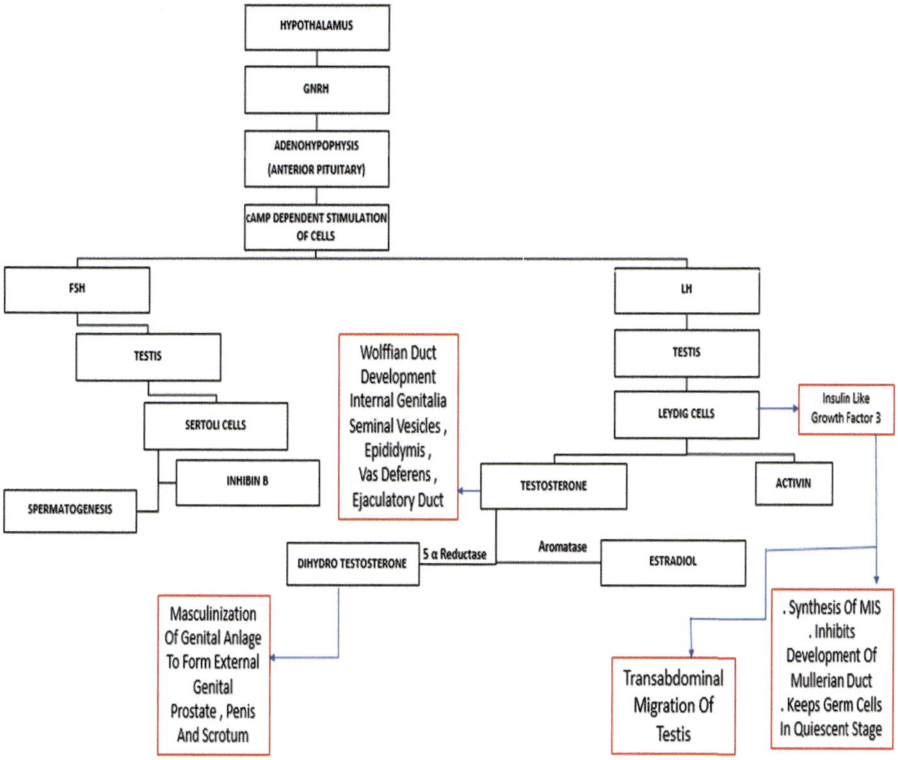

Fig. 2.4 Role of male reproductive hormones in utero

Distribution of Body Hair

It causes growth of hair over the pubis, upward along the linea alba to the umbilicus or above, on face, chest, and less often on the back, except on the crown of head—testosterone esp. DHT decreases growth of hair on the top of head and is one of the factors causing male pattern baldness.

Effect on Larynx

It causes hypertrophy of laryngeal mucosa and enlargement of the larynx. This results into cracking of voice but it gradually changes into typical adult masculine voice (probably due to protein anabolic effect).

	Stage	Testicular	Penile	Scrotum	Pubic Hair
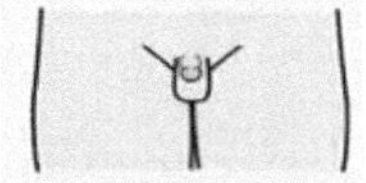	1	< 4 cc	Prepubertal	Prepubertal	None
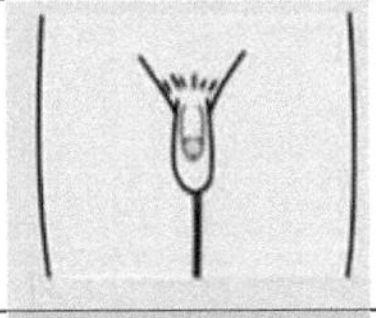	2	>= 4cc	-	Enlargement and Skin reddens and change in texture	Sparse , long &straight
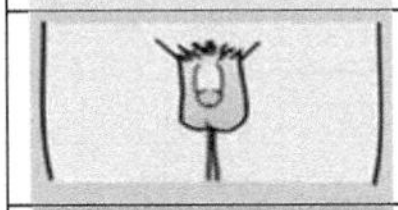	3	Further increase in volume	Enlargement in length	Further changes	Dark, coarse & curled
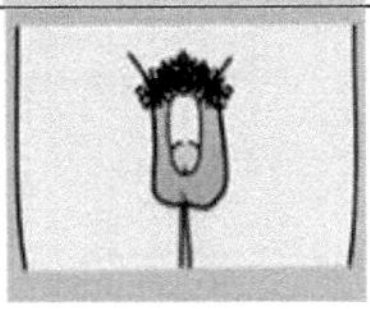	4	Increase in volume	Enlargement in length and breadth with glans development	Scrotal skin darkens	Dark, coarse & curled but covering small area compared to adults
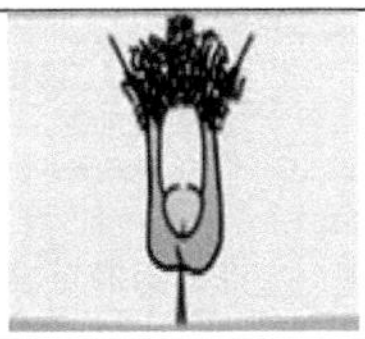	5	Adult Genitalia			Dark, coarse & curled extending towards umbilicus

Fig. 2.5 Tanner staging for male:

Effect on Skin

It increases the thickness of the skin. It also increases the secretion by sebaceous glands. Excess secretion of sebaceous glands on face causes development of acne.

Effect on Musculature

Because of increased protein synthesis, muscles hyperplasia and hypertrophy resulting in increase in muscle mass.

Effect on Bones

It causes bones to increase in thickness and increases deposition of calcium salts. It increases the quantity of bone matrix due to protein anabolic effect. Testosterone has a specific effect on pelvis. It narrows the pelvic outlet, lengthens it making the pelvis funnel shaped. It also greatly increases the strength of the entire pelvis for load bearing. However, testosterone causes the epiphyses of long bones to unite with the shafts at an early age in life. Therefore, in spite of rapidity of growth, uniting of epiphyses prevents the person from growing as tall as he would have grown if testosterone had not been secreted at all.

Effect on BMR

It increases BMR during adolescence by 5–10%. Increased BMR is the indirect effect of increased protein anabolism causing increased quantity of enzymes.

Effect on RBCs

It causes increase in RBC count partly due to increased metabolic rate and partly due to direct effect of testosterone in red cell formation via production of erythropoietin in the kidneys.

Water and electrolytes:

It causes minor increase in salt and water retention by kidneys.

Sexual Effects

Testosterone plays a vital role in men's sexual cycle. It enhances sexual desire and libido in addition to its local effects on erectile function via expression of androgen-dependent NOS and PDE5 gene expression in penile tissue. Recent data demonstrates blunted PDE5i efficacy in patients with hypogonadism. The molecular pathophysiology of ED shows, testosterone deficiency produces metabolic, structural, and functional alterations in the corpus cavernous resulting in endothelial dysfunction, arterial stiffness, and veno-occlusive dysfunction.

Mood and General Well-being

Physiological testosterone levels are needed for general and mental well-being (data relating mood to serum testosterone divergent). Recent epidemiologic data showed depressed mood inversely related to bioavailable testosterone.

Central Nervous System

Androgens can affect the release of neurotransmitters and modulate neuronal nicotinic receptors. It may interact with acetylcholine binding and thus affect cognition by enhancing hippocampal acetylcholine release and modulating nicotinic acetylcholine receptors. In castrated rats, there is reduced total spontaneous release of acetylcholine. Thus, serum testosterone correlates with cognitive function and spatial ability in men.

Mechanism of Action of Testosterone

Testosterone increases the rate of protein formation in the target cells (Fig. 2.6). After entering the target cell, testosterone is converted to dihydrotestoterone, which binds with cytoplasmic receptor protein. Hormone protein complex migrates to the nucleus and binds with nuclear protein, where it induces DNA-RNA transcription process. Within 30 min, RNA concentration begins to increase. There is progressive increase in cellular protein. After several days, quantity of DNA is also increased. Some target tissues do not possess the enzyme that converts testosterone to dihydrotestoterone. In such tissues testosterone has a direct effect usually with half the potency, e.g., in the male fetus for development of epididymis, vas deferens, and seminal vesicles, and in adults it has an effect on skeletal muscles and larynx.

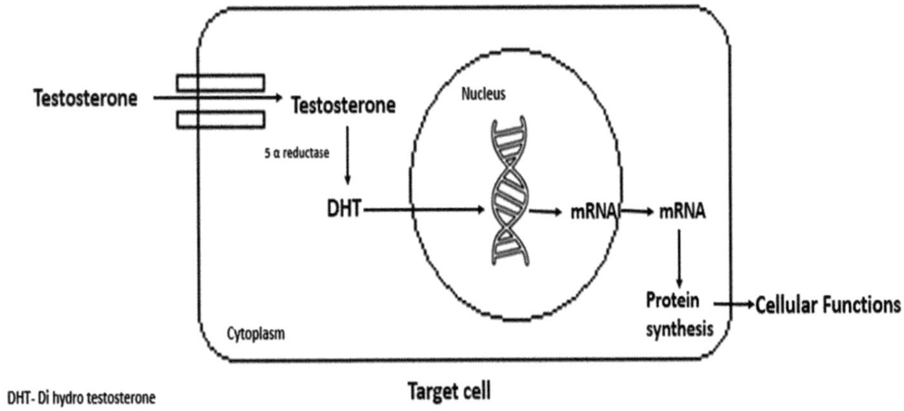

Fig. 2.6 Mechanism of action of testosterone

Testosterone Transportation and Metabolism

Physiological State of Testosterone

The majority of testosterone is bound to a carrier protein, rendering the hormone inactive. Fifty percent is tightly bound to sex hormone-binding globulin (SHBG) and about 45% less tightly bound to albumin. Some dissociation is possible from the latter fraction, which may possess some biological activity. Only the remaining 3–4% is unbound, also termed free testosterone (FT), which is biologically active. The frequently performed total testosterone (TT) assay measures all three fractions:

Total Testosterone = [SHBG bound testosterone] + [Albumin bound testosterone] + Free Testosterone.
Bioavailable Testosterone = [Albumin bound testosterone] + Free Testosterone.

Testosterone that does not become fixed to the tissues is rapidly converted into androsterone and dihydroepiandrosterone in liver, which are immediately conjugated as glucuronides and sulpftes. They are excreted through gut (in the bile) or in urine.

Natural History of Testosterone

Fetal Life

Early development of gonads and genitalia during the first 6 weeks of intrauterine life is undifferentiated.

By the 9th to 13th week, post activation of SRY gene on Y chromosome, there is sequential activation SOX- 9 and DAX −1 gene. The mesenchymal cells in the developing testis (intermediate plate mesoderm) form testosterone producing Leydig cells. The testosterone secretion is initially independent and peaks at 13 weeks. From 13th to 16th week it is under the influence of maternal HCG. Post 16th week onwards the production is under influence of LH via fetal pituitary (Fig. 2.7).

At Birth

Due to withdrawal of maternal gonadotropins, there is a surge in the testosterone levels resulting in a "mini Puberty" at 2 months (Fig. 2.7). This results in priming of cells for hormonal influence, puberty, gender-oriented behavior and elongation of penis.

At Puberty

At puberty 12–17 years, due to various factors, namely the kisspeptins, leptins, neurokinin, melatonin, there is pulsatile release of GnRH, where a phase of adrenarche is preceded by pubarche resulting in development of a phenotypic adult male.

Adulthood

The testosterone secretion becomes nyctohemeral, i.e., cyclic event occurring during both day and night. Testosterone is produced in range 6-7 g/day in damped irregular and pulsatile manner. It usually peaks and nadirs at fall and spring and morning and evening respectively. It peaks at second and third decade of life (Fig. 2.7).

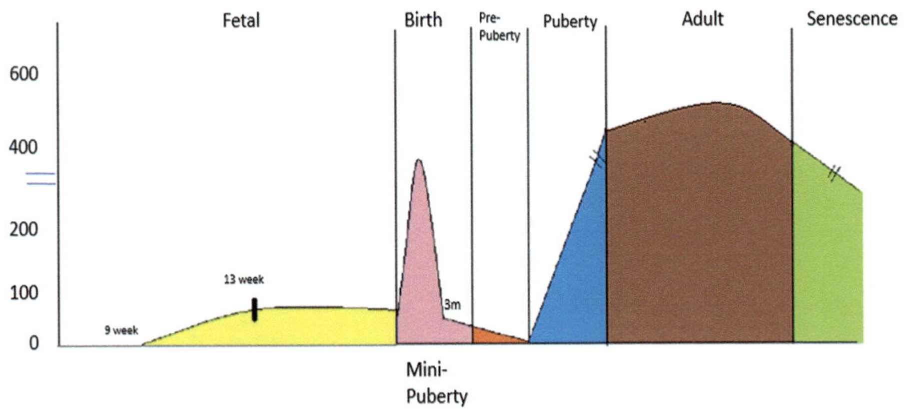

Fig. 2.7 Natural history of testosterone

Senescence

Association of aging in healthy men with decreased serum testosterone concentrations has long been a controversial issue. Several studies have shown that there is fall in serum testosterone levels from fourth to fifth decade of life at 1–2% per year. It has been observed that the mean serum testosterone at 75 years is about two-thirds of those at age 25 years. The exact decline and symptom development is highly variable unlike menopause in females.

Adult Onset Hypogonadism

Synonyms:
Definition:

Studies have shown Androgen deprivation therapy (ADT) for Carcinoma prostate (CaP) have shown detrimental effects of androgen deprivation on overall male health.

Androgen deficiency is associated with increase with mortality, quality of life (QOL) deterioration in terms of sexual, mental, and metabolic health.

With advancement of age, androgen deficiency in aging male is known as "Late/Adult Onset Hypogonadism" (LOH/AOH).

In the nineteenth century, Professor Brown Sequard was the first to define LOH. Over years, there has been various definitions but the exact definition is yet to be established.

According to International Society for the Study of Aging Male, androgen deficiency syndrome (AD) is defined as, "A biochemical syndrome associated with advancing age and characterized by deficiency in serum androgen levels with or without decrease in genetic sensitivity to androgens. It may result in significant alterations in QOL and adversely affect the function of multiple organ system."

Epidemiology of AOH

Table 2.2 mentions landmark studies in epidemiology of androgen deficiency.

Table 2.2 Studies in epidemiology of LOH

Study	Study type	Study design	Results	Advantage	Disadvantage
Hypogonadism in male study (USA)	Cohort study	Male >45 year, visiting PHC morning testosterone measurement Threshold <300 ng/dl as AD	52.4% of obese and 50% of diabetics have AD		Even though AD symptoms were assessed, only biochemical definition of AD was used
Massachusetts male aging study (MMAS)	Longitudinal cohort study	Men 40–70 years. with >= 3 AD symptoms* Testosterone cutoff <200 ng/dl	Prevalence of AD 6% Crude incidence = 1.3/100 person years	On follow-up after 8.8 months prevalence of AD 12.3% AD symptoms & biochemical definition of AD were assessed with follow-up	
European male aging study (EMAS)	Longitudinal cohort study	Men 40–79 years with > = 3 AD symptoms* Testosterone cutoff <320 ng/dl	Biochemical prevalence of AD 17%	AD symptoms & biochemical definition of AD were assessed separately	

*Reduced Libido: A noticeable decrease in sexual desire
Erectile Dysfunction: Difficulty achieving or maintaining an erection suitable for sexual activity
Sleep Disturbances: Issues such as insomnia or disrupted sleep patterns
Depressed Mood: Feelings of sadness, hopelessness, or a general lack of interest in activities
Lack of Energy: Persistent fatigue or a significant decrease in energy levels
Diminished Physical Performance: Reduced strength, endurance, or physical capability
Memory Problems: Difficulties with concentration, memory, or cognitive function
Irritability: Increased agitation, mood swings, or heightened sensitivity

Prevalence of AOH

Several studies have shown that mean serum testosterone levels in the adult male population decrease with age. At the same time there is a large interindividual variability of serum testosterone levels in all age groups. Some elderly men may have significant low serum testosterone levels while many others have perfectly preserved testosterone secretion, with serum levels well within the normal range as for young adults. With advancing age, a progressively larger proportion of men present with subnormal values relative to those in young adults.

Table 2.3 shows prevalence of AOH in various studies.

Table 2.3 Studies in prevalence of AOH

	Study	Study design	Conclusion	
1.	Vermeulen et al. 1996	300 healthy men aged 20 to 100 years	Subnormal testosterone level: (a) <1% below 40 years (b) >20% older than 60 years	
2.	Rohrmann et al. 2011	Unselected, population-based sample of NHANES III; USA*	Prevalence of men with low serum testosterone defined as <300 ng/dl (10.4 nmol/l) was 25%	
3.	Araujo et al. 2007	Unselected, population-based sample	Prevalence of men over 60 years with low serum testosterone defined as <300 ng/dl (10.4 nmol/l) was >20%	In this study, the prevalence was rather similar in younger men aged 40 to 60 years, which can be explained by the presence of comorbidity and mainly a high prevalence (>30%) of obesity in this study population
4.	Orwoll et al. 2006	MROS study includes large population of men over 65 years		Serum testosterone below 300 ng/dl, without further age-related changes in this age-group, was reported for large unselected population
5.	Schneider et al. 2009	Unselected German population of primary care patients with mean age of 59 years		20% presented with serum testosterone below 300 ng/dl

Causes of AOH

Studies have shown that in an aging male there is progressive decline in serum testosterone but serum LH levels almost remain the same. In fact, there is change in LH release frequency and amplitude, which may affect testosterone production by Leydig cells.

Hence, it might be safe to conclude the following major causes of low testosterone in an aging male:

1. Decrease in the number of Leydig cells in testis. (Low steroidogenesis).
2. Decrease in the androgenic activity of Leydig cells. (Low responsiveness to LH).
3. Decreased availability of free/bioavailable testosterone. (Increase in SHBG causes reduced availability of bioavailable testosterone). Because of the more rapid decline of free testosterone, the prevalence of elderly men with low free testosterone is greater than for low total testosterone.
4. Decrease in the number of androgen receptors.
5. Androgen receptor polymorphism and sensitivity:

   AR gene Xq11–12 has polyglutamine CAG repeats, which varies over length resulting in polymorphism, these repeats are determined by race (normally in range of 11–31). Studies have shown that the more the repeats, the less the sensitivity of androgen receptor, resulting in LOH.
6. Reduction in amplification pathway from testosterone to DHT.
7. Increase in diversification pathway from testosterone to estrogen.
8. Systemic illness: burns, trauma, respiratory disorders, surgical stress, chronic liver disease, chronic opioid exposure, HIV, cardiovascular accidents, septicemia, malignancy, and chronic renal failure obesity are common diseases associated with AD.

The above factors which either change testosterone pharmacokinetics or pharmacodynamics lead to the following physiological changes (Fig. 2.8) in male.

Conclusion

Adult-onset hypogonadism is a distinct physiological response that needs considerable acknowledgment and research. Clinical evidence supports its authenticity and its relevance in aging male. Research must be directed towards its epidemiology, pathophysiology, molecular pharmacotherapeutics, health-related outcomes, diagnosis, management , and treatment.

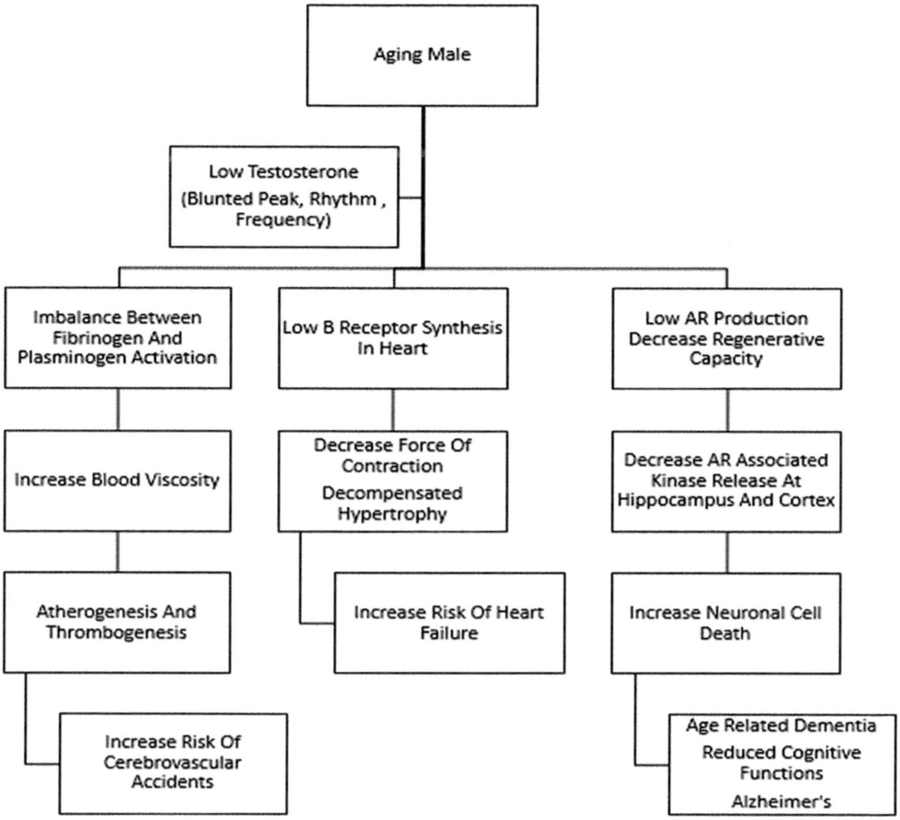

Fig. 2.8 Physiological changes in aging male

Further Reading

Araujo AB, Esche GR, Kupelian V et al. Prevalence of symptomatic androgen deficiency in men. JCEM. 2007;92(11):4241–7.

Hall JE. Guyton and Hall textbook of medical physiology. In: Guyton physiology. 13th ed. London: W B Saunders; 2015.

Kaplan HS. The New Sex Therapy: Active Treatment of Sexual Dysfunctions. New York: Brunner/Mazel. 1976.

Orwoll E, Lambert LC, Marshall LM et al. Testosterone and estradiol among older men. JCEM. 2006;91(4):1336–44.

Rohrmann S, Shiels MS, Lopez DS et al. Body fatness and sex steroid hormone concentrations in US men: results from NHANES III. CCC. 2011;22(8):1141–51.

Schneider HJ, Sievers C, Klotsche J et al. Prevalence of low male testosterone levels in primary care in Germany: cross-sectional results from the DETECT study. Clin Endocrinol. 2009;70(3):446–54.

Vermeulen A, Kaufman JM, Giagulli VA. Influence of some biological indexes on sex hormonebinding globulin and androgen levels in aging or obese males. JCEM. 1996;81(5):1821–6.

Wein AJ, Kavoussi LR, Partin AW, Peters CA. Campbell-Walsh urology: 4-Volume set. 11th ed. Philadelphia: Elsevier; 2016.

Chapter 3
Testosterone Assays: Current Techniques and Pitfalls

Fahim L. H. Rajiwate

Testosterone plays a pivotal role in regulating various physiological processes in males, encompassing metabolic, sexual, cardiovascular, and bone health. Accurate measurement of serum testosterone levels is indispensable for clinical assessment, management, and monitoring by healthcare providers.

Accurate measurement of serum testosterone levels is crucial across different clinical contexts, such as testosterone replacement therapy (TRT) for testosterone deficiency of puberty or late onset hypogonadism and transgender rehabilitation management of endocrine abnormalities. The contemporary clinical approach to diagnosing male hypogonadism relies on accurate serum testosterone levels. Consensus guidelines for testosterone replacement therapy hinge on two main criteria: firstly, the presence of low serum testosterone levels, and secondly, the manifestation of symptoms and signs such as fatigue, cognitive dysfunction, reduced body hair, and mood alterations (Fig. 3.1). Regular laboratory monitoring is essential for patients undergoing testosterone therapy to ensure safety, efficacy, and proper titration to target levels.

Multiple laboratory assays and protocols are available for measuring testosterone, with variations in technologies, protocols, and target ranges among clinical or commercial laboratories. However, standardization of recommended diagnostic and therapeutic ranges remains lacking. Obtaining precise testosterone assays faces challenges due to variations throughout the day, a broad spectrum of normal values, and technical and logistical intricacies during assay execution.

Ensuring the accuracy of serum testosterone level is vital for diagnosing hypogonadism across diverse clinical settings. However, numerous challenges arise, such as inconsistencies in laboratory standardization, reference range variations, and the expenses linked with top-tier equipment. Additionally, technical and logistical

F. L. H. Rajiwate (✉)
Ankur Healthcare / Raja Rajeswari Medical College and Hospital,
Bengarluru, Karnataka, India

Vasan S S et al. (eds.), *Men's Health*,
https://doi.org/10.1007/978-3-031-76898-9_3

Which of the following symptoms apply to you at this time? Please, mark the approprite box each symptom. For symptoms that do not apply, please mark "none"

	Symptoms	None	Mild	Moderate	Severe	Extremely severe
	Score =	1	2	3	4	5
1	**Decline in your feeling of general well-being** (general state of health, subjective feeling)	☐	☐	☐	☐	☐
2	**Joint pain and muscular ache** (lower back pain, joint pain, pain in a limb, general back ache)	☐	☐	☐	☐	☐
3	**Excessive sweating** (unexpected/sudden episodes of sweating, hot flushes independent of strain)	☐	☐	☐	☐	☐
4	**Sleep problems** (difficulty in falling a sleep, difficulty in sleeping through, waking up early and feeling tired, poor sleep, sleeplessness)	☐	☐	☐	☐	☐
5	**Increased need for sleep, often feeling tired**	☐	☐	☐	☐	☐
6	**Irritability** (feeling aggressive, easily upset about little things, moody)	☐	☐	☐	☐	☐
7	**Nervousness** (inner tension, restlessness, feeling fidgety)	☐	☐	☐	☐	☐
8	**Anxiety** (feeling panicky)	☐	☐	☐	☐	☐
9	**Physical exhaustion/lacking vitality** (general decrease in performance, reduced activity, lacking interest in leisure activities, feeling of getting less done, of achieving less, of having to force oneself to undertake activities)	☐	☐	☐	☐	☐
10	**Decrease in muscular strength** (feeling of weakness)	☐	☐	☐	☐	☐
11	**Depressive mood** (feeling down, sad, on the verge of tears, lack of drive, mood swings, feeling nothing is of any use)	☐	☐	☐	☐	☐
12	**Feeling that you have passed your peak**	☐	☐	☐	☐	☐
13	**Feeling burnt out, having hit rock-bottom**	☐	☐	☐	☐	☐
14	**Decrease in beard growth**	☐	☐	☐	☐	☐
15	**Decrease in ability/frequency to perform sexually**	☐	☐	☐	☐	☐
16	**Decrease in thenumber of morning erections**	☐	☐	☐	☐	☐
17	**Decrease in sexual desire/libido** (lacking pleasure in sex, lacking desire for sexual intercours	☐	☐	☐	☐	☐
	Have you got any other major symptoms?	Yes	☐	No	☐	
	If Yes, please describe:					

Ageing Male Symptom(AMS) score

Assesses sexual, psychological & somatic complaints

Severity does not necessarity correlate with testosterone level.

No single symptom pathonomonic of hypogonadism

www.issam.ch

Fig. 3.1 Aging male symptom score questionnaire. (Reproduced with permissions from Heinemann et al. [1]. Copyright © 2003 Heinemann et al.; licensee BioMed Central Ltd. Open Access)

obstacles further complicate assay procedures. This chapter aims to explore the diverse array of testosterone assays and their interpretation to provide clarity in clinical practice.

The Testosterone Equation

Total testosterone levels encompass testosterone bound to several proteins, including sex hormone-binding globulin (SHBG), albumin, corticosteroid-binding globulin, and orosomucoid, as well as a fraction of unbound hormone. The free hormone hypothesis proposes that the unbound fraction is the biologically active component, although this concept is debated. Some studies indicate that the bioavailable fraction, consisting of free testosterone and nonspecifically bound testosterone, more accurately reflects biological activity compared to free testosterone alone.

Total Testosterone = [SHBG bound testosterone] + [Albumin bound testosterone] + [Free Testosterone].

Bioavailable Testosterone = [Albumin bound testosterone] + [Free Testosterone].

Testosterone Measurements

Testosterone measurement poses significant challenges in standard clinical settings, with various methods available for assessing total testosterone levels, including immunoassays and mass spectrometry. Immunoassays, although cost-effective and technically straightforward, are surpassed by mass spectrometry, considered the gold standard despite its higher cost and technical complexity. Free testosterone measurement methods include equilibrium dialysis, immunoassays, or calculations using algorithms based on total testosterone, SHBG, and albumin levels. However, equilibrium dialysis, while the gold standard, is limited by technical demands and time constraints, making it impractical in most laboratories. Research highlighted significant disparities in assay accuracy and precision among laboratories, mainly due to calibration inaccuracies and insufficient analytical specificity. Programs like the CDC Hormone Standardization Program seek to accredit laboratories and assays, promoting uniformity and dependability in testosterone measurements. Addressing these challenges, the American Urological Association (AUA) recommends consistent total testosterone assessment at one laboratory using the same assay repeatedly, ideally with morning samples, to ensure result consistency and comparability.

Total Testosterone Measurements

Immunoassays

Immunoassays are commonly used to measure total testosterone levels, utilizing tracer-linked testosterone molecules that compete with native testosterone for binding to testosterone antibodies. These tracer molecules can be enzymes, radioisotopes, and chemiluminescent or fluorescent compounds. (Fig. 3.2). Despite their prevalence, immunoassays present drawbacks, necessitating technical proficiency, involving time-intensive extraction/chromatography procedures, and exhibiting diminished accuracy at extreme testosterone concentrations. Moreover, radioimmunoassay entail the generation of radioactive waste, further complicating their utilization.

Mass Spectrometry

The Liquid Chromatography-Tandem Mass Spectrometry (LC-MS/MS) technique involves several key steps (Fig. 3.3) in analyzing testosterone-containing samples. Initially, the samples undergo preprocessing and enrichment to enhance the concentration of testosterone. Following this, the testosterone compounds are separated using liquid chromatography (LC). Subsequently, ionization occurs either directly

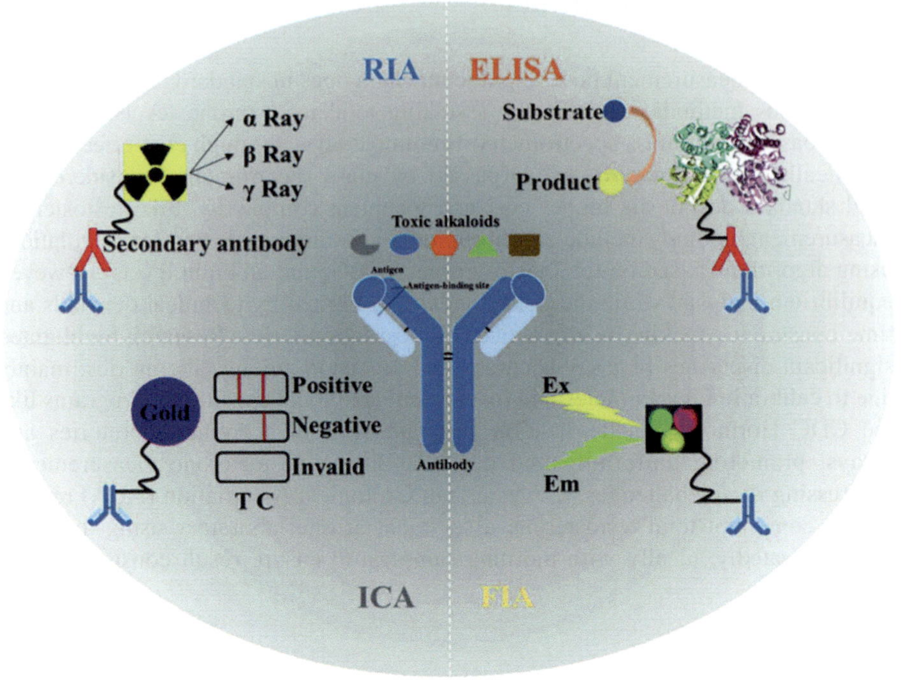

Fig. 3.2 Application and schematic diagram of four types of immunoassays for testosterone immunoassay. *RIA* radioimmunoassay, *ELISA* enzyme-linked immunosorbent assay, *ICA* immunochromatography assay, *FIA* fluoroimmunoassay, *Ex* excitation, *Em* emission, *T* test line, *C* control line. (With permissions from Ren et al. [3]. This article is an open access article distributed under the terms and conditions of the Creative Commons Attribution (CC BY) license (https://creativecommons.org/licenses/by/4.0/))

through electrospray ionization (ESI) or via spotting with matrix-assisted laser desorption ionization (MALDI). In the first mass analyzer (ion trap), precursor ions are selected and then fragmented using methods such as collision-induced dissociation (CID) or higher energy collisional dissociation (HCD). The resulting ions proceed to the second mass analyzer (e.g., orbitrap), where they undergo high-resolution measurement using bioinformatics tools. This comprehensive process ensures accurate and detailed analysis of testosterone levels in the sample.

Liquid Chromatography-Tandem Mass Spectrometry (LC-MS/MS) has risen as the favored method for total testosterone level measurement, establishing itself as the gold standard in clinical settings. Despite its higher cost, LC-MS/MS offers superior sensitivity and specificity compared to immunoassays, especially in detecting both low and high testosterone levels where IAs may show considerable variability. The adoption of LC-MS/MS assays has experienced substantial growth recently, highlighting the increasing recognition of its advantages in clinical practice. Despite some inter-laboratory variability; MS signifies a significant

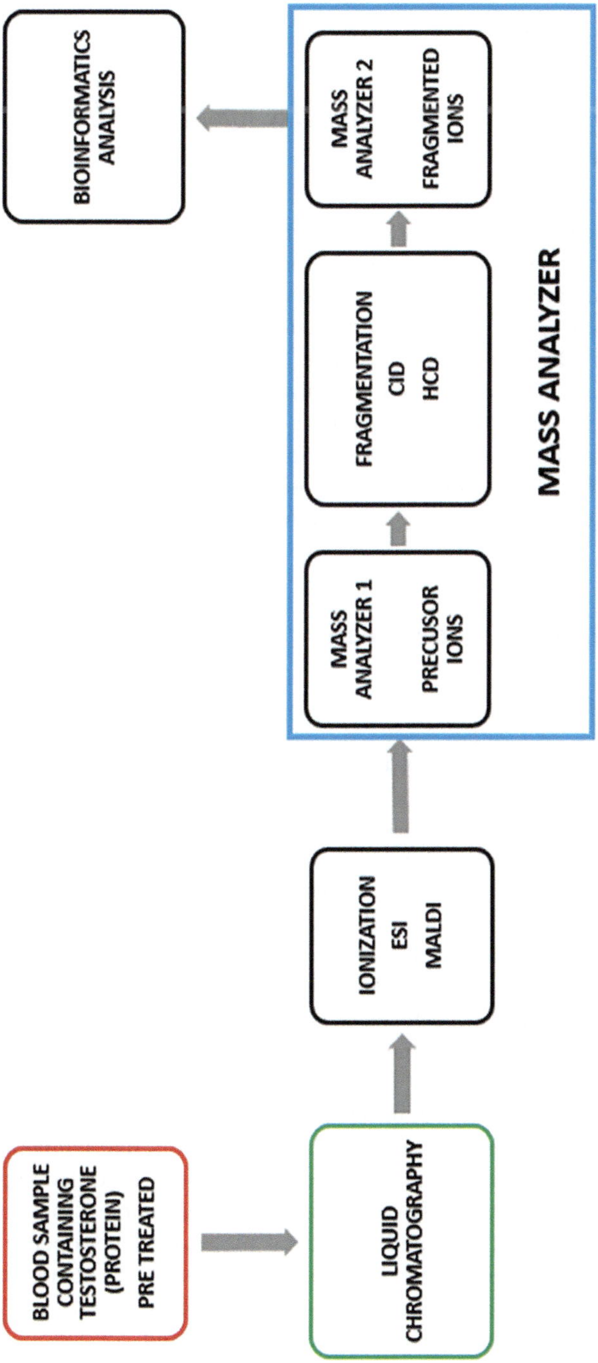

Fig. 3.3 Principle of Liquid Chromatography-Tandem Mass Spectrometry (LC-MS/MS)

advancement over commercially available immunoassays in terms of reliability and accuracy.

Immunoassay Vs. Mass Spectrometry for Measuring Total Testosterone

Research conducted by Wang et al. and Taieb et al. assessed the precision of various automated and manual Immunoassay methods, contrasting them with the gold standard liquid chromatography-tandem mass spectrometry. Neither study concluded that Immunoassay techniques were adequately precise at detecting low serum testosterone levels. Despite these limitations, specific Immunoassay methods might remain appropriate for diagnosing hypogonadism and guiding treatment choices in adult males with decreased testosterone levels. Some studies indicate that Immunoassay methods lack consistency in measuring low testosterone levels in women and children compared to mass spectrometry analysis, underscoring challenges in their suitability across diverse patient demographics.

Free Testosterone Measurements

Equilibrium Dialysis

Equilibrium dialysis stands out as the gold standard technique for free testosterone detection. This method employs a semi-permeable dialysis membrane (Fig. 3.4) to separate two compartments: one containing plasma with protein-bound and free testosterone, and the other containing phosphate buffered saline (PBS). The dialysis membrane serves as a molecular sieve, permitting free testosterone to pass through while retaining plasma proteins and testosterone-protein complexes in the donor compartment. The calculation of free testosterone can then be conducted through either direct methods, such as LC-MS/MS or immunoassays, or indirect methods involving a small quantity of testosterone radiotracer. The accuracy of this measurement significantly hinges on the analytical performance during the measurement step.

Challenges associated with equilibrium dialysis include extensive time for sample dilution and processing and susceptibility to factors like temperature and pH, emphasizing the need for a standardized environment. A modified approach called ultrafiltration, utilizing centrifugation to expedite the sample's movement through the membrane, has been developed. While this method reduces operating times significantly and offers comparable analytical performance to standard equilibrium dialysis, it may encounter issues such as sample adsorption to the ultrafiltration filter, which varies depending on the commercial filter used.

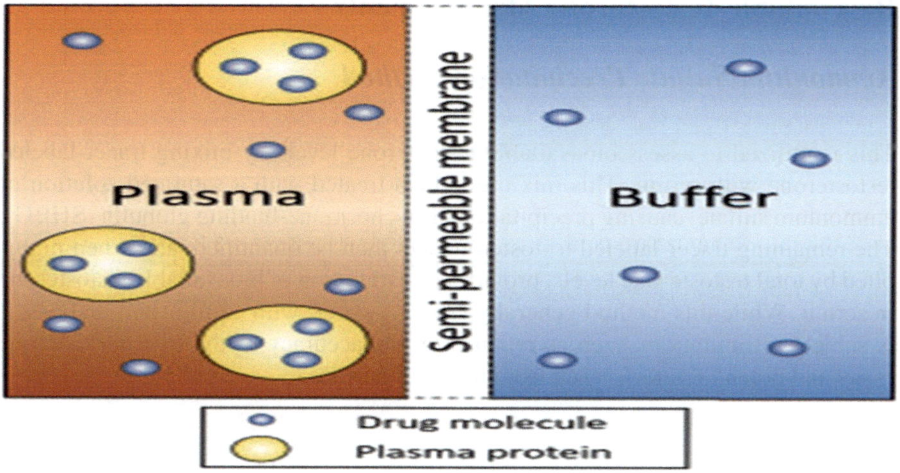

Fig. 3.4 Principle of equilibrium dialysis. (Permission from: Hann et al. [4])

Analog Immunoassays

Analog Immunoassays (IAs) offer similar advantages as discussed previously, being readily available in both large and small laboratories, cost-effective, and quick to perform. However, despite their accessibility, IAs may yield inaccurate measurements of free testosterone due to fluctuations in SHBG levels, especially considering the relatively low concentrations of free testosterone. Consequently, utilizing IAs for free testosterone measurement is generally discouraged.

Calculated Free Testosterone

Indirect methods for assessing free testosterone involve utilizing established algorithms to estimate bioavailable testosterone, free androgen index (FAI), and free testosterone index (FTI). These algorithms, including the Sodergard, Nanjee-Wheeler, Vermeulen, and Ly-Handelsman approaches, utilize measured concentrations of testosterone, albumin, and sex hormone-binding globulin (SHBG) to calculate free testosterone levels. Despite some scrutiny regarding their predictive accuracy, studies such as that conducted by Morris et al. have demonstrated their efficacy in assessing biochemical hypogonadism. Through regression analysis, Morris et al. derived an equation for bioavailable testosterone that showed a strong correlation with true values.

The precision of the calculated free testosterone value depends on the accuracy of total testosterone, SHBG, and albumin measurements. Several algorithms have been developed based on equilibrium binding principles or empirical modeling using known concentrations of analytes.

Bioavailable Testosterone Measurements

Ammonium Sulfate Precipitation Method

This is utilized to assess bioavailable testosterone levels by mixing tracer-labeled testosterone with serum. This mixture is then treated with a saturated solution of ammonium sulfate, causing precipitation of sex hormone-binding globulin (SHBG). The remaining tracer-labeled testosterone can then be quantified, and when multiplied by total testosterone levels, provides an estimation of bioavailable testosterone in serum. While this method generally correlates well with equilibrium dialysis, it is subject to limitations such as reliance on the accuracy of the total testosterone assay and potential interference from tracer impurities.

Concanavalin A Separation Method

An alternative method to SHBG precipitation using ammonium sulfate is concanavalin A separation. This approach is suggested as a more specific alternative, aiming to address issues related to nonspecific albumin precipitation in poorly controlled assay conditions. A study conducted by Giton et al. compared bioavailable testosterone measurements using both techniques and found comparable results. However, further assessment is necessary before considering the widespread adoption of concanavalin a separation in routine clinical practice.

Testosterone Reference Ranges

The absence of a universally recognized standard reference range for testosterone levels in healthy men highlights the variability and lack of consensus regarding lower testosterone thresholds. Precise reference ranges are essential for the accurate diagnosis of conditions such as hypogonadism. Table 3.1 outlines the recommended cutoff ranges suggested by medical societies.

Age-Specific Reference Ranges

The association between aging in healthy men and declining serum testosterone concentrations has been a topic of debate for some time. Numerous studies indicate a decrease in serum testosterone levels from the fourth to fifth decade of life, declining by approximately 1–2% per year. Research suggests that the mean serum

Table 3.1 Different medical societies propose varying lower threshold limits for testosterone levels

Medical society	Testosterone cutoff value
American Society of Andrology (ASA) International Society for the Study of Aging Male (ISSAM) International Society of Andrology (ISA) European Association of Urology (EAU) European Academy of Andrology (EAA)	230 ng/dl (8 nmol/L)
Endocrine Society	280–300 ng/dl (9.7 to 10.4 nmol/L)
American Urological Association (AUA)	<300 ng/dl (<10.4 nmol/L)

testosterone levels at 75 years of age are roughly two-thirds of those observed at 25 years of age.

In a study conducted by Zhu et al. in 2022, researchers analyzed the testosterone levels of 1486 men aged between 20 and 44. Their approach involved defining normal testosterone levels by selecting the middle third of the data range, aligning with the American Urological Association's definition of normal testosterone levels. However, this method of determining normal ranges might result in overly narrow reference intervals. As more data accumulates, it's anticipated that testosterone reference ranges will evolve to incorporate age-specific values.

In a cross-sectional cohort study by Zitzmann et al. in 2006 involving 434 men, it was observed that specific symptoms were more prevalent as testosterone levels declined below certain thresholds:

Reduced energy levels were more likely when testosterone levels fell below 15 nmol/L.
Weight gain became more prevalent with testosterone levels below 12 nmol/L.
Low mood was more commonly reported when testosterone levels dropped below 10 nmol/L.
Erectile dysfunction was observed to increase when testosterone levels fell below 8 nmol/L.

Nevertheless, focusing on the overall trend of testosterone levels and the presence of associated symptoms may hold greater significance. Even if an individual falls within the lower end of the normal range without experiencing symptoms, it could still be considered normal for them.

Utilizing a uniform reference range for all age brackets might lead to an overestimation of low testosterone prevalence among older individuals when contrasted with age-specific criteria. Laboratory standards frequently fail to account for age-related fluctuations in testosterone consistently. This inconsistency is further complicated by the age-linked elevation in sex hormone-binding globulin (SHBG), intensifying the decline in bioavailable testosterone among aging men. Notably, findings from the Massachusetts Male Aging Study revealed a 2–3% annual reduction in bioavailable testosterone. Hence, the establishment of age-specific reference ranges is imperative for precisely evaluating testosterone levels across diverse age cohorts.

Standardization of Reference Ranges

Establishing consistent reference ranges for testosterone levels presents challenges due to variations influenced by biological, environmental, and methodological factors. Discrepancies between assays and laboratories further complicate this process, along with the impact of diseases and medications on testosterone levels.

Efforts to standardize assay technologies aim to address these challenges by minimizing differences between systems. Normalizing equations, calibrated to a reference method, help reduce variation between cohorts, facilitating the calculation of unified reference ranges applicable across different laboratories. However, setting standardized reference ranges requires a comprehensive understanding of the biological and social factors influencing testosterone distribution.

Validation through data from randomized trials and longitudinal studies is essential to ensure the clinical suitability and reliability of standardized reference ranges. This rigorous approach ensures that reference ranges accurately reflect testosterone levels across diverse populations, supporting effective clinical decision-making.

What Time to Suggest for Laboratory Testing?

The testosterone secretion becomes nyctohemeral in adulthood, i.e., cyclic event occurring during both day and night. Testosterone is produced in the range of 6–7 g/day in a damped irregular and pulsatile manner. It usually peaks and nadirs at fall and spring and morning and evening respectively, and it peaks at the second and third decade of life.

The fluctuation of testosterone levels throughout the day exhibits a less pronounced pattern in older men compared to their younger counterparts. Research indicates a significant difference of 20–25% in testosterone levels between morning and afternoon among younger men aged 30–40, whereas this difference diminishes to about 10% in men aged 70.

For precise assessment of peak morning levels, it has been recommended to collect testosterone samples between 07:00 and 09:00. This timing optimizes the assessment of testosterone status, facilitating reliable diagnosis and monitoring of conditions associated with testosterone levels.

Frequency/Follow-Up Laboratory Testing

Ensuring the accuracy of testosterone level assessments involves validating laboratory values with at least two readings. This step is crucial because many men initially diagnosed with low testosterone levels were later found to have normal values upon retesting, emphasizing the need for confirmation.

It is worth noting that repeat measurements can exhibit significant variability, ranging from 65% to 153%, depending on the assay used. Therefore, performing two or more repeat measurements can help reduce some of this variability and offer a more precise evaluation of testosterone status.

Conclusions

In conclusion, diagnosing hypogonadism and optimization of testosterone therapy requires precise measurement of serum testosterone levels. Despite challenges such as inconsistencies in assay standardization, variations in reference ranges, and technical complexities, notable advancements have been achieved in improving our understanding and approach to testosterone measurement.

Various methods, including immunoassays and mass spectrometry, are available for quantifying total testosterone levels, each with its advantages and limitations. While immunoassays are widely accessible and relatively cost-effective, mass spectrometry is recognized as the gold standard due to its superior accuracy and specificity, particularly at extreme testosterone levels. Furthermore, the measurement of free testosterone, although technically demanding, is essential for a comprehensive evaluation of androgen status.

Efforts to standardize reference ranges and harmonize assay technologies have enhanced the consistency and reliability of testosterone measurements across different laboratories and populations. However, ongoing research and validation are necessary to ensure the clinical relevance and applicability of standardized reference ranges, especially in diverse demographic groups and clinical settings.

Additionally, considerations such as the timing of laboratory testing and the importance of repeat measurements play a vital role in accurately interpreting testosterone levels and making informed clinical decisions.

In summary, despite the complexities and challenges involved in testosterone measurement, continued advancements in technology, standardization efforts, and research endeavors contribute to improving the accuracy and utility of testosterone assays in clinical practice. By addressing these challenges and leveraging emerging technologies, healthcare providers can effectively diagnose and manage testosterone-related conditions, ultimately enhancing patient care and outcomes.

Further Reading

1. Heinemann LA, Saad F, Zimmermann T, Novak A, Myon E, Badia X, Potthoff P, T'Sjoen G, Pöllänen P, Goncharow NP, Kim S, Giroudet C. The Aging Males' Symptoms (AMS) scale: update and compilation of international versions. Health Qual Life Outcomes. 2003;1:15. https://doi.org/10.1186/1477-7525-1-15. PMID: 12747807; PMCID: PMC155679
2. Wein AJ, Kavoussi LR, Partin AW, Peters CA. Campbell-Walsh urology: 4-volume set. 11th ed. Philadelphia: Elsevier; 2016.

3. Ren Z, Zhang H, Wang Z, Chen X, Yang L, Jiang H. Progress in immunoassays of toxic alkaloids in plant-derived medicines: a review. Toxins. 2022;14(3):165. https://doi.org/10.3390/toxins14030165.
4. Hann E, Malagu K, Stott A, et al. The importance of plasma protein and tissue binding in a drug discovery program to successfully deliver a preclinical candidate. In: Witty DR, Cox B, editors. Progress in medicinal chemistry, vol. 61. Philadelphia: Elsevier; 2022. p. 163–214.

Chapter 4
Testosterone Therapy: Challenges, Concerns, and Controversies

Fahim L. H. Rajiwate

In recent years, testosterone therapy has emerged as a significant intervention, proving to be a boon for some and a bane for others. The medical application of testosterone has spanned a diverse range of conditions, from addressing puberty disorders to assisting hypogonadal men and managing andropause. However, the multifaceted nature of testosterone's effects has led to a dual narrative in its usage.

For many individuals, testosterone therapy has been a transformative and positive force, offering relief from various health challenges. It has been a cornerstone in the management of conditions affecting puberty and hypogonadal men, contributing to improved well-being and overall quality of life.

On the other side, the misuse of testosterone in the pursuit of muscle aesthetics has gained recognition as a concerning trend. The allure of achieving enhanced physical performance and appearance has led to its misuse in certain sectors, raising questions about the potential risks and consequences associated with such practices. This misuse not only poses a threat to individual health but also has broader implications for the overall quality of life.

In navigating the complex landscape of testosterone therapy, it becomes imperative to strike a balance between its legitimate medical applications and the potential hazards linked to its misuse. This delicate equilibrium is crucial in ensuring that the benefits of testosterone therapy are harnessed responsibly, promoting health and well-being without compromising individual safety or the integrity of the field.

Testosterone therapy has been a subject of ongoing debate and controversy, particularly concerning its potential impact on cardiovascular health. Some studies have suggested a link between testosterone therapy and increase in cardiovascular risk [1, 2], while others have not definitively established this association [3, 4]. The uncertainty surrounding the cardiovascular risk of testosterone therapy has led to

F. L. H. Rajiwate (✉)
Ankur Healthcare / Raja Rajeswari Medical College and Hospital,
Bengarluru, Karnataka, India

Vasan S S et al. (eds.), *Men's Health*,
https://doi.org/10.1007/978-3-031-76898-9_4

conflicting perspective among experts [5, 6]. Moreover, the use of testosterone therapy in individuals with prostate cancer remains contentious due to potential stimulation of cancer growth stimulation [7].

Testosterone and Cardiovascular Health

Numerous clinical studies and investigations into surrogate markers have provided compelling evidence linking low testosterone levels to cardiovascular disease (CVD). Longitudinal epidemiological studies and clinical trials consistently report increased cardiovascular mortality in men with testosterone deficiency, with a major focus on the role of CVD as a leading cause of death.

Association with Cardiovascular Risk Factors

Research highlights a significant association between low total testosterone (TT) and various cardiovascular risk factors, including central obesity, insulin resistance, hyperglycemia, elevated blood pressure, and dyslipidemia. Some studies demonstrate the inverse relationship between endogenous testosterone levels and body mass index (BMI), waist–hip ratio, and prevalence of type 2 diabetes. Additionally, interventions aimed at normalizing testosterone levels have shown promising effects on survival rates.

Inflammatory Markers and Coronary Heart Disease (CHD)

Clinical and biochemical markers associated with increased CVD risk, such as CRP (C-reactive protein), show a notable correlation with testosterone concentrations. Furthermore, the severity of CHD, as assessed by vessel stenosis, is linked to altered interleukin levels and lower testosterone levels. Atherosclerosis, particularly in the carotid arteries, is prevalent in individuals with decreased testosterone levels, as evidenced by carotid intima media thickness studies.

Subclinical Markers and Treatment Effects

Carotid intima media thickness serves as a reliable subclinical marker for atherosclerosis progression, with studies demonstrating a direct association between low testosterone levels and increased CIMT. Testosterone replacement therapy (TRT) has shown promise in reducing CIMT and improving cardiovascular outcomes over time.

Clinical Outcomes in Acute Settings

Low testosterone levels on admission for acute myocardial infarction are independently associated with higher mortality rates after 30 days. Prospective cohort studies further emphasize the relationship between low testosterone and increased mortality from major adverse cardiovascular events.

Association with Metabolic Conditions

Low testosterone levels are closely associated with insulin resistance, metabolic syndrome, and type II diabetes mellitus. Experimental evidence supports the direct impact of testosterone on insulin sensitivity, with studies demonstrating increased mortality risk in men with low testosterone levels and type II diabetes.

Androgen Deprivation Therapy (ADT) and Cardiovascular Risks

ADT, a standard treatment for advanced prostate cancer, induces hypogonadism and is linked to changes in body composition. Large-scale studies highlight the increased risk of incident DM, CHD, MI, and sudden death in men undergoing ADT, particularly in those with comorbid diabetes. Metabolic changes induced by ADT contribute to the pathophysiology of CVD.

Testosterone Replacement Therapy (TRT) as a Therapeutic Intervention and Cardiovascular Health

While low testosterone is associated with heightened cardiovascular risks, recent studies suggest that TRT may have potential benefits. Improved sexual function, bone mineral density, body composition, and potential cardio-protective effects, including vasodilation, have been reported. Survival benefits in hypogonadal men, especially those with type II diabetes, further underline the potential positive impact of TRT on cardiovascular outcomes.

Controversies and Contradictions

Controversies surround recent reports linking TRT to increased cardiovascular events. Two retrospective studies have sparked debates, with one suggesting increased CV events among TRT recipients and the other reporting an elevated risk of nonfatal myocardial infarctions post-TRT prescriptions. However, critical analysis reveals methodological flaws, including assumptions of treatment continuity and inadequate consideration of confounding variables, challenging the validity of these findings.

Meta-Analyses and Contradictory Findings

Systematic meta-analyses present conflicting results regarding the cardiovascular risks associated with TRT. While some reports link TRT to increased CVD, others, including recent meta-analyses of substantial sample sizes, refute these claims. Methodological discrepancies, selective inclusion of events, and the disproportionate impact of specific studies underscore the complexity of drawing definitive conclusions regarding TRT and cardiovascular outcomes.

Conclusion

The intricate interplay between testosterone levels and cardiovascular health unveils a complex narrative. While evidence supports the association between low testosterone and cardiovascular risks, the role of TRT in mitigating or exacerbating these risks remains contentious. Further research, incorporating rigorous methodologies and long-term follow-ups, is essential to delineate the nuanced relationship between testosterone interventions and cardiovascular outcomes. A cautious approach is warranted, considering individual patient characteristics and potential confounding factors in clinical decision-making.

Impact of Testosterone Replacement Therapy (TRT) on Benign Prostatic Hyperplasia (BPH)

A pivotal randomized, double-blind, placebo-controlled trial by Marks et al. [8] involving 44 hypogonadal men demonstrated that 6 months of TRT improved serum androgen levels without significantly affecting prostate tissue androgen levels, tissue biomarkers, or gene expression. While testosterone supplementation has been associated with a 12% increase in prostate size, the crucial aspect is that lower urinary tract symptoms (LUTS) and urinary retention do not exacerbate in men undergoing testosterone therapy was shown by Sih R. et al. 1997 [9].

Schatzl G et al. in 2000 [10] and Kenny AM et al. in 2010 [11] surprisingly reported hypogonadism in men with reportable LUTS did not predict a worsening of International Prostate Symptom Scores (IPSS) or maximal urinary flow rates.

On the contrary, to concerns, some studies and Ko YH et al. 2013 [12] even suggested an improvement in LUTS after 1 year of TRT. In a randomized controlled trial by Shigehara K in 2011 [13], where 52 men receiving TRT, specifically 250 mg of testosterone enanthate every 4 weeks, reported significant enhancements in IPSS and maximal urinary flow rates compared to baseline and controls after 1 year. Importantly, none of the participants in this trial required additional medication or experienced urinary retention.

Although older men on TRT exhibit an increase in overall prostate size, this increment aligns with the prostatic hypertrophy observed in elderly men not undergoing testosterone therapy as shown by Behre HM et al. [14].

In summary, existing evidence indicates that TRT does not significantly exacerbate LUTS and is not considered contraindicated for men diagnosed with BPH. As practitioners navigate the complexities of TRT in an aging population, these findings provide valuable insights for informed patient counseling and decision-making. Taken together, TRT does not appear to grossly worsen LUTS and is not contraindicated in men diagnosed with BPH.

Testosterone Therapy and Prostate Cancer Risk

Endogenous Testosterone and Prostate Cancer Risk: Fact or Fiction

Endogenous testosterone's involvement in prostate cancer (PrCa) has been a longstanding subject of investigation, rooted in both historical and contemporary data, commonly known as the "androgen hypothesis." The seminal work of Huggins and Hodges in 1941 [15] first proposed the link between androgens and PrCa growth, based on observations of the benefits of castration in PrCa patients. Modern laboratory findings support this hypothesis, revealing that many well-differentiated PrCa cell lines exhibit responsiveness to androgens and undergo programmed cell death when androgens are withdrawn [16–18].

Bladou et al. in 1996 [19] and Ahmad et al. in 2008 [20] have shown in animal models about the androgen–prostate cancer connection, with androgens promoting tumorigenesis and xenograft growth, while tumor regression occurs with androgen deprivation. Clinically, androgen deprivation therapy (ADT) continues to be a cornerstone in PrCa treatment, particularly for advanced cases [Rove and Crawford, 2014] [21]. Despite robust basic science evidence supporting androgens' role in PrCa pathogenesis, clinical data on the impact of endogenous testosterone on de novo human PrCa development present conflicting perspectives.

A comprehensive review of literature examining PrCa development in PrCa-naive patients reveals diverse findings. Some studies implicate elevated testosterone levels, while others suggest lower testosterone levels as a potential risk factor. Notably, there are studies reporting no significant association between testosterone levels and PrCa risk. This variability in clinical data underscores the complexity of the relationship between endogenous testosterone and the initiation of prostate cancer in humans.

Elevated Testosterone and Prostate Cancer Risk

Numerous longitudinal studies have delved into the intricate relationship between elevated testosterone levels and the subsequent development of prostate cancer. Gann et al. in 1996 [22] conducted an analysis using data from the Physicians' Health Study [23], revealing that men in the highest quartile of serum testosterone were more likely to develop PrCa compared to controls (odds ratio 2.6, 95% CI 1.34–5.02, $p = 0.004$). Pierorazio et al. [24] further in 2010 explored this connection in a cohort of 781 patients, finding that high-risk PrCa was associated with free testosterone index (FTI) and calculated free testosterone. Shaneyfelt et al. [25] performed a meta-analysis, consolidating data from multiple studies and demonstrating an increased risk of PrCa for men in the highest quartile of serum testosterone in 2000.

Lower Testosterone and Prostate Cancer Risk

Conversely, smaller yet well-designed studies have presented contrasting evidence, associating lower testosterone levels with an increased risk of PrCa. In 2006 Morgentaler and Rhoden [26] observed a relationship between low testosterone and PrCa in untreated hypogonadal men with PSA <4.0 ng/ml (odds ratio 2.02, 95% CI 1.10–3.72)]. Another prospective cohort Korean study by Shin et al. [27] in 2010 in men undergoing prostate biopsy revealed that low testosterone levels were associated with PrCa risk (odds ratio 1.99, 95% CI 1.25–3.16, $p = 0.003$).

No Association of Testosterone and Prostate Cancer Risk

Robust data from the placebo arm of the Reduction by Dutasteride of Prostate Cancer Events (REDUCE) trial [28] challenged the association between testosterone and PrCa risk. Muller in 2012 [29] Analyzed 3242 patients; the study found no significant association between testosterone or dihydrotestosterone (DHT) levels and PrCa incidence or Gleason grade. Similarly, a meta-analysis by Roddam et al. [30] in 2008 involving data from the Endogenous Hormones and Prostate Cancer Collaborative Group [31], including 3886 PrCa patients and 6438 controls, identified an inverse association of PrCa with sex hormone-binding globulin (SHBG), but not with serum testosterone.

Conclusion

The complex relationship between testosterone levels and PrCa risk is underscored by conflicting evidence from various studies. While elevated testosterone levels have been associated with increased PrCa risk in some investigations, others have found the opposite or no significant association. Further research, considering factors such as study design and patient characteristics, is crucial to unravel the nuances of this intricate connection and guide clinical understanding.

Testosterone Replacement Therapy in Prostate Cancer

The acceptance of TRT in men who have undergone definitive treatment for prostate cancer is growing. Studies show that TRT does not increase cancer recurrence in hypogonadal men following radical prostatectomy [32]. In a 2013 study by Pastuszak et al. [33], men treated with TRT post-radical prostatectomy exhibited twice as many cancer recurrences in the control group after 36 months of follow-up.

For men with untreated prostate cancer on active surveillance, the stance on TRT remains debated. While some studies indicate that TRT is not associated with progression of prostate cancer, evidenced by stable PSA and Gleason grade on repeat biopsy, caution is urged. In a study by Morgentaler et al. [1], 13 men with symptomatic hypogonadism and untreated prostate cancer received TRT for a median of 2.5 years with no observed local prostate cancer progression or distant disease.

However, there have been anecdotal reports of metastatic prostate cancer in older men on testosterone therapy; the overall, consensus is that TRT does not cause the development of prostate cancer. However, administering TRT to hypogonadal men previously treated for high-risk prostate cancer demands caution. Regular PSA monitoring is recommended for men on TRT, and any significant PSA change within the first 3–6 months may indicate preexisting cancer, warranting cessation of therapy. Practice Committee of the American Society for Reproductive Medicine [34] has shown that current guidelines on the frequency of PSA monitoring and the role of pretreatment transrectal ultrasound-guided prostate biopsy remain inconclusive.

Conclusion

While the consensus denies TRT as a direct cause of prostate cancer development, its administration to hypogonadal men previously treated for high-risk prostate cancer requires careful consideration. Ongoing research and adherence to vigilant monitoring practices will continue to shape our understanding of the intricate interplay between TRT and prostate health.

Testosterone and Its Potential Link to Male Breast Cancer

While there is no established physiologic connection between testosterone and the direct development of breast cancer in males, there exists a theoretical proposition. It suggests that elevated testosterone levels might contribute to increased aromatization, leading to the active derivative of estrogen. This, in turn, could potentially stimulate breast tissue receptors, thereby elevating the risk of male breast cancer.

The precise role of testosterone in the initiation and progression of male breast cancer remains a subject of ongoing investigation. Currently, a few case reports by Thomas et al. in 2008 [35] and a retrospective review by Medras et.al [36] in 2006 citing an incidence of 11% in 45 men undergoing long-term TRT over a decade contribute to the existing body of evidence. However, definitive conclusions are hampered by the limited scope of existing studies.

To gain a comprehensive understanding of the potential association between testosterone replacement therapy (TRT) and male breast cancer, future research endeavors should focus on prospective studies with extended follow-up periods. These investigations will play a pivotal role in elucidating whether a substantial link between TRT and male breast cancer truly exists, providing crucial insights for clinical practice and patient counseling.

Testosterone's Impact on Red Blood Cell Count and the Cautionary Note of Polycythemia

Testosterone administration is associated with a notable increase in hemoglobin levels, typically ranging from 5% to 7%. The following is the pathophysiology (Fig. 4.1).

Despite the beneficial impact on baseline anemia, TRT introduces the potential side effect of polycythemia, a condition characterized by an abnormal increase in red blood cell count. Although studies addressing the occurrence of polycythemia in men undergoing TRT are limited, it is acknowledged as a recognized risk. Polycythemia may affect more than 20% of men on TRT, raising concerns about a potential heightened risk of vascular events such as stroke, myocardial infarction, and deep vein thrombosis, with the added risk of pulmonary embolus. It is crucial to note that while these complications are theoretically associated with polycythemia; concrete evidence linking them to TRT remains elusive.

In light of the potential risk, vigilant monitoring becomes paramount for men engaging in TRT. Regular complete blood count (CBC) assessments should be an integral part of the monitoring protocol throughout the therapy. Additionally, a baseline CBC before initiating testosterone therapy is advisable. Should the hematocrit (HCT) surpass 54% during TRT, a cautious approach is warranted. Temporarily halting testosterone therapy until HCT normalizes is recommended. If reinitiated, it should be done so at a lower dose, accompanied by continued meticulous

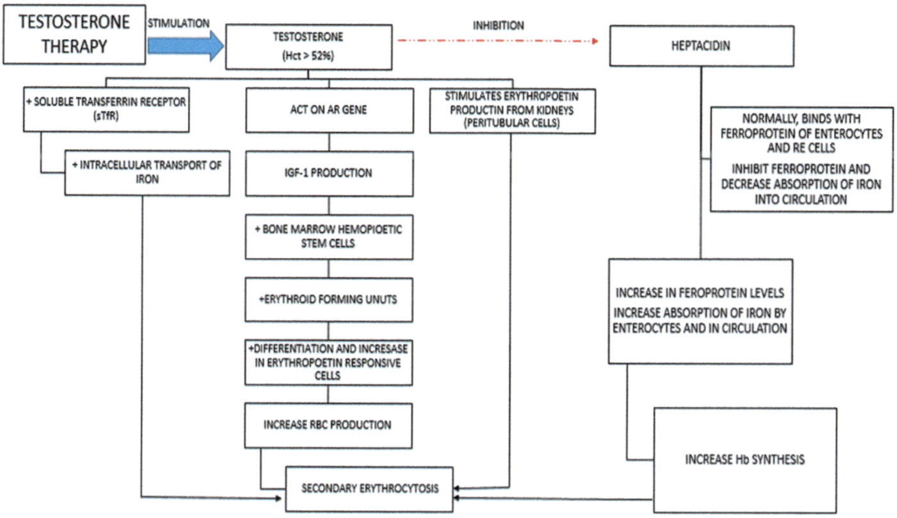

Fig. 4.1 Pathophysiology of secondary erythrocytosis in testosterone therapy

monitoring. This review underscores the importance of vigilance and proactive management to mitigate potential complications associated with red blood cell count alterations during testosterone replacement therapy.

The Relationship between Obstructive Sleep Apnea (OSA) and Testosterone Replacement Therapy

The association between OSA and TRT in men presents a complex landscape, lacking a comprehensive understanding of its etiology. Conflicting perspectives in existing studies contribute to the ambiguity surrounding this relationship. Some studies suggest an absence of a clear association, while others indicate the occurrence of OSA in men undergoing TRT, with its resolution observed upon cessation of supplementation.

The limited clarity in this association necessitates careful counseling for men initiating TRT. A proactive approach involves monitoring patients for potential symptoms indicative of OSA, such as increased snoring or heightened fatigue. Importantly, individuals commencing TRT with a preexisting OSA diagnosis should receive thorough counseling regarding the possibility of exacerbated symptoms.

While OSA stands as a relative contraindication for initiating TRT, the nuanced nature of this relationship prompts a call for more comprehensive research. A deeper understanding of the etiological factors, if any, linking OSA and TRT is essential to inform clinical decision-making and enhance the safety and efficacy of testosterone replacement therapy. Future research endeavors will play a crucial role in unraveling the intricacies of this association and providing valuable insights for clinical practice.

Medical Misuse of Androgens in Men with Fertility Issues

A common misapplication of androgens involves prescribing them to men experiencing fertility problems, often due to a misunderstanding of the hormonal intricacies governing spermatogenesis. Spermatogenesis, the process of sperm production, relies on follicle-stimulating hormone (FSH) from the pituitary gland and a high concentration of testosterone within the testes. However, administering exogenous testosterone does not achieve the necessary testicular testosterone levels required for spermatogenesis; instead, it is counterproductive.

Exogenous testosterone, once converted to estradiol, suppresses FSH, essential for initiating spermatogenesis, as well as luteinizing hormone (LH), necessary for synthesizing testicular testosterone—essential for later stages of spermatogenesis. It is universally accepted in medical practice that testosterone administration is ineffective in treating male fertility problems.

Determining the appropriate use of testosterone replacement therapy (TRT) presents a challenge, balancing the legitimate need for androgen treatment in many men with the risk of overprescribing to those with dubious indications. Indications for androgen replacement should be based on clinical signs of androgen deficiency supported by laboratory evidence of testosterone levels below reference values. Notably, in elderly men, clinical signs of androgen deficiency may be less apparent than in younger men, complicating diagnosis. Additionally, laboratory diagnosis of testosterone deficiency faces challenges such as lack of standardization in testosterone measurement methods, as detailed in the section on laboratory diagnosis of testosterone deficiency.

Nonmedical Use of Testosterone and Its Derivatives

A prominent form of misuse involving testosterone and its derivatives is their unauthorized use to enhance athletic performance, particularly in power sports where increased muscle mass equates to greater strength. Additionally, these substances are utilized in sports requiring quick reflexes and endurance to combat muscle fatigue. Some unethical medical practitioners offer guidance to elite athletes regarding the use of androgens and other performance-enhancing substances, though often these preparations are illegally obtained. Illicit manufacture or production by unknown entities in countries with lax drug enforcement laws is common, with the chemical composition frequently differing from what is indicated on the label. Sometimes, these substances are intended for veterinary use.

A more widespread misuse occurs within bodybuilding circles, where men seek to achieve an imposing muscular physique and enhance strength. Among these individuals, there exists a significant amount of misinformation regarding androgen preparations, with many acquiring these drugs through illegal means as previously described. Recently, anabolic steroid use has extended beyond men to include female users. Unfortunately, adolescents dissatisfied with their body image often resort to using these substances, hoping for rapid muscle growth and strength gains to excel in sports and improve their chances of attracting a sexual partner.

Medical professionals may identify misuse in men exhibiting unusually high muscle mass, engaging in excessive gym workouts, often with obsessive tendencies. Physically, signs such as acne, gynecomastia, and testicular atrophy may be evident due to suppression of follicle-stimulating hormone (FSH) and subsequent atrophy of the spermatogenetic epithelium. Those using testosterone derivatives may also have low endogenous testosterone levels. Recovery from the suppression of endogenous luteinizing hormone (LH) and FSH caused by these drugs may take several months or even years, complicating efforts to break the cycle of abuse. Discontinuation of anabolic steroids can result in low endogenous testosterone production, leading to negative psychological and sexual effects, as well as potential fertility issues requiring normal FSH and LH production.

Anabolic steroids share similarities with other drugs of abuse and are often used illicitly alongside them, leading to various physiological and behavioral consequences, including violence and aggression. Their use may lead to addiction, dependence, and withdrawal effects, prompting continued use despite known health risks. While some speculate on the hedonic effects of androgens, the exact neurobiological mechanisms are not fully understood. Withdrawal from androgens can manifest in a range of psychiatric symptoms.

Several medical organizations and legal systems now prohibit the prescription of these substances for nonmedical purposes. In some jurisdictions, testosterone is classified as a controlled substance, requiring medical documentation justifying its use.

Conclusion: Navigating the Complex Landscape of Testosterone Replacement Therapy

In the realm of testosterone replacement therapy (TRT), a delicate balance emerges between its numerous benefits and potential adverse effects. While TRT can significantly enhance the quality of life for patients, concerns regarding its association with prostate cancer, benign prostatic hyperplasia (BPH), polycythemia, and obstructive sleep apnea (OSA) warrant careful consideration.

Despite the lack of specific safety data for the aging population, the existing links between TRT and certain health conditions underscore the need for vigilant monitoring and a nuanced approach to patient selection. A comprehensive assessment of TRT's morbidity ideally requires a large-scale, randomized, controlled trial.

The question of whether testosterone promotes prostate cancer pathogenesis in humans remains elusive, with evidence pointing in conflicting directions. While androgens exhibit a promotional role in animal models, the human scenario lacks a clear association between higher endogenous testosterone and prostate cancer development. Paradoxically, lower testosterone levels seem to correlate with increased prostate cancer severity.

The controversy deepens in the context of TRT for men with diagnosed prostate cancer. Despite growing evidence suggesting safety in well-selected cases, the small patient cohorts and the clinical heterogeneity of prostate cancer necessitate cautious consideration. Future randomized controlled trials are crucial for precisely defining the influence of testosterone on prostate cancer progression.

In this current landscape, TRT should be approached with circumspection, offered exclusively to select patients under meticulous monitoring. A comprehensive understanding of the potential risks and benefits is essential for both informed decision-making by patients and prudent guidance from healthcare providers. As research unfolds, a clearer path will emerge, guiding the judicious use of TRT for optimal patient outcomes.

References

1. Morgentaler A, Traish A, et al. Testosterone therapy and prostate cancer: an historical and modern perspective. Eur Urol. 2015;68(3):328–33.
2. Baillargeon J, Urban RJ, et al. Risk of myocardial infarction in older men receiving testosterone therapy. Ann Pharmacother. 2014;48(9):1138–44.
3. Mulhall JP, Trost LW, Brannigan RE, et al. Evaluation and management of testosterone deficiency: AUA guideline. J Urol. 2018;200(2):423–32.
4. Lee JH, Kim SY, et al. Long-term safety of testosterone replacement therapy: evidence from observational and controlled studies. J Clin Endocrinol Metab. 2021;106(1):61–70.
5. Yeap BB, Wu FCW. Clinical practice update on testosterone therapy for male hypogonadism: contrasting perspectives to optimize care. Clin Endocrinol. 2018;89(1):3–22.
6. Park SY, Lee BS, et al. A meta-analysis on the effects of testosterone therapy on cardiovascular events. J Men's Health. 2019;15(2):3–11.
7. Pastuszak AW, Pearlman AM, Katz DJ. Testosterone replacement therapy in the new era of specialty pharmacy. Trends Urol Men's Health. 2013;4(5):10–5.
8. Marks LS, Mazer NA, Mostaghel E, et al. Effect of testosterone replacement therapy on prostate tissue in men with late-onset hypogonadism: a randomized controlled trial. JAMA. 2006;296(19):2351–61. https://doi.org/10.1001/jama.296.19.2351.
9. Sih R, Morley JE, et al. Testosterone replacement in older hypogonadal men: a 12-month randomized controlled trial. J Clin Endocrinol Metab. 1997;82(6):1661–7.
10. Schatzl G, Madersbacher S, et al. Impact of testosterone replacement therapy on prostate-specific antigen and prostate cancer incidence. Eur Urol. 2000;38(1):18–27.
11. Kenny AM, Bellantonio S, et al. Effects of transdermal testosterone on cognitive function and health perception in older men. J Gerontol Med Sci. 2010;65A(1):82–8.
12. Ko YH, et al. Role of testosterone in the pathophysiology of aging male hypogonadism. Aging Male. 2013;16(1):1–9.

13. Shigehara K, et al. Treatment outcomes of testosterone replacement therapy in Japanese hypogonadal men with metabolic syndrome. Int J Impot Res. 2011;23(3):60–5.
14. Behre HM, et al. Investigation of male reproductive function by testosterone administration. Endocr Rev. 1996;17(4):280–303.
15. Huggins C, Hodges CV. Studies on prostate cancer: the effect of castration, estrogen, and androgen injection on serum phosphatases in metastatic carcinoma of the prostate. Cancer Res. 1941;1(4):293–7.
16. Kyprianou N, et al. Biochemical changes associated with androgen-dependent and independent prostate cancer cell lines. Cancer Res. 1990;50(22):7149–54.
17. Webber MM, Waghray A, et al. In vitro progression of human prostatic epithelial cells to androgen independence. Cancer Res. 1996;56(24):5764–72.
18. Schwab TW, et al. Effects of testosterone on prostate cancer cells: a systematic review. J Androl. 2000;21(4):456–62.
19. Bladou F, et al. Predictive factors in the treatment of metastatic prostate cancer with castration and chemotherapy. J Urol. 1996;155(1):195–200.
20. Ahmad I, et al. Testosterone and prostate health: the paradox of prostate cancer. J Men's Health. 2008;5(4):354–62.
21. Rove KO, Crawford ED. Androgen deprivation therapy for prostate cancer: impacts and management. J Clin Oncol. 2014;32(8):808–11.
22. Gann PH, Hennekens CH, et al. Prospective study of sex hormone levels and risk of prostate cancer. J Natl Cancer Inst. 1996;88(16):1118–26.
23. Physicians' Health Study. A study on the relationship between testosterone levels and prostate cancer. N Engl J Med.
24. Pierorazio PM. et al. Clinical practice guidelines for prostate cancer: insights and recommendations.
25. Shaneyfelt T, et al. The role of testosterone therapy in men with prostate cancer. Ann Intern Med. 2000;132(2):1–10.
26. Morgentaler A, Rhoden EL. Clinical safety of testosterone therapy in men with hypogonadism: evidence-based data on adverse effects and safety. Int J Clin Pract. 2006;60(7):762–70. https://doi.org/10.1111/j.1368-5031.2006.00950.x.
27. Shin D, et al. Testosterone levels and metabolic syndrome in Korean men: a longitudinal study. Korean J Men's Health. 2010;8(4):256–64.
28. REDUCE Trial. Randomized controlled trial on testosterone reduction for prostate cancer prevention.
29. Muller M. Testosterone therapy in aging men: a review of clinical outcomes. Endocrinol Metab Clin. 2012;41(2):417–32.
30. Roddam AW, et al. Meta-analysis of testosterone and prostate cancer risk. Cancer Epidemiol Biomark Prevent. 2008;14(9):2255–60.
31. Endogenous Hormones and Prostate Cancer Collaborative Group. Collaborative study on hormone levels and cancer risk. Cancer Res, 20(3):511–21.
32. Leibowitz S, et al. Testosterone and prostate cancer: a clinical review. Curr Opin Endocrinol. 2010;19(3):263–71.
33. Pastuszak AW, et al. Long-term safety and efficacy of testosterone therapy. BJU Int. 2013;112(3):392–9.
34. Practice Committee of the American Society for Reproductive Medicine. Evidence-based guidelines for testosterone therapy. Fertil Steril 103(5):1319–27.
35. Thomas EJ, et al. Risks and benefits of testosterone therapy in older men. J Androl. 2008;29(5):488–95.
36. Medras M, et al. Testosterone and cardiovascular health in aging men. Aging Male. 2006;9(4):245–51.

Chapter 5
Traditional Asian Herbs: Potential Use for Late-Onset Hypogonadism?

Peter Huat Chye Lim

Introduction

Sexual herbs throughout the ages have been eagerly consumed no matter how unappetizing or bizarre. In our never-ending search for better sex, humans have ingested such diverse items as elephant tusks, lion blood, bull testicles, rhino horn, ram penis, pig genitals, and the dried remains of the Mediterranean Cantharis beetle, otherwise known as "Spanish fly." The motivation to use these herbs has been largely to improve sexual function. Can they be used to treat hypogonadism? The Bomos (village doctors) in Malaysia and Indonesia and Chinese Traditional Medical Practitioners (in China and elsewhere) have been using these herbs for centuries. Some of these work purportedly by apparently restoring testosterone levels directly, by releasing it from testosterone-binding globulin, or by enhancing their action at the receptor sites. If these claims can be proven then surely the aging male suffering from andropause may derive benefit from their consumption. Generations of Asians taking them have either really improved physically or at least psychologically from a placebo effect. These herbals can be found throughout Asia and range from Tongkat Ali, Ginseng, to Tribulus, etc. I will discuss only those herbs that claim to increase testosterone levels by increasing its actual level or its free fraction or cause

P. H. C. Lim (✉)
Department of Andrology, Urology Continence Center, Gleneagles Hospital, Singapore, Singapore

H.T. Naval Medical School, Surabaya, Indonesia

Edith Cowan University, Joondalup, WA, Australia

Society for Men's Health Singapore, Midview City, Singapore

Singapore Gleneagles Medical Centre, Singapore, Singapore

Department of Urology, Changi General Hospital, Singapore, Singapore
e-mail: tphphcl@pacific.net.sg

Vasan S S et al. (eds.), *Men's Health*,
https://doi.org/10.1007/978-3-031-76898-9_5

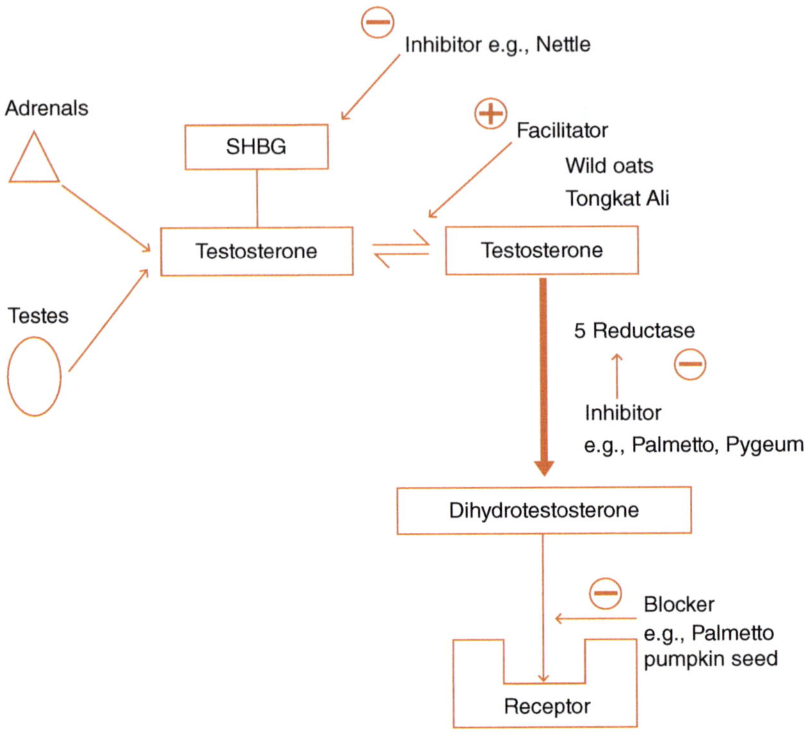

Fig. 5.1 Action sites of phytotherapies-examples

existing testosterone to be more effective by blocking its aromatization (see Fig. 5.1).

Only the common varieties easily found ubiquitously in Asia will be covered by this author to give readers an idea of the homeopathic medical remedies used in the region.

Tribulus terrestris

This plant has long been used as a folk medicine in several parts of Asia and most widely in Eastern Europe and Bulgaria for sexual deficiency. The properties of this herb have been associated with increased sperm production, sexual endurance, and testosterone levels. Since testosterone plays a huge role for men, systemically, the use of this herb could be useful. However, it is not a hormone as some believe. In Bulgaria, the "hormone-balancing effects" of *Tribulus terrestris* are being used for premenstrual syndrome and menopausal syndrome.

There are three groups of active phytochemicals in *Tribulus terrestris*, i.e.: (1) dioscin, which may help sexual energy by increasing the free testosterone level for men and modulating pregnenolone, progesterone, estrogen, etc.; (2) sterols, this group could protect the prostate from swelling and in combination with the X steroidal saponins; and (3) steroidal saponins, which can influence the immune system and also possess antimicrobial properties (against herpes).

Tongkat Ali (*Eurycoma longifolia*)

This native plant found throughout Southeast Asia is used as an aphrodisiac since 1996. It has to be used regularly, and it apparently works by enhancing testosterone and cGMP production. Benefits are felt gradually over a period of time, mainly because it enhances the natural biological synthesis of testosterone. When this hormone level is increased, health and vitality are restored. In studies on mice, Tongkat Ali increased the frequency and duration of sexual performance by enhancing testosterone levels increasing up to 440%. In a recent study on humans, 62% of the subjects showed an increase of the free testosterone index indicating its possible role in the biosynthesis of steroids. Thus, its mode of action is increasing free testosterone from SHBG. It has also been shown to increase sperm concentration and motility.

Epimedium Extract (Horny Goat Weed)

The Chinese refer to this herb as "Yin Yang Huo," a "licentious goat plant"; hence, its common name is well known as "horny goat weed" in many Western cultures. Scientifically, studies have shown that Epimedium may restore low levels of both testosterone and thyroid hormone, which may account for some of its claimed benefits in improving sexual libido. It also apparently blocks conversion of testosterone into estradiol and blocks estrogen receptors in the body.

Aswaganda—2 mode of action: possibly blocks conversion of testosterone into estradiol. The bioactive plant component also purportedly fills up and blocks estrogen receptors in the body.

Pimpinella alpina (*Purwoceng*) from Java and *Lunasia amara Blanco* (*Sanrego*) from South Sulawesi in Indonesia are androgenic herbs with androgenic properties used as aphrodisiacs.

Muira Puama

The herb *Ptychopetalum olacoides* extracted from this is otherwise called "potency wood," and it is the best-known Amazonian folk medicine to increase libido and penile hardness. It purportedly acts as a nerve stimulant to heighten receptiveness to sexual stimuli and physical sensation of sex. Rich in sterols, e.g., sitosterol, campesterol, and lupol, it is postulated to activate the body's receptors for testosterone to heighten libido and enhance performance. Another purported action is an increase of free testosterone from its bound state to SHBG. The other ingredients present are volatile oils like camphor which are used by homeopathics to restore sex drive, inner depth of libido, and mental ability to be aroused.

Pumpkin Seed

Besides having a pleasant flavor, pumpkin seeds are known to possess antidepressant properties in Chinese history. More importantly, pumpkin seed ingestion can influence positively prostate health, which is very important for male sexual health. It is commonly used to strengthen the prostate gland and promote healthy hormone function in men. Myosin, an amino acid found in pumpkin seeds, is known to be essential for muscular contractions and increasing free testosterone from SHBG plus blocking DHT linking to DHT receptors.

Nettle Leaf

Among its many properties, nettle leaf has lately been shown to influence prostate health and prevention of prostate conditions, especially prostatitis, which is an inflammation of the prostate gland. Besides, there is also speculation that nettle leaf may help with male pattern baldness. Irrespective of the age, prostate health is essential for men. Prostate problems can interfere with a healthy sex life. Nettle is also considered to be an overall energizer of the body, as well as a natural diuretic and anti-inflammatory remedy. It is rich in iron, zinc, and chlorophyll. The claims are that it increases free testosterone from SHBG.

Ginseng (*Panax Ginseng*)

This is an adaptogenic herb touted to have boosted the potency of Ottoman sultans. Used to increase the body's ability to handle environmental stresses and combat biochemical imbalances, it energizes when one is fatigued and controls anxiety. It may also increase sex-related hormones like testosterone and enhances sexual responses in both sexes. It thus acts as a tonic, stimulant, and aphrodisiac. The most commonly used type is Chinese Ginseng renowned for increasing sexual vitality.

Wild Oats

Avena sativa is a biologically standardized green oats extract. A study in 1986 by the Institute for Advanced Study of Sexuality in San Francisco reported effects like heightened sexual awareness, increased sexual thoughts, more orgasms (36% in men and 29% in women), and some male subjects showed increased levels of testosterone attributed to unbinding of testosterone from SHBG. Oats supply steroidal saponins which modulate hormonal balance. A Singapore study done in the 1990s showed that EXSAIVA—a Swiss version of wild oats—released up to 28% of testosterone from SHBG in a cohort of 90 volunteers tested.

Others

Saw palmetto, rye grass, and pygeum are claimed to be effective in increasing free testosterone from SHBG and inhibiting 5-alpha reductase thus preventing testosterone from becoming active DHT. Saw palmetto apparently can additionally block DHT linking to DHT receptors.

Conclusion

This chapter is intended to demonstrate the other side of medicine in Asia where use of traditional phytotherapies abounds. It serves to introduce the reader to what is essentially Asian homeopathic practices focusing on the therapies that have been claimed to increase available testosterone in the subjects using them or enhancing its utilization in the tissues by stimulatory or inhibitory bioactions. Whether these claims can be substantiated remains to be proven as few if any placebo-controlled trials have been done on them. Also the mechanism of action needs to be convincingly elucidated before the theories behind each of these herbs can be accepted as fact and not fiction. Notwithstanding the lack of complete scientific documentation, we will continue to see these herbs being used for the management of sexual hypofunction and currently for late-onset hypogonadism generated by a burgeoning interest in using testosterone replacement therapy in the aging male in Asia.

Bibliography

1. Ang HH, Cheang HS, Yusof AP. Effects of *Eurycoma longifolia* J (Tongkat Ali) on the initiation of sexual performance of inexperienced castrated male rats. Exp Anim. 2000;49:35–8. PubMed CrossRef

2. Benny Tan KH, Victor Ong YC, Peter Lim HC. Chapter 10: Singapore experience. In: Park NC, et al., editors. Modern oriental phytotherapy in sexual medicine EDS. Seoul: Publ Koon Ja Publishing Inc; 2010. p. 111–32. ISBN 978-89-6278-304-9.
3. Bucci LR. Selected herbals and human exercise performance. Am J Clin Nutr. 2000;72:624S–36S. PubMed
4. Carey MP, Johnson BT. Effectiveness of yohimbine in the treatment of erectile disorder: four meta-analytic integrations. Arch Sex Behav. 1996;25:341–60. PubMed CrossRef
5. CHEMEXCIL. *Tribulus terrestris* L. (N.O. Zygophyllaceae). Selected medicinal plants of India. A monograph of identity, safety and clinical usage. Bombay: Tata Press; 1992. p. 323–6.
6. Ernst E. The desktop guide to complementary and alternative medicine—an evidence-based approach. St Louis: Mosby; 2001.
7. Garg SK. Evaluation of safety & efficacy of "Tentax Royal" in management of ED. Med Update. 2004;12(8):51–5.
8. Hryb DJ, Kahn MS, Romas NA, Rosner W. The effect of extracts of the roots of the stinging nettle (Urtica dioica) on the interaction of SHBG with its receptor on human prostatic membranes. Planta Med. 1995;61:31–2. PubMed CrossRef
9. Komesaroff PA, Black CV, Cable V, Sudhir K. Effects of wild yam extract on menopausal symptoms, lipids and sex hormones in healthy menopausal women. Climacteric. 2001;4:144–50. PubMed
10. Kuang AK, Chen JL, Chen MD. Effects of yang-restoring herb medicines on the levels of plasma corticosterone, testosterone and triiodothyronine. Zhong Xi Yi Jie He Za Zhi. 1989;9(737–8):–710. PubMed
11. Liang P, Li H, Peng X, Jiao J, Liu J, Ye Z. Effects of Astragalus membranaceus injection on sperm abnormality in Cd-induced rats. Zhonghua Nan Ke Xue 2004;10:42–5,48.21.PubMed
12. PHC L. Traditional Asian folklore medicines in sexual health. Indian J Urol. 2006;22:241–5. 5th World Congress on the Aging male 9–12 Feb 2006, Salzburg, Austra
13. Malo AF, Roldan EF, Garde J, Soler AJ, Gomendio M. Antlers honestly advertise sperm production and quality. Proc Biol Sci. 2005;272:149–57. PubMed CrossRef
14. Meletis CD. Better sex naturally. Dean of Medical Affairs, Chief Medical Officer, National College of Naturopathic Medicine.
15. Natural Medicines Comprehensive Database. Compiled by the Editors of Prescriber's Letter and Pharmacist's Letter.
16. Natural Medicines Comprehensive Database. http://www.naturaldatabase.com/pda
17. PDR Herbal and Nutritional Supplement editions. 2002, 2003.
18. Rowland DL, Tai W. A review of plant-derived and herbal approaches to the treatment of sexual dysfunctions. J Sex Marital Ther. 2003;29:185–205. PubMed CrossRef
19. Wang KY, Dahlen M. Chinese herbal medicine. Hong Kong: Workman Press; 1994.
20. Wong KY, Daylen M. Chinese herbal medicines-60 common herbs: principles and practice. Hong Kong: Wokman Press 1994/1999. ISBN 962-7316-02-4.
21. Wong K-Y, Martha D. Chinese herbal medicine. Hong Kong: Publ Wokman Press; 1999. ISBN 962-7316-02-4
22. Zhu J, Halpern G, Jones K. The scientific rediscovery of a precious ancient Chinese herbal regimen: Cordyceps sinensis: part II. J Alternat Complement Med. 1998;4:429–57. CrossRef

Part II
Ejaculatory Dysfunction

Chapter 6
Introduction, Definition, and Classification of Premature Ejaculation

Peter Huat Chye Lim

Introduction

In the past, it was thought that premature ejaculation is mainly psychogenic in nature. In fact, when premature ejaculation is part of the symptoms of erectile dysfunction, it has been inferred that the etiology of erectile dysfunction is more likely to be psychogenic in nature. However, with improving knowledge of the male sexual physiology, it is believed now that premature ejaculation has an organic basis (e.g., penile hypersensitivity and serotonin receptor dysfunction) rather than being just indicative of the patient's anxious state in approaching sexual intercourse.

Definition

The simple definition is the following: Delayed ejaculation, also called retarded ejaculation, is the difficulty in ejaculating, even with a firm erection and sufficient sexual arousal and stimulation.

P. H. C. Lim (✉)
Department of Andrology, Urology Continence Center, Gleneagles Hospital, Singapore, Singapore

H.T. Naval Medical School, Surabaya, Indonesia

Edith Cowan University, Joondalup, WA, Australia

Society for Men's Health Singapore, Midview City, Singapore

Singapore Gleneagles Medical Centre, Singapore, Singapore

Department of Urology, Changi General Hospital, Singapore, Singapore
e-mail: tphphcl@pacific.net.sg

Vasan S S et al. (eds.), *Men's Health*,
https://doi.org/10.1007/978-3-031-76898-9_6

The Second International Consultation on Sexual and Erectile Dysfunction defines premature ejaculation (PE) as "ejaculation with minimal stimulation and earlier than desired before or soon after penetration, which causes bother or distress, and over which the sufferer has little or no voluntary control". The International Society for Sexual Medicine has defined *lifelong PE* as, "Premature ejaculation is a male sexual dysfunction characterized by ejaculation which always or nearly always occurs prior to or within about 1 min of vaginal penetration; and inability to delay ejaculation on all or nearly all vaginal penetrations; and negative personal consequences, such as distress, bother, frustration and/or the avoidance of sexual intimacy". The common themes in these definitions include:

Classification

If the patient has always had PE from the time he began coitus, then he has primary PE. If he had successful coitus in the past and developed PE with the current relationship, then he has secondary premature ejaculation. In most cases, secondary PE is easier to treat and has a better prognosis.

- *Primary Premature Ejaculation* [1]
  - *Prior psychological difficulties*, as psychiatric conditions are more common in males with primary PE in the general population.
  - *Patient's early sexual experiences*. Any traumatic sexual episode as a child or teenager? For example, parental discovery of masturbation, with guilt feelings or punishment/threats for masturbation.
  - *Family relationships* while growing up. What was the relationship with mother, father, brother(s), and sister(s)? Any history of incest or sexual assault? Males can be sexually assaulted by other males and, in rare instances, by females, including siblings.
  - *Peer relationships*—male friends, female friends? *Self-regard* with respect to peers (e.g., inferior, superior, athletic, frail, more intelligent, less intelligent)?
  - *Difficulties at work* (or school, if still a student)?
  - General *attitude toward sex* (i.e., regarded as dirty), and what is the patient's sexual preference, fantasy, and arousal pattern?
  - Strict *religious upbringing*? If so, what was he taught about sex?
  - *Guilt feelings* when PE began with earlier nonmarital relationship.
  - If PE started from first coital marital relationship, ask about *premarital, noncoital sexual play* between the partners.
  - Sexual attitude and *response of the female partner*; any dyspareunia which could relate to the male's problem or may have preceded it.
  - *Nonsexual part of the relationship*—fights, power struggles?
  - If sexual partner is not present, ask why (i.e., *partner not supportive* or blaming him).
  - Clues from these and similar questions usually point toward causation factors.

- *Secondary Premature Ejaculation* [1]
  - Prior relationships when PE was not present and any prior relationships in which transient episodes of PE occurred.
  - In the current relationship, *was PE always a problem*, or did it start after an initial time frame when coitus was OK to both partners?
  - Quality of the relationship vis-a-vis *nonsexual factors*. Partners get along mostly or conflict present? Who is dominant, and is the relationship equal?
  - If *female sexual partner who accompanies him* did not come with him, ask why. She may regard the problem as only his rather than a couple issue.
  - Does he have *impotence*? If he has erectile dysfunction (ED), did it begin after the PE or before? If no ED, what is the general timing for PE for the male—intromission, or what stage later?
  - Was actual *coitus achieved or prevented by PE*?
  - Is PE present at self-stimulation (i.e., masturbation), with nonintercourse stimulation by the partner, or *just with coitus*?
  - *Time required for the female partner to reach climax*. Climax with intercourse, or requires direct clitoral stimulation (oral or manual) to be able to climax?
  - If *ED began after the PE*, then treatment of both conditions may be required; ED may resolve when confidence in controlling ejaculation is restored. If ED started initially, PE may be a secondary sexual dysfunction, which resolves upon successful treatment of ED.

Reference

1. Benson A, Ost LB, Noble MJ, Lakin M. Premature ejaculation: over view of presentation and treatment. http://emedicine.medscape.com/article/435884-overview. Accessed on 6 Dec 2012.

Chapter 7
Etiology and Pathophysiology of Ejaculatory Dysfunction

Sitaram Mummalaneni

Introduction

Ejaculation is a physiological biphasic process, mediated by a complex interplay between neurological and hormonal pathways. A normal antegrade ejaculation happens in two distinct but interrelated stages:

- Emission—corresponds to the deposition of seminal fluid from testis and accessory sex glands into posterior urethra while the bladder neck and external urethral sphincter close simultaneously.
- Expulsion—corresponds to the intense burst of pelviperineal striated muscle contraction and antegrade propulsion of the seminal fluid.

Anatomical Structures Involved in Emission and Expulsion

Epididymis

The epididymis is a single, 3- to 4-m-long, convoluted tubule of epithelial cells consisting of three parts: the caput (head), the corpus (body), and the cauda (tail). The basal epithelial cells are surrounded by connective tissue partly composed of smooth muscle cells. Nerve fibers reside in the connective tissue and are predominantly sympathetic, which play an important role in basal peristaltic activity along with estrogen-dependent factors, oxytocin, and endothelin-1. On sexual arousal, the mature spermatozoa in the tail (cauda) get released into the contiguous ductus deferens.

S. Mummalaneni (✉)
Andrology & Urology, Androcare Andrology Institute, Hyderabad, India

Vasan S S et al. (eds.), *Men's Health*,
https://doi.org/10.1007/978-3-031-76898-9_7

Vas Deferens

Vas deferens (ductus deferens) is 25–45 cm in length from its origin at cauda epididymis to the fusion with seminal vesicles. The strong peristatic contractions of vas deferens smooth muscle cells propel sperms into the ejaculatory duct during the phase of emission. Burnstock and Verkhratsky [1], noted that both divisions of ANS (autonomic nervous system) supply the vas deferens but sympathetic plays the predominant role with norepinephrine being the key neurotransmitter.

Seminal Vesicles

The seminal vesicles are paired tubular glands situated between the bladder base and rectum. Each seminal vesicle measures 2 cm (width) × 4 cm (length) × 1.5 cm (Antero posterior diameter) in a nondilated state. The epithelial cell of seminal vesicles contributes 50–80% of the total ejaculatory volume, and during the phase of emission, seminal vesicle secretions are expelled into the prostatic urethra via the excretory duct. The neural innervation of seminal vesicles is similar to that of ductus deferens and supplied by both sympathetic and parasympathetic.

Ejaculatory Ducts

Ejaculatory ducts are paired structures measuring around 2 cm in length with a luminal dimeter of 1.7 ± 0.3 mm proximally, 0.6 ± 0.1 in the middle and 0.3 ± 0.1 mm in the distal-part [2]. Ejaculatory ducts originate at the confluence of ampullary vas with the excretory duct of seminal vesicle and then pass through the prostate in an oblique posterior anterior plane to open into the prostatic urethra.

Bladder Neck and External Urethral Sphincter (EUS)

Bladder neck acts as a physiological sphincter during the phases of emission and ejaculation.

Closure of the bladder neck is mediated by sympathetic system (alpha-1 adrenergic). The EUS belongs to the transverse perineal muscle group and is under the control of somatic nervous system. The bladder neck closure along with the synchronized opening of the EUS helps antegrade propulsion of semen.

Perineal Striated Muscles

The bulbospongiosus muscle arises from perineal body and encompasses the corpus spongiosum and urethra. The ischiocavernosus muscles originate from ischial tuberosity and encompass the lateral roots of the penis (crura). The intense rhythmic contractions of these muscles during the phase of expulsion have a major role in pulsatile expulsion of semen from the urethra and mediated via a branch of the perineal nerve (arises from pudendal nerve, S2-S4).

Neurophysiology

Spinal Ejaculation Generator (SEG)

The spinal ejaculation generator, also referred to as the ejaculatory reflex center, is located at L3-L4 level of spinal cord. SEG integrates neural input from peripheral sensory afferents, higher cerebral centers with efferent sympathetic, parasympathetic outflow, and somatic system, coordinating the process of ejaculation. SEG comprises of specialized neural cells known as LSt cells (lumbar spinothalamic) and glutamate being the main activating neurotransmitter, acting via N-methyl-d-aspartic acid (NMDA) receptors on LSt cells [3] (Image 7.1).

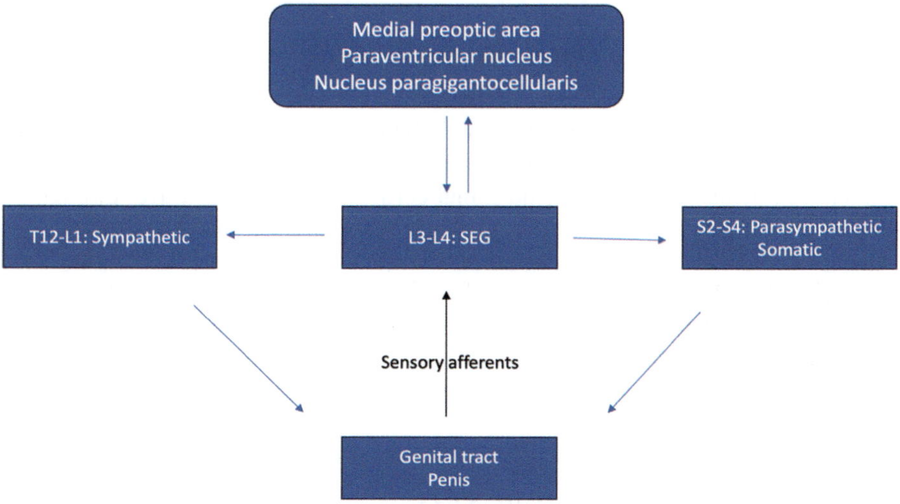

Image 7.1 SEG control of ejaculation

Table 7.1 Cerebral control over SEG

Higher center	Role	Neurotransmitter
MPOA (Medial preoptic area)	Excitatory	Dopamine
PVN (Paraventricular nucleus)	Excitatory	Oxytocin
nPGi (Nucleus paragigantocellularis)	Inhibitory	Serotonin

Afferent Input to SEG

The main sensory input from the penis passes via the pudendal nerve to the S2-S4 spinal cord region and from there to the spinal ejaculation generator. Increase in ejaculatory latency is noted when there is an interruption in the afferent fibers from the penis but not loss of the ejaculatory response. As long as higher cerebral pathways and the sympathetic outflow are intact, ejaculation can happen.

Cortical Input to the SEG

SEG is under both augmentory and inhibitory influence from higher cerebral centers, which include but not restricted to the following (Table 7.1).

The cortical input to the SEG is mediated via the anterolateral columns of the cord. It is important to remember that the ejaculatory reflex can still be elicited in the absence of cortical influence as seen in certain spinal cord injuries.

Efferent Sympathetic Output from the SEG

The cell body of the preganglionic sympathetic neurons are located in the dorsal gray column and in the intermediolateral cell column of lower thoracic and upper lumbar segments (T12 - L1) of the spinal cord, and their axons travel through the ventral roots to the paravertebral sympathetic chain. Most of the axons without synapsing heads to superior hypogastric plexus at the level of L4-L5. Postganglionic fibers then travel to their target organs: bladder neck, seminal vesicles, prostate, and vas deferens to mediate sympathetic control of the emission phase. Emission phase of ejaculation is predominantly mediated by sympathetic system and the specific role of parasympathetic system is yet to be fully elucidated.

Efferent Somatic Output from SEG

The expulsion phase is mainly commanded by the somatic nervous system. Somatic fibers passing from the ventral horn of S2-S4 (Onuf nucleus) innervate bulbospongiosus and ischiocavernosus via the perineal branch of pudendal nerve. Stimulation of this nerve triggers a synchronous activation of bulbospongiosus, ischiocavernosus, levator ani muscles and external urethral sphincter. The contractions of muscles are rhythmic and occur at an interval of 0.8 s with a frequency of 3–7 contractions at time of orgasm (Image 7.2).

Neurophysiology

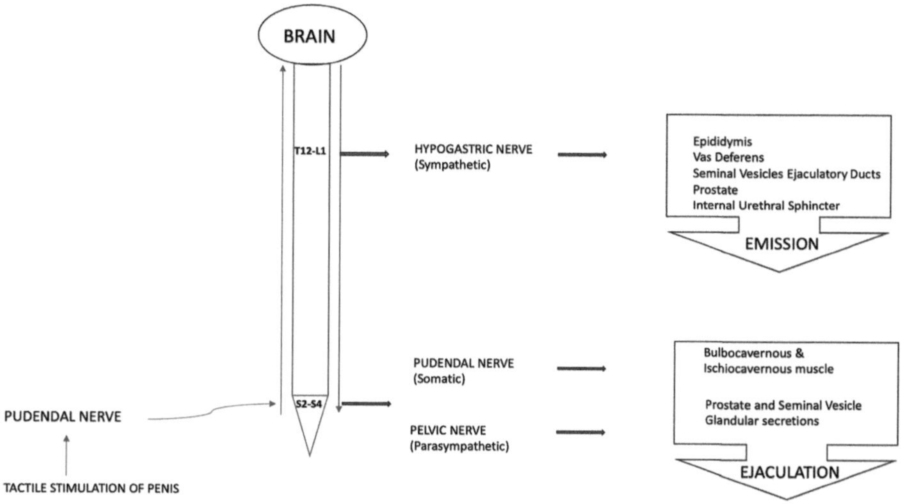

Image 7.2 Neurophysiology of ejaculation

Definition and Classification of Ejaculatory Dysfunction

The quest for perfect sexual experience and the ability to control the timing of ejaculation eludes none but ejaculatory dysfunction remains one of the most common and difficult-to-treat male sexual disorders.

The spectrum of ejaculatory dysfunction (EjD) extends from premature ejaculation to anejaculation and includes delayed ejaculation, retrograde ejaculation, painful ejaculation, ejaculatory anhedonia, and post-orgasmic illness syndrome. But with time, it became evident that ejaculation and orgasm are two different phenomena and in 2018, ICD-10 was revised (to include a modified classification of EjD (ICD-11):

1. Male early ejaculation (HA03.1)
2. Male delayed ejaculation (HA03.2)
3. Retrograde ejaculation (MF40.3)

4. Other specified ejaculatory dysfunctions (HA03.Y)
5. Ejaculatory dysfunctions, unspecified (HA03.Z).

Premature Ejaculation (PE)

PE is one of the most common male sexual disorders affecting 20–30% of men [4]. Most men experience premature ejaculation at least once in their lives. The lack of universally accepted definitions, criteria of PE, different methodology and reluctance of men with PE to report the complaint due to concerns of social stigmatization makes it difficult to assess the real prevalence of PE.

Classification of Premature Ejaculation

Taxonomy (Image 7.3)

Thus, with addition of variable and subjective PE, PE can be classified [5] as in Table 7.2.

Defining Premature Ejaculation

There is still, no universally accepted definition of PE, but in 2013, ISSM (International Society for Sexual Medicine) proposed the first evidence based, Unified definition for lifelong and acquired PE [6]. This definition can help guide a clinician in diagnosis and classification of PE and also forms the basis for future clinical trials. The definition intentionally mentions intravaginal ejaculation latency

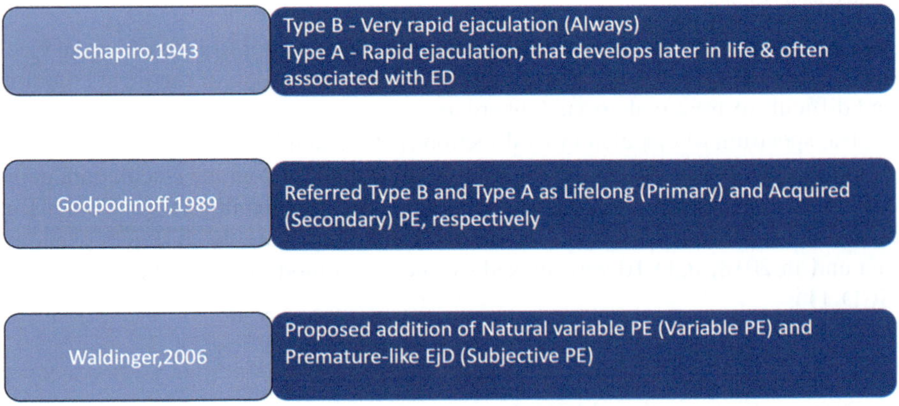

Image 7.3 Taxonomy

Table 7.2 Classification of premature ejaculation.

Variable	Lifelong PE	Acquired PE	Variable PE	Subjective PE
Possible Etiology	Neurobiological and Genetic	ED, prostatitis Medications Psychological/ Performance anxiety/ Relationship Problems	Natural variation	Psychological
IELT	<1–1.5 min (Very short IELT)	<1.5–2 min (Short IELT)	Inconsistent (short or normal, 3–8 min)	Normal or long (3–30 min)
Onset	From first sexual encounter	Develops later in life	Irregular and Inconsistent	Subjective Perception
Control over ejaculation	No ability to control	Diminished control	Control over ejaculation (+)/ diminished	Control over ejaculation (+)/ diminished

time (IELT) cut-off as "within about 1 minute," to provide some diagnostic flexibility as some men can present with IELT as long as 90 seconds.

A Unified Definition of Lifelong and Acquired PE

(i) Ejaculation that always or nearly always occurs prior to or within about 1 min of vaginal penetration from the first sexual experience (lifelong PE) or a clinically significant and bothersome reduction in latency time, often to about 3 min or less (acquired PE);
(ii) The inability to delay ejaculation on all or nearly all vaginal penetrations;
(iii) Negative personal consequences, such as distress, bother, frustration, and/or the avoidance of sexual intimacy.

Pathophysiology

Lifelong PE

Waldinger et al. hypothesized that neurobiological factors could contribute to lifelong PE. Serotonin (5 Hydroxytryptamine, 5-HT) is a key neurotransmitter involved in the process of ejaculation. 5-HT inhibits ejaculations reflex and hence prolongs the ejaculation latency time. From neurobiological point of view, hypersensitivity of 5-HT1A receptor or hyposensitivity of 5-HT2c receptor/low levels of 5-HT cause PE.

The serotonin reuptake from the synapse is facilitated by a specific protein transporter—the 5-HTT. With its high affinity for serotonin, 5-HTT regulates the availability, duration, and signaling capacity of 5-HT in the synapse and it can be argued that an increased function of the 5-HTT is related to PE. In 2009, Janssen et al [7], published the first research article suggesting that the genetic polymorphism of 5-hydroxytryptamine transporter-linked promoter region [5-HTTLPR] is associated with occurrence of lifelong PE. The 5-HTTLPR gene has two variant alleles, a short (S) and a long (L) allele, and the genotypes composed of these alleles are known as SS, LL, and SL. Janssen et al., postulated that men LL genotype have shorter IELT (geometric mean IELT 13.2 s) when compared to man with SS genotype (geometric mean IELT 26 s) and SL genotype (25.3 s).

Acquired PE

The pathophysiology of acquired PE seems to be both organic and nonorganic in origin.

Acquired PE has long been correlated to psychological, urological, hormonal, and neurological diseases [8]. The risk factors associated with acquired PE are listed in Table 7.3:

Acquired PE and Psycho-Relational Factors

Since ages, anxiety has been mentioned as a cause of PE. It is suggested that anxiety triggers sympathetic nervous system, reducing the ejaculatory threshold and in return decreasing the IELT. In Hypoactive sexual desire, the unconscious desire of the man to abbreviate the sexual act may lead to PE. Similarly female sexual dysfunctions like hypoactive sexual desire, arousal disorders, anorgasmia, and vaginismus also contribute to acquired PE.

Acquired PE and Erectile Dysfunction

Data from studies [9, 10] demonstrate that nearly half of subjects with erectile dysfunction also suffer from PE. Men with ED may intentionally rush intercourse to avoid early detumescence of partial erection and these men are often under pressure of performance, leading to brief latency.

Table 7.3 Acquired PE—risk factors

Risk factors	
Psychorelational	Anxiety, relationship problems
Urologic diseases	Prostatitis
Endocrine	Hyperthyroidism
Neurological	Penile Hypersensitivity
Other sexual conditions	Associated with erectile dysfunction, hypoactive sexual desire, female sexual dysfunction

Acquired PE and Prostate Disease

It is presumed that the inflammation of prostate may lead to altered sensation and modulation of the ejaculatory reflex [11].

Fasolo et al. [9], noted that men with prostatic inflammation had a twofold higher risk of PE than those who do not have prostatic inflammation. Rowland eta al [12], .did an analysis about ejaculatory latency using multiple sources of information and reported that PE was the main sexual dysfunction complaint in men with CPPS or chronic prostatitis with a prevalence of 26% to 77%.

In line with these observations, El-Nashar and Shamloul [13] noted that in treated patients of confirmed bacterial prostatitis, IELT has improved by 2.6-fold and improved ejaculatory control was reported by 83.9% subjects.

Acquired PE and Hyperthyroidism

The impact of thyroid hormones on male sexual dysfunction has been studied only recently. The possible ways by which hyperthyroidism can affect ejaculatory latency are the following [14]:

- Activation of sympathetic nervous system as an effect of thyrotoxicosis.
- Alteration at central serotonergic pathway.
- Hyperthyroidism can increase SHBG, leading to relative hyperestrinism and upregulation of oxytocin activity and in turn decreasing ejaculatory latency.

Carani et al. [15], noted that the prevalence of PE in men with hyperthyroidism fell from 50% to 15% after treatment and normalization of thyroid hormone levels. This supports the idea of endocrine system involvement in ejaculatory function.

Delayed Ejaculation and Anejaculation

Delayed ejaculation (DE) is probably the least reported, least studied, and least understood male sexual dysfunction. Studies [16, 17] suggest the prevalence of DE around 3%. Terms like retarded ejaculation, inhibited ejaculation, primary impotentia ejaculations, idiopathic anejaculation are used as synonyms for DE and the spectrum of DE can extend from varying latency times to complete inability to ejaculate (anejaculation). Subtle variations in meaning do exist between the existing terms and also noting that ejaculation and orgasm are two distinct entities, we focus on classification and definition of delayed ejaculation (encompassing any and all of EjD resulting in delay or absence of ejaculation), hereafter.

Definition and Classification of DE

Delayed ejaculation can result in significant distress, anxiety, and lack of sexual confidence and impairment of both the sexual and nonsexual aspects of their relationships, and the negative effects get compounded when procreation is considered.

The criteria for "DELAYED" ejaculation in terms of IELT (intravaginal ejaculation latency time) threshold is not clearly defined. The IELT of most men range within about 4–10 min as noted from population-based studies [18, 19]. Extrapolating the data an IELT threshold of 20–25 min can be assumed by a clinician as delayed, which represents about 2 standard deviations above the mean IELT found in studies [20].

ICD-11 Definition and Classification of Male DE [21]

> Inability to achieve ejaculation or an excessive or increased latency of ejaculation, despite adequate sexual stimulation and the desire to ejaculate. The pattern of delayed ejaculation has occurred episodically or persistently over a period at least several months , and is associated with clinically significant distress.

Classification

Male delayed ejaculation, lifelong, generalised (HA03.10)
Male delayed ejaculation, lifelong, situational (HA03.11)
Male delayed ejaculation, acquired, generalised (HA03.12)
Male delayed ejaculation, acquired, situational (HA03.13)
Male delayed ejaculation, unspecified (HA03.1Z)

The fourth International Consultation on Sexual Medicine definition & classification of Male DE [22]:

Lifelong (or Primary) DE

> Lifelong experience or inability to ejaculate in all of almost all (75%-100%) occasions of coital activity, associated with distress. Voluntary cessation of coital activity may subsequently occur after a variable time to avoid frustration, physical exhaustion, or genital irritation of self or partner. Men with lifelong DE might or might not be able to achieve ejaculation by subsequent non-coital activity, including masturbation.

Acquired (or Secondary) DE

> Distressing lengthening of ejaculatory latency that occurs in most (>50%) coital experiences after a period of normal ejaculatory function or a clinically meaningful change that results in distress. Voluntary cessation of coital activity may subsequently occur after a variable time to avoid frustration, physical exhaustion, or genital irritation of self or partner.

Anejaculation

Anejaculation is a rare presentation and difficulty for many men to truly distinguish between ejaculation and orgasm, making it difficult to access the prevalence through epidemiological studies. As per Kinsey et al. [23], 0.14% of general population suffer from anejaculation.

EAU, describes anejaculation as

> Complete absence of antegrade or retrograde ejaculation. It is caused by the failure of semen emission from the seminal vesicles, prostate, and ejaculatory ducts into the urethra.

SMSNA [24] classifies anejaculation as:

- Primary—when a man has never experienced an ejaculation in his lifetime.
- Secondary—A man, losing the ability to ejaculate after being able to do so normally for a period of time.
- Situational.
- Total (anorgasmic anejaculation, orgasmic anejaculation).

Anejaculation not only causes bother, distress, and sexual dissatisfaction for male partner but also affects the female partner. Burri et al [25], in a study of 240 sexually active heterosexual women noted that >94% considered partner ejaculation as an important component during sexual encounters and 56% of participants agreed that they had a more intense orgasm when their partner ejaculated during vaginal penetration.

The common causes of DE/AE seen in practice are—Psychogenic, diabetic autonomic neuropathy, SSRI sequalae, pelvic/radical prostatic surgeries.

Psychogenic Factors

Psychogenic DE is often related to a man's sexual performance anxiety, which may draw his attention away from erotic cues. There are various proposed psychogenic factors causing DE and Althof [26], which are summarized into four theories.

1. Insufficient Sexual Stimulation:

   This theory suggests that DE is due to insufficient mental or penile stimulation and was proposed by Masters & Johnson and Bancroft [27]. In support of this theory, Rowland et al., from their study noted that men with DE had no organic etiology but experienced less sexual arousal than other men. Xia et al., noted that patients with primary DE have penile shaft hyposensitivity. Furthermore, Nelson et al., confirmed the theory of insufficient penile stimulation leading to secondary DE, as he could treat 72% of patients with penile vibratory stimulus [28–30].

2. Unusual Masturbatory Pattern and Styles:

   Unusual masturbatory styles and fantasies that cannot be replicated during heterosexual intercourse can lead to DE/AE. Perelman and Rowland [31] identified three factors that characterized patients with such patterns.

- High-frequency masturbation (age-based average of more than three times a week).
- Idiosyncratic masturbation.
- Disparity between masturbatory fantasy and real-life sex with a partner.

3. The third theory—Apfelbaum [32] conceptualized DE as a disguised sexual desire disorder, where the individual prefers solo masturbation, rather than intercourse with a partner.
4. The fourth theory describes DE as psychodynamic in origin, as a consequence of psychic conflict. The conflicts can be—hostility towards partner, guilt from a rigid religious upbringing, fear of "spilling seed," fear of pregnancy, fear of exposure of the problem, and further shame and fear of rejection.

Diabetes Mellitus

Autonomic neuropathy is a sequela of long-standing diabetes mellitus and eventually leads to ejaculatory dysfunction. Although the real prevalence of diabetes affecting ejaculation is unknown, research indicate that it may be as high as 40% [33]. The spectrum of ejaculatory dysfunction progresses from retrograde ejaculation (preserved seminal vesicle and vasal contraction, but incompetent bladder neck closure) to failure of seminal vesicle and vasal contraction leading to reduced/absent sperm in the ejaculate.

Drug Induced

Prescribed drugs or recreational drugs that can alter the levels of neurochemicals such as dopamine, serotonin, or oxytocin and can affect ejaculatory latency times. Antipsychotic medications probably by dopamine antagonistic activity or by elevating prolactin levels lead to delayed ejaculation (Table 7.4) [34].

Prostate cancer Treatment and Effect on Ejaculation

Prostate cancer is the most common non-skin malignancy in men in the United States. Radical prostatectomy (open or robotic) and radiotherapy (external beam and brachytherapy) are the most effective and common treatment options for localized disease but sexual side effects remain an Achilles' heel. Following radical prostatectomy, men no longer ejaculate, as the prostate and seminal vesicles are removed and vas disconnected, but can maintain a sense of orgasm. 89% of patients reported a lack of ejaculation after external beam radiotherapy and 25–60% reported sexual life dissatisfaction following radiation therapy [35].

Table 7.4 Antipsychotics and their relation to sexual dysfunction.

Drugs	Mechanism of action	Sexual dysfunction prevalence
Tricyclic antidepressants: Imipramine, amitriptyline, doxepin	Inhibits serotonin and norepinephrine reuptake	30%
Selective serotonin reuptake inhibitors (SSRIs): Fluoxetine, paroxetine, sertraline, citalopram, escitalopram	Inhibits reuptake of serotonin	Up to 73%
Serotonin norepinephrine reuptake inhibitors (SNRIs): Venlafaxine, duloxetine	Inhibits norepinephrine and serotonin reuptake	Up to 70%
Monoamine oxidase inhibitors (MAOIs) phenelzine	Blocks MAOI which inactivates serotonin, dopamine, norepinephrine	40%

Retroperitoneal Lymph Node Dissection (RPLND)

RPLND plays an integral role in the overall treatment strategy of carcinoma testis. The lymphatic drainage of testis is close to and admixed with tissues carrying the thoracolumbar sympathetic outflow, and damage to the peripheral sympathetic innervation of vas, seminal vesicles, prostate, and bladder neck leads to ejaculatory failure. With the modified nerve sparing techniques, an antegrade ejaculation is attained in 80–100% cases [36]. However, Basiri et al. [37], noted that only 61% of their patients had antegrade ejaculation post RPLND, reminding that perfect results are not always possible.

Spinal Cord Injury

Ejaculatory failure is a common sequalae of spinal cord injury and the effect on sexual life and fertility cannot be overemphasized. The nature of erectile and ejaculatory failure depends on the level and completeness of spinal cord lesion. In contrast to erectile capacity, the ability to ejaculate improves with descending levels of spinal cord injury. Commar et al. [38], in their study noted that only 1% and 22% of patients retained ejaculation with complete and incomplete upper motor neuron lesion respectively. Whereas, 15% and 100% of patients retained ejaculation with complete and incomplete lower motor lesion respectively. In lower motor lesion, an intact spinal ejaculation generator and adequate cognitive augmentation is enough of a stimulus to trigger the ejaculation sequence but the force of expulsion can be reduced or normal, depending on the extent of motor output damage to the periurethral musculature [39].

Aging The age-related increase in prevalence of DE is attributed to the degenerative age-related changes in the penile receptors, leading to decreased penile sensitivity. Other factors like diabetes, late-onset hypogonadism, and slower bulbospongiosus reflexes also contribute to DE.

Ejaculatory duct obstruction (EDO) EDO can be a sequalae of pathologies like prostatitis, seminal vesiculitis, midline prostatic cysts, and ejaculatory duct malformations. EDO can present with ejaculatory pain coexisting with infertility.

Retrograde Ejaculation

During the ejection phase of ejaculation, the bladder neck closes to prevent any reflux of semen into the bladder. The bladder neck closure is under the control of sympathetic system and failure of closure, results in backward flow of semen into bladder known as retrograde ejaculation (RE). The incidence of RE in fertility clinics is around 0.3–2% [40] and the incidence in type-1-diabetic population and post-TURP cases is 8.8% [41] and 68% [42] respectively.

ICD-11 defines RE as:

> The condition in which semen is not ejected antegrade but rather flows into the bladder during climax. This is typically due to failure of the bladder neck to close during the emission phase and may be idiopathic or secondary to bladder neck surgery, pharmacological agents, or neurologic lesion. In most cases of retrograde ejaculation, orgasm occurs and feels pleasurable. Some men with retrograde ejaculation may report that their experience of orgasm is qualitatively different."

Ejaculation is a complex coordinated process between sympathetic, parasympathetic system and structures involved in emission and expulsion. The sympathetic system via the hypogastric nerve coordinates the bladder neck closure and seminal emission, whereas the parasympathetic nervous system via pelvic nerves coordinates the seminal vesicle, prostatic secretions, and also bulbospongiosus, ischiocavernosal, and pelvic floor muscle contraction. Any alteration of reflux that inhibits bladder neck closure can lead to retrograde ejaculation.

The aetiological factors leading to retrograde ejaculation are described in Table 7.5.

Alpha-blockers: Lower urinary tract symptoms (LUTS) associated with benign prostatic hyperplasia (BPH) is a common, bothersome condition affecting up to

Table 7.5 Aetiology of retrograde ejaculation

Aetiology	
Neurogenic	Diabetes mellitus, autonomic neuropathy, spinal cord injury, multiple sclerosis, Prostate, colorectal surgeries, retroperitoneal lymphadenectomy, Parkinson's
Anatomic causes	Urethral stricture, ectopic ureterocele, bladder neck resection, congenital bladder neck defects & incompetence
Endocrine	Hypogonadism, hypothyroidism
Drugs	Aplha-1 adrenoreceptor antagonists, thiazide diuretics, antipsychotic and antidepressants

50% of men aged 50–60 years, 60% of men between 60–70 years, and in 90% of men aged greater than 80 years [43].

Alpha-blockers are offered as first-line treatment for most of these patients to help relax the prostatic smooth muscle and improve the urinary flow. Alpha-1a receptors are also present in the bladder neck, seminal vesicles, and vas, and they conversely cause relaxation of the smooth muscle, leading to a range of ejaculatory dysfunctions from retrograde ejaculation, decreased ejaculatory volume, or anejaculation. Despite, the hope that super selective alpha blockers would minimize the side-effect, ejaculatory dysfunction is noted across all alpha-blockers.

Painful Ejaculation

Painful ejaculation is also referred to as dysejaculation, post-orgasmic pain, dysorgasmia, and odynorgasmia. The prevalence ranges between 1–10% [44] and may even rise up to 30–75% in men with chronic prostatitis/chronic pelvic pain syndrome (CP/CPPS) [45]. Painful ejaculation can have both psychogenic and organic pathology and should be evaluated for lower urinary tract dysfunction and CP/CPPS.

EAU describes painful ejaculation as the following:

"Painful ejaculation is a condition in which a patient feels mild discomfort to severe pain during or after ejaculation" and pain may occur anywhere in the pudendal territory and usually lasts between 2 and 24 h [46].

In painful ejaculation, a patient can present with mild discomfort to severe pain during or following ejaculation involving the penis, scrotum, or perineum. Painful ejaculation has a detrimental effect on a patient's self-esteem and quality of life. Its etiology can range from a simple urinary tract infection to post-radical prostatectomy, and due the sensitive nature of issue, it is an underreported symptom.

Etiopathogenesis

There are various factors that can result in painful ejaculation, and below we discuss some common possible causes.

Infection and inflammation In a community-based study conducted by Blanker et al., conditions like urethritis, epididymitis, orchitis are found to be associated with painful ejaculation [47].

Benign prostate hyperplasia (BPH) Litwin et al., noted that patients with BPH had more painful ejaculation [48]. BPH with varying degrees of lower urinary tract symptoms and prostatitis like-symptom of painful ejaculation differentiates a group of men with both BPH and chronic prostatitis, the evaluation and management of painful ejaculation should address in that line, rather than being ignored.

Seminal vesicle stone conditions like, chronic infection, reflux of urine, diabetes, prostate malignancy can cause seminal vesicle stone. The majority of patients with seminal vesicle stone complain of painful ejaculation and hematospermia [49].

Medications Painful ejaculation can be seen in patients on anti-depressant drugs like imipramine, clomipramine, fluoxetine, and venlafaxine, and stopping the medications has shown positive results in patients [56].

Other conditions like ejaculatory duct obstruction, sexually transmitted diseases, pelvic radiation, prostate surgery, and herniorrhaphy can also lead to painful ejaculation.

Post-Orgasmic Illness Syndrome (POIS)

POIS is a rare ejaculatory disorder, where an affected man experiences a cluster of bothersome symptoms post-ejaculation, which include flu-like malaise, severe fatigue, feverishness, irritability, burning eyes, nasal congestion [50]. The symptoms may start within few minutes of ejaculation and can last between 2 and 7 days. Waldinger and Schweitzer first described post-orgasmic illness syndrome in 2002, and they hypothesized that POIS is likely "a hypersensitivity reaction against autologous semen expressed as a combined Type-I and IV allergic reaction, triggered by ejaculation."

Classification of POIS

- Primary: POIS manifests from the first ejaculation.
- Secondary: POIS starts later in life.

Further, Waldinger et al. [51], noted that the presentation of POIS can be variable but meets these five criteria which point towards an "immunogenic" origin:

> Criterium 1. One or more of the following symptoms: sensation of a flu-like state, extreme fatigue or exhaustion, weakness of musculature, experiences of feverishness or perspiration, mood disturbances and/or irritability, memory difficulties, concentration problems, incoherent speech, congestion of nose or watery nose, itching eyes;
>
> Criterium 2. All symptoms occur immediately (e.g., seconds), soon (e.g., minutes), or within a few hours after ejaculation that is initiated by coitus, and/or masturbation, and/or spontaneously (e.g., during sleep);
>
> Criterium 3. Symptoms occur always or nearly always, e.g., in more than 90% of ejaculation events;
>
> Criterium 4. Most of these symptoms last for about 2 to 7 days;
>
> Criterium 5. The symptoms disappear spontaneously.

In 2015, Waldinger observed the POIS phenomena in three men before and after sterilization. This phenomenon suggests "that the antigen is most likely not bound to the spermatozoa but associated with the seminal fluid."

To conclude, POIS is a new and rare phenomenon in the group of ejaculatory disorders. The exact etiology is not very clear but most probably an autoimmune-mediated disease where specific cytokines are produced against the man's seminal fluid.

References

1. Burnstock G, Verkhratsky A. Vas deferens–a model used to establish sympathetic cotransmission. Trends Pharmacol Sci. 2010;31(3):131–9.
2. Nguyen HT, Etzell J, Turek PJ. Normal human ejaculatory duct anatomy: a study of cadaveric and surgical specimens. J Urol. 1996;155(5):1639–42.
3. Staudt MD, de Oliveira CV, Lehman MN, McKenna KE, Coolen LM. Activation of NMDA receptors in lumbar spinothalamic cells is required for ejaculation. J Sex Med. 2011;8(4):1015–26.
4. Jannini EA, Lenzi A. Epidemiology of premature ejaculation. Curr Opin Urol. 2005;15(6):399–403.
5. Waldinger MD, Schweitzer DH. The use of old and recent DSM definitions of premature ejaculation in observational studies: a contribution to the present debate for a new classification of PE in the DSM-V. J Sex Med. 2008;5(5):1079–87.
6. Serefoglu EC, McMahon CG, Waldinger MD, Althof SE, Shindel A, Adaikan G, Becher EF, Dean J, Giuliano F, Hellstrom WJ, Giraldi A. An evidence-based unified definition of lifelong and acquired premature ejaculation: report of the second international society for sexual medicine ad hoc committee for the definition of premature ejaculation. Sex Med. 2014;2(2):41–59.
7. Janssen PK, Bakker SC, Réthelyi J, Zwinderman AH, Touw DJ, Olivier B, Waldinger MD. Serotonin transporter promoter region (5-HTTLPR) polymorphism is associated with the intravaginal ejaculation latency time in Dutch men with lifelong premature ejaculation. J Sex Med. 2009;6(1):276–84.
8. Donatucci CF. Etiology of ejaculation and pathophysiology of premature ejaculation. J Sex Med. 2006;3:303–8.
9. Fasolo CB, Mirone V, Gentile V, Parazzini F, Ricci E. Andrology Prevention Week centers. Premature ejaculation: prevalence and associated conditions in a sample of 12,558 men attending the andrology prevention week 2001—a study of the Italian Society of Andrology (SIA). J Sex Med. 2005;2(3):376–82.
10. Laumann EO, West S, Glasser D, Carson C, Rosen R, Kang JH. Prevalence and correlates of erectile dysfunction by race and ethnicity among men aged 40 or older in the United States: from the male attitudes regarding sexual health survey. J Sex Med. 2007;4(1):57–65.
11. Shamloul R, Nashaar AE. Chronic prostatitis in premature ejaculation: a cohort study in 153 men. J Sex Med. 2006;3(1):150–4.
12. Rowland DL, Strassberg DS, de Gouveia Brazao CA, Slob AK. Ejaculatory latency and control in men with premature ejaculation: an analysis across sexual activities using multiple sources of information. J Psychosom Res. 2000;48(1):69–77.
13. El-Nashaar A, Shamloul R. Antibiotic treatment can delay ejaculation in patients with premature ejaculation and chronic bacterial prostatitis. J Sex Med. 2007;4(2):491–6.
14. JP B. The influence of hyperthyroidism and hypothyroidism on alpha-and beta-adrencrgic receptor systems and adrenergic responsiveness. Endocr Rev 1983;4:378–388.
15. Carani C, Isidori AM, Granata A, Carosa E, Maggi M, Lenzi A, Jannini EA. Multicenter study on the prevalence of sexual symptoms in male hypo-and hyperthyroid patients. J Clin Endocrinol Metabol. 2005;90(12):6472–9.
16. Simons JS, Carey MP. Prevalence of sexual dysfunctions: results from a decade of research. Arch Sex Behav. 2001;30:177–219.

17. Laumann EO, Paik A, Rosen RC. Sexual dysfunction in the United States: prevalence and predictors. JAMA. 1999;281(6):537–44.
18. Waldinger MD, Quinn P, Dilleen M, Mundayat R, Schweitzer DH, Boolell M. A multinational population survey of intravaginal ejaculation latency time. J Sex Med. 2005;2(4):492–7.
19. Patrick DL, Althof SE, Pryor JL, Rosen R, Rowland DL, Ho KF, McNulty P, Rothman M, Jamieson C. Ejaculatory disorders: premature ejaculation: an observational study of men and their partners. J Sex Med. 2005;2(3):358–67.
20. Rowland D, McMahon CG, Abdo C, Chen J, Jannini E, Waldinger MD, Ahn TY. Disorders of orgasm and ejaculation in men. J Sex Med. 2010;7(4_Part_2):1668–86.
21. World Health Organization. International Classification of Diseases and Related Health Problems 11th Revision. 2018.
22. McCabe MP, Sharlip ID, Atalla E, Balon R, Fisher AD, Laumann E, Lee SW, Lewis R, Segraves RT. Definitions of sexual dysfunctions in women and men: a consensus statement from the Fourth International Consultation on Sexual Medicine 2015. J Sex Med. 2016;13(2):135–43.
23. Kinsey AC, Pomeroy WR, Martin CE. Sexual behavior in the human male. Am J Public Health. 2003;93(6):894–8.
24. Vosbergen M. Anejaculation and anorgasmia [Internet]. SMSNA. Available from:https://www.smsna.org/patients/conditions/anejaculation-and anorgasmia.
25. Burri A, Buchmeier J, Porst H. The importance of male ejaculation for female sexual satisfaction and function. J Sex Med. 2018;15(11):1600–8.
26. Althof SE. Psychological interventions for delayed ejaculation/orgasm. Int J Impot Res. 2012;24(4):131–6.
27. Masters WH, Johnson VE. Human sexual inadequacy. Boston: Little, Brown & Company; 1970.
28. Rowland DL, Keeney C, Slob AK. Sexual response in men with inhibited or retarded ejaculation. Int J Impot Res. 2004;16(3):270–4.
29. Xia JD, Han YF, Pan F, Zhou LH, Chen Y, Dai YT. Clinical characteristics and penile afferent neuronal function in patients with primary delayed ejaculation. Andrology. 2013;1(5):787–92.
30. Nelson CJ, Ahmed A, Valenzuela R, Parker M, Mulhall JP. Assessment of penile vibratory stimulation as a management strategy in men with secondary retarded orgasm. Urology. 2007;69(3):552–5.
31. Perelman MA, Rowland DL. Retarded ejaculation. World J Urol. 2006;24:645–52.
32. Apfelbaum B. Retarded ejaculation: a much-misunderstood syndrome. Principles and practice of sex therapy, 2nd end.
33. Dunsmuir WD, Holmes SA. The aetiology and management of erectile, ejaculatory, and fertility problems in men with diabetes mellitus. Diabet Med. 1996;13(8):700–8.
34. Higgins A, Nash M, Lynch AM. Antidepressant-associated sexual dysfunction: impact, effects, and treatment. Drug Healthc Patient saf. 2010;9:141–50.
35. Incrocci L. Sexual function after external-beam radiotherapy for prostate cancer: what do we know? Crit Rev Oncol Hematol. 2006;57(2):165–73.
36. Van Basten JP, Jonker-Pool G, Van Driel MF, Sleijfer DT, Droste JH, Van De Wiel HB, Koops HS, Molenaar WM, Hoekstra HJ. Sexual functioning after multimodality treatment for disseminated nonseminomatous testicular germ cell tumor. J Urol. 1997;158(4):1411–6.
37. Basiri A, Ghaed MA, Simforoosh N, Tabibi A, Danesh A, Nouralizadeh A, Parizi MK. Is modified retroperitoneal lymph node dissection alive for clinical stage I non-seminomatous germ cell testicular tumor? Urol J. 2013;10(2):873.
38. Comarr AE. Sexual function among patients with spinal cord injury. Urol Int. 1970;25(2):134–68.
39. Phillips E, Carpenter C, Oates RD. Ejaculatory dysfunction. Urol Clin. 2014;41(1):115–28.
40. Jefferys A, Siassakos D, Wardle P. The management of retrograde ejaculation: a systematic review and update. Fertil Steril. 2012;97(2):306–12.
41. Hylmarova S, Stechova K, Pavlinkova G, Peknicova J, Macek M, Kvapil M. The impact of type 1 diabetes mellitus on male sexual functions and sex hormone levels. Endocr J. 2020;67(1):59–71.
42. Emberton M, Neal DE, Black N, Fordham M, Harrison M, McBrien MP, Williams RE, McPherson K, Devlin HB. The effect of prostatectomy on symptom severity and quality of life. Br J Urol. 1996;77(2):233–47.

43. Miner M, Rosenberg MT, Perelman MA. Treatment of lower urinary tract symptoms in benign prostatic hyperplasia and its impact on sexual function. Clin Ther. 2006;28:13–25.
44. Blanker MH, Bosch JR, Groeneveld FP, Bohnen AM, Prins AD, Thomas S, Hop WC. Erectile and ejaculatory dysfunction in a community-based sample of men 50 to 78 years old: prevalence, concern, and relation to sexual activity. Urology. 2001;57(4):763–8.
45. Mo MQ, Long LL, Xie WL, Chen S, Zhang WH, Luo CQ, Deng LW. Sexual dysfunctions and psychological disorders associated with type IIIa chronic prostatitis: a clinical survey in China. Int Urol Nephrol. 2014;46:2255–61.
46. Parnham A, Serefoglu EC. Retrograde ejaculation, painful ejaculation and hematospermia. Transl Androl Urol. 2016;5(4):592.
47. Blanker MH, Bohnen AM, Groeneveld FP, Bernsen RM, Prins A, Thomas S, Bosch JR. Correlates for erectile and ejaculatory dysfunction in older Dutch men: a community-based study. J Am Geriatr Soc. 2001;49(4):436–42.
48. Litwin MS, McNaughton-Collins M, Fowler FJ, Nickel JC, Calhoun EA, Pontari MA, Alexander RB, Farrar JT, O'leary MP. The National Institutes of Health chronic prostatitis symptom index: development and validation of a new outcome measure. J Urol. 1999;162(2):369–75.
49. Zaidi S, Gandhi J, Seyam O, Joshi G, Waltzer WC, Smith NL, Khan SA. Etiology, diagnosis, and management of seminal vesicle stones. Curr Urol. 2019;12(3):113–20.
50. Waldinger MD, Meinardi MM, Zwinderman AH, Schweitzer DH. Postorgasmic illness syndrome (POIS) in 45 Dutch Caucasian males: clinical characteristics and evidence for an immunogenic pathogenesis (part 1). J Sex Med. 2011;8(4):1164–70.
51. Waldinger MD. Post orgasmic illness syndrome (POIS). Transl Androl Urol. 2016;5(4):602.

Chapter 8
Clinical Assessment and Evaluation of Ejaculatory Dysfunction

Pookkan Dhinaharan

Chapter Overview

Ejaculatory dysfunction encompasses a broad spectrum of disorders that affect a significant portion of the male population. These conditions, including premature ejaculation, delayed ejaculation, and anejaculation, not only compromise fertility but also profoundly impact the psychological well-being and quality of life for both individuals and couples. This chapter aims to provide a comprehensive evaluation of ejaculatory dysfunction, exploring the various types, underlying physiological mechanisms, and associated comorbidities.

Creating a supportive and nonjudgmental environment is crucial during the evaluation process to ensure open communication and effective management of premature ejaculation.

Evaluation of Premature Ejaculation

When men present with self-reported premature ejaculation (PE), a thorough evaluation is crucial to understand the underlying causes and determine appropriate treatment strategies. The evaluation process should encompass a comprehensive medical/sexual history, a focused physical examination, assessment of erectile function, and any necessary investigations based on the findings.

The medical/sexual history is the cornerstone of the evaluation process. Healthcare professionals (HCP) should sensitively inquire about the patient's sexual experiences, concerns, and overall health. Additionally, the history-taking process provides an opportunity for patients to discuss their sexual complaints, as they may

P. Dhinaharan (✉)
Consultant Urologist and Andrologist, Chennai, India

Vasan S S et al. (eds.), *Men's Health*,
https://doi.org/10.1007/978-3-031-76898-9_8

be hesitant or embarrassed to raise such concerns without prompting. By creating an open and non-judgmental environment, HCPs can facilitate a more comprehensive understanding of the patient's condition and associated health risks.

Involving the partner in the treatment process can be a valuable aspect of managing PE. While some patients may not immediately grasp the importance of including their partners, a cooperative partner can play a crucial role in enhancing the patient's self-confidence, skills, self-esteem, and sense of masculinity. Moreover, partners can assist in the development of ejaculatory control, leading to improvements not only in the couple's sexual relationship but also in broader aspects of their partnership. While involving the partner in the management process is not mandatory, it can significantly contribute to treatment success.

The impact of involving partners in treating PE has not been extensively studied through controlled research. However, evidence from studies on erectile dysfunction (ED) suggests that addressing interpersonal factors can significantly influence treatment success. Inquiring about the patient's sexual health not only allows for a more accurate diagnosis but also screens for associated health risks, such as cardiovascular issues and ED. Thus, discussing sexual health is an important part of the evaluation process, granting patients permission to express their concerns and seek appropriate treatment [1].

To aid in the evaluation, specific questions should be asked when patients complain of PE. The recommended questions are essential for establishing the diagnosis and guiding treatment decisions, while the optional questions help gather additional details for implementing a tailored treatment plan.

Diagnosis of PE

The process of diagnosing premature ejaculation (PE) involves a thorough assessment of the patient's medical and sexual history. It is essential to determine whether the PE is lifelong or acquired and whether it occurs only under specific circumstances or with a specific partner or consistently in all situations. Various factors should be taken into account, including the time it takes for ejaculation to occur, the level of sexual stimulation required, the impact of PE on sexual activity and the individual's quality of life, as well as any history of drug use or abuse.

It is crucial to distinguish between PE and erectile dysfunction (ED), as sometimes patients with ED may develop secondary PE due to anxiety related to their difficulty in achieving and maintaining an erection. Additionally, some individuals may mistakenly complain of ED when the actual problem is PE because they are unaware that it is normal to lose an erection after ejaculation.

Different definitions of PE exist, but they typically share four common factors:

1. the assessment of time to ejaculation using intravaginal ejaculation latency time (IELT),
2. perceived control over ejaculation,

3. the level of distress, bother, frustration, and
4. interpersonal difficulties related to the ejaculatory dysfunction.

Taking into consideration these multiple dimensions ensures a comprehensive and accurate diagnosis of PE.

The International Society for Sexual Medicine (ISSM) definition of Premature Ejaculation (PE) serves as the basis for diagnosing PE.

Premature Ejaculation Assessment Questionnaires

To effectively diagnose and manage PE, healthcare professionals rely on various assessment questionnaires. Several PE measures have been described in the literature, although only a small number have undergone extensive psychometric testing and validation. Five validated questionnaires have been developed and published to date.

Premature Ejaculation Diagnostic Tool (PEDT)

The Premature Ejaculation Diagnostic Tool (PEDT) is one of the first and most widely used questionnaires for assessing PE [2]. Developed through focus groups and interviews in the USA, Germany, and Spain, the PEDT consists of five items that evaluate the following aspects:

- Time to ejaculation
- Control over ejaculation
- Sexual satisfaction
- Distress related to PE
- Interpersonal difficulty

Each question is scored on a 5-point Likert scale, with higher scores indicating a higher likelihood of PE. The total score ranges from 0 to 20, with a score above 11 suggesting a diagnosis of PE, 9 or 10 indicating a probable diagnosis, and below 8 indicating a low likelihood of PE (Fig. 8.1).

Index of Premature Ejaculation (IPE)

The Index of Premature Ejaculation (IPE) is another widely used questionnaire developed by Althof et al., which assesses various domains related to PE [3]. It consists of five questions, scored on a 5-point Likert scale, which evaluate the following aspects:

	Not difficult at all	Somewhat difficult	Moderately difficult	Very difficult	Extremely difficult
1. How difficult is it for you to delay ejaculation?	0	1	2	3	4

	Never or almost never (0%)	Less than half the time (25%)	About half the time (50%)	Over half the time (75%)	Always or almost always (100%)
2. Do you ejaculate before you want to?	0	1	2	3	4
3. Do you ejaculate with very little stimulation?	0	1	2	3	4

	Not at all	Slightly	Moderately	Very	Extremely
4. Do you feel frustrated because of ejaculating before you want to?	0	1	2	3	4
5. How concerned are you that your time to ejaculation leaves your partner unfulfilled?	0	1	2	3	4

Fig. 8.1 PE diagnostic tool questionnaire

Question	Strongly Agree (5)	Agree (4)	Neutral (3)	Disagree (2)	Strongly Disagree (1)
1. I ejaculate too quickly during...					
2. I am bothered by how quickly I...					
3. My partner is bothered by how...					
4. I feel anxious about how quickly...					
5. I feel satisfied with my sexual...					
Total Score (5-25)					

Fig. 8.2 Scoring of the Index of Premature Ejaculation (IPE)

- Ejaculatory control
- Sexual satisfaction
- Personal distress related to PE
- Partner's distress related to PE

The IPE provides a total score ranging from 0 to 20, with higher scores indicating a higher likelihood of PE (Fig. 8.2).

Fig. 8.3 Scoring of the Premature Ejaculation Profile (PEP)

Domain	Score
Time to ejaculation	
Control over ejaculation	
Satisfaction with sexual intercourse	
Personal distress related to PE	
Partner's distress related to PE	
Total Score (0-30)	

The PEP questionnaire (Fig. 8.3) has become a standard tool in the evaluation and management of premature ejaculation. Its development was based on extensive research, and its application has been validated in numerous clinical studies. The utilization of tools like the PEP questionnaire underscores the importance of patient-reported outcomes in the effective management of sexual health conditions like PE.

Other questionnaires for characterizing PE include the Premature Ejaculation Profile (PEP), Index of Premature Ejaculation (IPE), and Male Sexual Health Questionnaire Ejaculatory Dysfunction (MSHQ-EjD), which are optionally used in daily clinical practice. The Masturbatory Premature Ejaculation Diagnostic Tool (MPEDT) has been proposed since PE patients report differing experiences with masturbation versus partnered sex, but further validation is needed for routine use.

Assessment of Coexisting ED

Comorbid ED in PE should be evaluated with instruments like the IIEF (International Index of Erectile Function) or IIEF-5, defined by specific criteria. Studies show that up to half of ED subjects also experience PE, with varying prevalence across regions. The relationship between ED and PE may involve factors like increased stimulation needs and performance anxiety, but caution must be exercised in diagnosis due to potential confusion and false-positive diagnoses, as indicated by specific research [4].

Physical Examination

Physical examination in the context of premature ejaculation (PE) remains primarily a supplementary tool for comprehensive evaluation. The diagnosis of lifelong premature ejaculation (L-PE) largely relies on medical history, given the absence of predictive physical findings or definitive tests [4]. Differentiating between L-PE and acquired premature ejaculation (A-PE) can be challenging, especially in younger men or those with limited sexual experience or few previous partners. In such cases, a physical examination is not only valuable but also highly recommended, serving as a pivotal opportunity for screening cardiovascular and gender-specific diseases.

In the clinical evaluation of premature ejaculation (PE), a meticulous examination encompassing the urological, endocrine, and neurological systems is paramount.

Such an examination is aimed at identifying potential underlying medical pathologies that might be concomitantly present with PE or other coexisting sexual dysfunctions.

This ensures the identification of concomitant medical conditions that may be causative or associative of PE or other sexual dysfunctions. Such conditions include endocrinopathies, Peyronie's disease, urethritis, and prostatitis. It is prudent to emphasize that laboratory or physiological testing should not be undertaken as a routine measure. Instead, the necessity for these tests should arise from particular findings gleaned from the patient's medical history or discerned during the physical examination.

For men diagnosed with A-PE, the physical examination becomes imperative to discern the root cause of the PE and address it effectively. Concurrently, the potential presence of erectile dysfunction (ED) should be assessed either through patient history or using a validated tool. While lab tests or imaging are occasionally requisitioned based on a patient's history, a digital prostate examination is a routine recommendation in andrological settings for men over 40, aiding in the identification of potential prostatic inflammation or infection [5].

Evaluation and Diagnosis of Delayed Ejaculation

Delayed ejaculation (DE) is one of the less common but potentially distressing male sexual dysfunctions. Its evaluation requires a systematic approach, integrating clinical, psychosocial, and, if necessary, laboratory findings.

Definition

Both the European Association of Urology (EAU) and the International Society for Sexual Medicine (ISSM) define DE as a marked delay, infrequency, or absence of ejaculation during sexual activity, despite the presence of adequate sexual stimulation and arousal. This dysfunction must cause marked distress or interpersonal difficulty to be considered pathological [6, 7].

Evaluation

Clinical History

A thorough sexual, medical, and psychosocial history is paramount. It should delve into:

- Duration and onset of DE (sudden vs. gradual).
- Specificity: Is the problem situational or generalized?

- Masturbation patterns and outcomes.
- Relationship and interpersonal dynamics.
- Medications, especially those known to affect ejaculatory function.
- Previous surgeries, particularly those in the pelvic region.

Physical Examination

While DE is often psychogenic, a physical examination is essential to rule out potential organic causes:

- Genital anatomical anomalies.
- Neurological assessment focusing on the perineal and penile sensation.
- Prostate examination, especially in older men or those with symptoms of prostatitis.

Laboratory Tests

These are not routinely recommended but might be considered based on clinical findings, such as suspected testosterone deficiency or hyperprolactinemia.

Questionnaires

While DE-specific validated questionnaires are limited compared to those for PE, there are instruments like the Male Sexual Health Questionnaire-Ejaculation Disorder (MSHQ-EjD) which assess ejaculation function and satisfaction [8].

Evaluation Algorithm

1. Begin with a comprehensive sexual, medical, and psychosocial history.
2. Conduct a targeted physical examination.
3. If the history and physical suggest an organic cause, proceed with pertinent laboratory tests.
4. Utilize the MSHQ-EjD or equivalent instruments to quantify the severity and impact of DE.
5. Differentiate between primary (lifelong) and secondary (acquired) DE.
6. Consider psychogenic causes, especially if the patient can ejaculate normally through masturbation or nocturnal emissions.

Conclusions

Evaluating DE demands a multifaceted approach that recognizes the often intricate interplay between organic and psychogenic factors. By adopting a methodical evaluation algorithm, clinicians can offer patients the most accurate diagnosis and thereby the most effective treatment.

Evaluation of Delayed Ejaculation

Delayed ejaculation (DE) or anejaculation (aspermia) is a challenging male sexual dysfunction to diagnose and manage. An effective evaluation is predicated on a holistic approach that amalgamates clinical, hormonal, and, at times, radiological insights.

Clinical Evaluation

Medical/Sexual History

- *Classification of DE:* It is essential to determine if DE is lifelong or acquired and whether it is global (occurring in all situations) or situational (specific to certain scenarios).
- *Ejaculatory Latency:* Document the frequency of successful ejaculation during intercourse and the intravaginal ejaculatory latency time (IELT)—the time elapsed from penetration to ejaculation.
- *Details of Failed Ejaculations:* If ejaculation does not occur, ascertain the duration of thrusting before intercourse is halted, reasons for stopping (like fatigue, loss of erection, sense of ejaculatory futility, partner's request), and the ability to achieve ejaculation through postcoital self- or partner-assisted masturbation.
- *Premonitory Sensation:* Determine if there's a sensation suggestive of approaching ejaculation during intercourse or masturbation. This gives insight into whether arousal levels near the ejaculatory threshold are achieved.
- *Arousal and Psychological Aspects:* Identify variables that may augment or diminish performance. Note the man's capacity to relax, sustain arousal, heighten arousal, and concentrate on erotic sensations. Investigate any patient-, partner-, or interpersonal-related negative psychological impacts like distress, frustration, or sexual avoidance. Assess the frequency of intercourse, initiator of sexual activity, and the quality of the nonsexual relationship.
- *In Acquired DE:* Delve into past medical history, surgeries, medication use, and significant life events or circumstances that might have precipitated DE. This may encompass various life stressors and psychological elements that affect arousal.

Physical Examination

- *Genital Examination:* Ensure the testes, epididymes, and vasa are normal.
- *Digital Rectal Examination:* Evaluate prostate size, anal sphincter tone, and the bulbocavernous reflex (BCR). This might be unnecessary for young men with clear psychogenic inhibited ejaculation.

Laboratory and Imaging

- *Testosterone Levels:* A screening morning total testosterone helps identify potential hormonal imbalances.
- *Neuropathy Investigation*: If a neuropathy is suspected, electrophysiologic evaluations like pudendal somatosensory, motor-evoked potentials, sacral reflex arc testing, and sympathetic skin responses are useful.
- *Assessment of Ejaculation:* An orgasm with either absent or low-volume ejaculation indicates possible retrograde ejaculation (RE) or ejaculatory duct obstruction. The presence of sperm in postmasturbation urine signifies RE, while azoospermic/oligospermic fluid with low viscosity, fructose, and pH on semen analysis hints at ejaculatory duct obstruction.
- *Exclusion of Pathology:* For ambiguous DE causes, prostatic secretion cultures, urine cytology, and serum prostate-specific antigen levels help rule out prostatitis, bladder, and prostate cancer.
- *Imaging:* In certain scenarios, transrectal ultrasound (TRUS), MRI, or ultrasonography of the testicles and epididymes can be instrumental in identifying localized pathologies.

In conclusion, a methodical evaluation encompassing a thorough history, clinical examination, and selective laboratory/imaging investigations forms the linchpin of DE diagnosis. This ensures not just the identification but also the management of this intricate sexual dysfunction.

Evaluation of Retrograde Ejaculation

Introduction

Retrograde ejaculation is a condition wherein seminal fluid travels backward into the bladder rather than being expelled through the urethra during ejaculation. While this is not a life-threatening condition, it can result in infertility and may significantly impact the quality of life. This chapter aims to provide a comprehensive overview of the evaluation methods for diagnosing retrograde ejaculation, which is crucial for management and potential treatment.

Physiology Overview

To understand retrograde ejaculation, it is essential to briefly review the normal physiology of ejaculation. The process is composed of two phases: emission and expulsion. During emission, the seminal fluid is transported from the seminal vesicles and combined with sperm from the testes. This mixture is then propelled toward the prostatic urethra. During expulsion, rhythmic contractions of the pelvic musculature push the semen out through the urethra and out of the penis.

In retrograde ejaculation, the bladder neck fails to close, allowing semen to flow backward into the bladder.

Clinical Presentation

Patients may present with:

1. Infertility
2. Absent or decreased ejaculate volume ("dry orgasm")
3. Cloudy urine post-orgasm

History and Physical Examination

Medical History

1. Diabetes Mellitus.
2. Prior surgeries such as retroperitoneal lymph node dissection, bladder neck surgery, or prostatectomy.
3. Medications: Some antihypertensives and psychotropic medications can lead to retrograde ejaculation.
4. Neurological conditions: Spinal cord injuries or multiple sclerosis.

Physical Examination

Generally, it is unremarkable unless other coexisting conditions like prostatitis or testicular disorders are present.

Diagnostic Evaluation

Semen Analysis

In a typical semen analysis, a very low volume or no ejaculate would raise suspicions.

Post-Ejaculatory Urinalysis

This is the definitive test. After ejaculation, a fresh urine sample is analyzed for the presence of sperm. If the sperm count is significantly high (5–10/HPF), this is diagnostic of retrograde ejaculation.

Imaging Studies

While not commonly used for the sole purpose of diagnosing retrograde ejaculation, imaging like ultrasound can be helpful in identifying structural issues affecting the bladder neck or other parts of the reproductive tract.

Additional Tests

Cystoscopy may be used in some cases to visualize the internal urethral orifice and bladder neck during the ejaculation process.

Differential Diagnosis

1. Anejaculation: No ejaculation.
2. Hypogonadism: Low testosterone levels can affect semen volume.
3. Obstructive causes: Ejaculatory duct obstruction can cause low ejaculate volume.

Summary

Evaluating retrograde ejaculation involves a combination of medical history, physical examination, and targeted diagnostic tests. Understanding the underlying physiology and ruling out other potential causes are crucial for proper management and treatment, which may involve pharmacotherapy or surgical interventions.

Evaluation of Painful Ejaculation

Introduction

Painful ejaculation, also known as dysorgasmia or orgasmalgia, is a relatively uncommon but distressing symptom that can significantly impact a man's sexual and psychological well-being. It is characterized by pain or discomfort during or following ejaculation. This chapter aims to provide a systematic approach to the evaluation of painful ejaculation, detailing its clinical presentation, differential diagnosis, and the variety of diagnostic tests used to pinpoint the cause.

Basic Physiology

Normal ejaculation is a complex process involving a myriad of physiological and psychological systems, including the nervous system, muscular contractions, and various reproductive glands. Painful ejaculation may be indicative of underlying conditions affecting these systems or secondary to medications and surgical procedures.

Clinical Presentation

Patients typically describe a range of symptoms such as:

1. Pain localized to the penis, perineum, or testicles
2. Pain that can be sharp, dull, or burning in character
3. Discomfort during or after ejaculation
4. Occasional blood in semen (hematospermia)

History Taking

A thorough history is paramount to identify potential causes:

1. Onset and duration of symptoms
2. Type of pain and localization
3. Relationship to ejaculation: before, during, or after
4. Medical history including prostate issues, urinary tract infections, sexually transmitted diseases, or recent surgeries
5. Medication history: Some antidepressants and antipsychotics can lead to painful ejaculation

Physical Examination

The physical exam should include a comprehensive genital examination, focusing on:

1. Penile abnormalities
2. Testicular or scrotal tenderness
3. Prostate examination through a digital rectal exam (DRE)

Diagnostic Tests

Urinalysis and Culture

Infections of the urinary tract or prostate can cause painful ejaculation. Urinalysis and culture can rule out these possibilities.

Semen Analysis and Culture

Assessment for infections or inflammatory markers can sometimes provide clues.

Transrectal Ultrasound (TRUS)

This can be used to visualize the ejaculatory ducts and prostate for signs of obstruction or inflammation.

Cystoscopy

In rare cases, a direct visual examination of the lower urinary tract may be needed.

Hormone Analysis

Tests to measure testosterone, luteinizing hormone, and other hormones may be necessary based on clinical suspicion.

Differential Diagnosis

1. Prostatitis: Chronic or acute inflammation of the prostate.
2. Orchitis: Inflammation of the testicles.
3. Urethritis: Inflammation of the urethra.
4. Pelvic muscle tension.
5. Neurological Causes: Certain neuropathies can cause painful ejaculation.
6. Psychological Factors: Anxiety or stress.
7. Medication-induced.

Painful ejaculation is a condition that demands thorough evaluation for effective management. A detailed history, focused physical examination, and appropriate diagnostic tests are the cornerstones of its evaluation. By employing a systematic approach, clinicians specializing in Andrology can not only accurately diagnose the underlying causes but also provide targeted treatments to alleviate the symptoms and improve the patient's quality of life.

Evaluation of Ejaculatory Anhedonia

The evaluation of ejaculatory anhedonia, a condition where an individual experiences an absence of pleasure or sensation during ejaculation, requires a multifaceted approach due to its complex nature. Ejaculatory anhedonia can have both psychological and physiological roots, and the diagnosis often involves ruling out other potential causes of sexual dysfunction.

An extensive history-taking process is crucial, focusing on sexual, medical, and psychological histories, as well as medication usage. Physical examinations including a genital examination and possibly a digital rectal exam (DRE) are typically carried out to assess for anatomical or pathological issues that might be contributing factors.

Diagnostic tests may include hormone panels to check for imbalances that could be affecting sexual response, as well as neurophysiological studies to rule out nerve damage. Advanced imaging techniques like MRI or ultrasound may be employed in rare cases.

Psychological evaluations are also essential, as mental health issues such as depression or anxiety can be underlying causes. Effective evaluation is crucial for targeted treatment, which may involve pharmacotherapy, psychosexual counseling, or a combination of both.

References

1. Patrick DL, Althof SE, Pryor JL, et al. Premature ejaculation: an observational study of men and their partners. J Sex Med. 2005;2(3):358–67.
2. Rosen RC, Cappelleri JC, Smith MD, et al. Development and evaluation of an abridged, 5-item version of the International Index of Erectile Function (IIEF-5) as a diagnostic tool for erectile dysfunction. Int J Impot Res. 1999;11(6):319–26.
3. Symonds T, Perelman MA, Althof S, et al. Development and validation of a premature ejaculation diagnostic tool. Eur Urol. 2007;52(2):565–73.
4. McMahon C. Current and emerging treatments for premature ejaculation. Sex Med Rev. 2005;3(3):183–202.
5. Jannini EA. Sexological approach to ejaculatory dysfunction. Int J Androl. 2006;29(5):513–9.
6. European Association of Urology. Guidelines on male sexual dysfunction: erectile dysfunction and premature ejaculation. EAU. 2020;
7. International Society for Sexual Medicine. Guidelines for the diagnosis and treatment of delayed ejaculation. ISSM; 2020.
8. Rosen RC, Catania J, Pollack L, et al. Male Sexual Health Questionnaire (MSHQ): scale development and psychometric validation. Urology. 2004;64(4):777–82.

Chapter 9
Management Strategies for Ejaculatory Dysfunction: Algorithms and Recent Advances

Sanjay Prakash Jayaprakash

Ejaculatory disorders are the most common disorders of sexual function in the male. The mechanisms leading to these dysfunction are poorly understood, hence no single drug is completely effective in reversing the dysfunction. Except for early ejaculation (premature ejaculation, old terminology), there are no specific guidelines and FDA-approved drugs available for the management of these conditions. Hence the treatment strategies adopted are also diverse. The aim of this chapter is to provide an insight into the different treatment protocols followed and share authors' suggestions and experiences for better office management of these conditions.

Early Ejaculation/Premature Ejaculation (PME)

PME is the commonest ejaculatory disorder in the male. An algorithmic approach to a patient presenting with PME is illustrated in Fig. 9.1.

Behavioral Therapy

Men with PME are anxious, less motivated, worried, with personality changes, and blame themselves for dysfunctional sexual response. Sometimes the partner expectations are higher, which causes further distress [1, 2]. The goals of psychosexual therapies (behavioral, cognitive, or couple focussed) are to teach methods to regulate or delay ejaculation, boost sexual performance and confidence, lessen anxiety,

S. P. Jayaprakash (✉)
Department of Andrology, Asian Institute of Nephrology and Urology, Chennai, Tamil Nadu, India

Vasan S S et al. (eds.), *Men's Health*,
https://doi.org/10.1007/978-3-031-76898-9_9

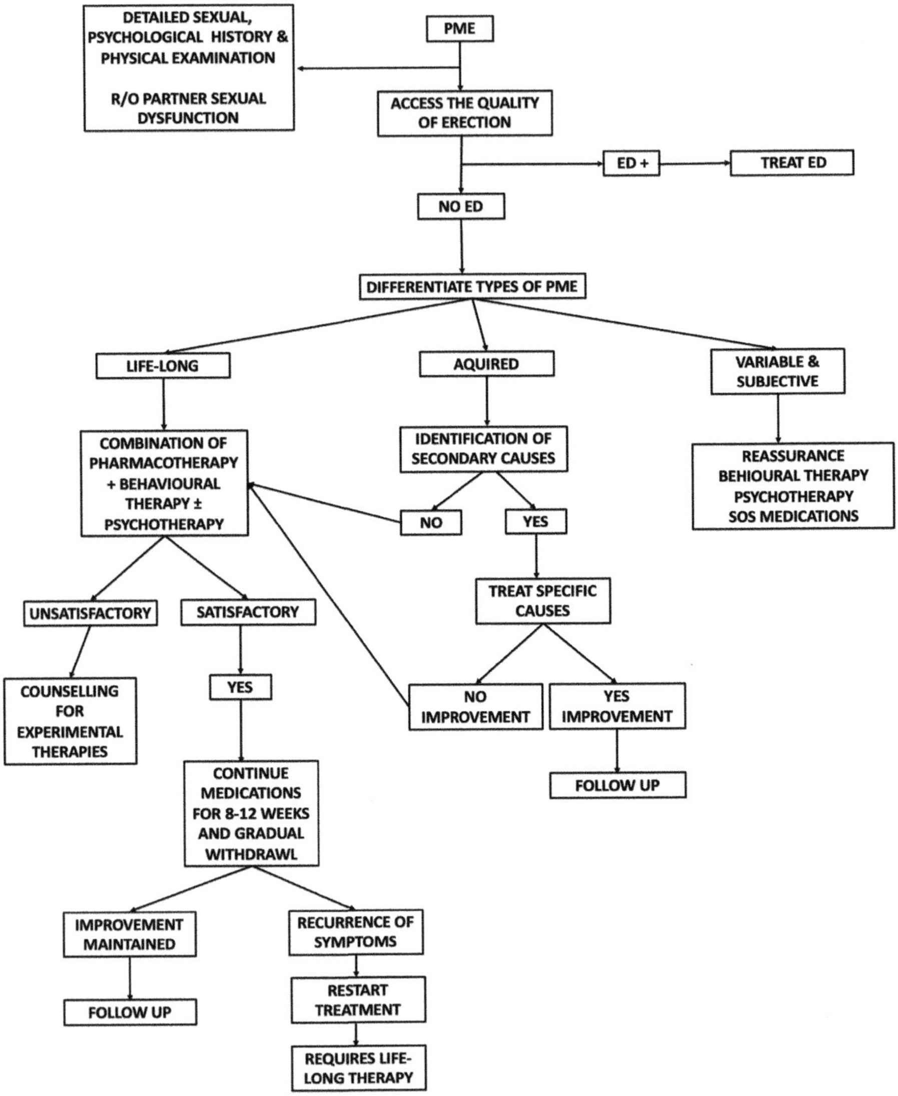

Fig. 9.1 Algorithmic approach to a patient presenting with PME. *PME* premature ejaculation, *ED* erectile dysfunction

and foster communication and problem-solving within the couple [3]. Psychosexual education with mindful techniques combined with behavioral modifications may improve PME symptoms and associated distress [4].

Some of the common practices in behavioral therapy are as follows.

1. The *stop-start technique*, described by Semans in 1954, the male/partner would stimulate the penis till the point where he has the urge to ejaculate, then imme-

diately stopped by the partner/self, till the sensation wears off and this is repeated until the satisfactory level of stimulation is achieved for final ejaculation. Later, the same steps are repeated with lubrication in order to mimic the moist vagina (Fig. 9.2) [5].

2. In the *penis squeezing technique*, described by Master and Johnson in the 1970s, the glans penis is squeezed between the thumb and the forefinger by the partner when there is an urge to ejaculate. This continuous squeeze causes contraction of the bulbospongiosus muscle via the bulbospongiosus reflex and results in diminished ejaculatory urgency, loss of desire with reduced penile sensations, thereby helping to prolong sexual activity. This squeeze is repeated multiple times before letting ejaculation to occur (Fig. 9.3) [6].
3. The *internal squeeze technique*, where the man contracts his pelvic muscles to control ejaculation and thereby can prolong sexual activity. Kegels exercises help in improving the strength of pelvic muscles.
4. Other techniques include extended foreplay, mindful distraction, using thick/ delay condoms to reduce the sensitivity, alternate sex positions (e.g. partner on top), interval sex, and increasing the frequency of intercourse, masturbating 2 hours before sex [7].

Although these techniques theoretically increase the threshold and delay ejaculations, the recent RCTs and guidelines provide weak recommendation for isolated

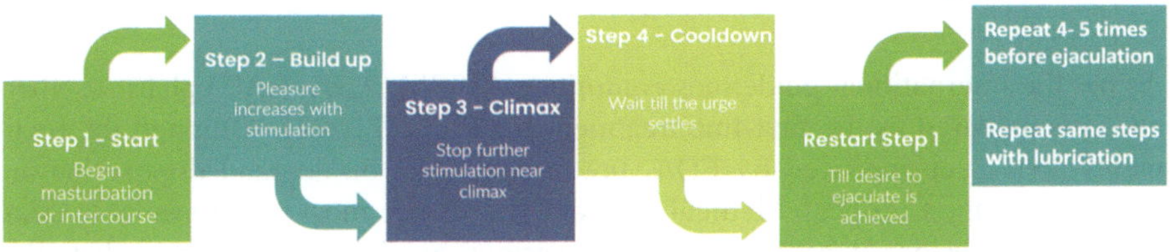

Fig. 9.2 The steps of start-stop technique

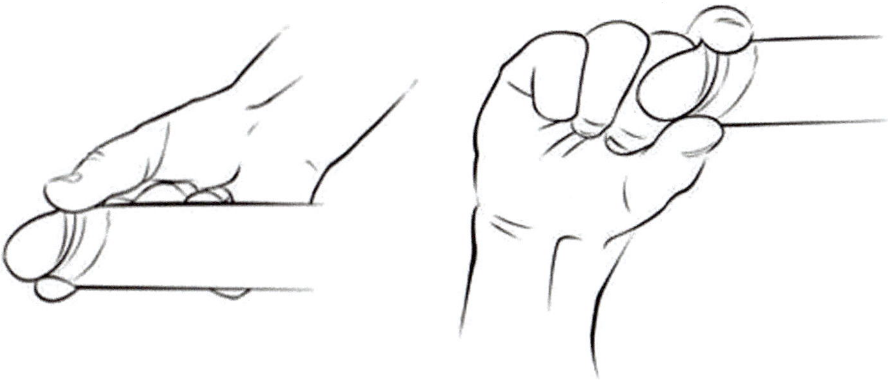

Fig. 9.3 The squeeze technique

treatment of PME [8]. However these therapies are more effective when used along with medical interventions. It has been reported that psychological and behavioral therapy when combined with a PDE5I and SSRI was more effective than monotherapies and in patients where other therapies have failed [9]. These techniques are difficult to follow as they require a lot of practice and coordination. Moreover, they may be helpful only in men with sensitivity at the glans penis and not the root of penis (bulbospongiosus muscle hyperactivity).

Partner Sexual Dysfunction

Partner sexual dysfunction is one of the disregarded and underrated cause of PME. Female sexual dysfunction (FSD) like vaginismus and dyspareunia are a few missed factors while evaluating PME and are responsible for anteportal ejaculation (ejaculation before penetration). Hence FSD should be ruled out in the management of PME. Sometimes the demand of the female partner will be high and hence men will end up ejaculating faster in an anxiety to fulfil the female partner's need, a state of false early ejaculation [10].

Pharmacotherapy

As per the international guidelines committees (ISSM, AUA, EAU) pharmacotherapy is considered as the first-line treatment for PME [11, 12]. Although the treatments aren't yet approved by FDA, few options like on-demand dopoxetine are approved by the European Medical Agency [13]. Hence most of the available treatments are considered as off-label. The various available drugs are enlisted in Fig. 9.4.

Dapoxetine

It is a short-acting selective serotonin reuptake inhibitor (SSRI). It is rapidly absorbed and metabolized in the body, and it reaches maximum plasma concentration in 1.5 h and 95% clearance occurs in 24 h. This property makes it suitable for on-demand use [14]. It is available in doses of 30 mg and 60 mg for use in the Asian and European countries but unavailable in the USA. It is recommended to consume it 1–2 h before intercourse and has been observed to not only increase IELT (2.5–3 fold) but also improve ejaculatory control, distress, and overall satisfaction [15]. The common treatment emergent adverse effects (TEAE) are nausea, diarrhea, headache, and dizziness. There is a very low chance of vasovagal syncope and no increased risk of suicidal ideation or SSRI syndrome [16]. Despite being the safest

PHARMACOTHERAPEUTIC DRUGS USED IN PME	
ON-DEMAND	**DAILY OFF-LABEL**
Dapoxetine (30mg, 60mg)	Paroxetine (20-40mg)
Metered-dose aerosol spray Lignocaine (150mg/ml)+Prilocaine (50mg/ml)	Sertraline (25-100mg)
ON-DEMAND OFF-LABEL	Fluoxetine (10-60mg)
Tramadol (50mg)	PDE5Is
Silodosin (4mg)	
Clomipramine (25mg, 50mg)	

Fig. 9.4 Pharmacotherapeutic agents used in early ejaculation. *PDE5Is* phosphodiesterase inhibitors

among the drugs used for the treatment of PME, the dropout rate is very high, close to 90% at 2 years. The primary reasons are cost, on demand nature of the drug and the TEAE [17].

Selective Serotonin Reuptake Inhibitors (SSRIs)

Increase in the central serotonin (5-HT) activity delays ejaculation. There are two groups of receptors of clinical importance, postsynaptic (5-HT_{1B} and 5-HT_{2C}) stimulation of which leads to delayed ejaculation and presynaptic (5-HT_{1A} and 5-HT_{1B}) stimulation facilitates ejaculation. SSRIs are administered either as on-demand or daily dosing.

The principle behind daily dosing, there is desensitization of the presynaptic receptors, resulting in increase in serotonin levels in the synaptic cleft which leads to subsequent stimulation of postsynaptic receptors and hence delay in ejaculation. It also blocks the reuptake of serotonin from the synaptic cleft by the serotonin transporters which further increases the ejaculatory latency [18]. The commonly used drugs in decreasing the order of efficacy are paroxetine (10–40 mg), sertaraline (25–200 mg), fluoxetine (10–60 mg), citalopram (20–60 mg), and fluvoxamine (50–100 mg). From the various studies conducted, it is reported that daily paroxetine treatment is associated with the strongest delay in ejaculation (upto 8.8 times delay in IELT over baseline) and both fluvoxamine and citalopram cause the least delay in ejaculation [19].

Daily treatment with SSRIs takes 1–3 weeks to induce a clinically significant delay in ejaculation. This period is necessary for the desensitization to occur. The efficacy may last for 6–12 months owing to tachyphylaxis beyond which there will be necessity to increase the dose or the patients will become unresponsive to medications [20]. The TEAE, nausea, vomiting, diarrhea, dry mouth, fatigue, drowsiness, and perspiration, is usually experienced with initiation of treatment and will gradually improve over 2–3 weeks. It can also cause mood disorders like mania, hypomania, agitation, abnormal behavior, and suicidal ideation. Hence it has to be used with extreme caution in patients with preexisting mental illness and young adolescents <18 years. Sudden withdrawal or rapid dose reduction leads to SSRI syndrome characterized by lethargy, dizziness, visual symptoms, irritability, and paresthesia. This has been reported in 21.2% men treated with daily SSRIs [21]. PME patients trying to conceive should avoid these drugs due to its deleterious effects on the sperm parameters. Studies have reported reduction in sperm counts, motility, morphology, and sperm DNA damage as well [22].

Considering the side effects, the overall dropout rate is close to 70% with the lowest discontinuation rate for paroxetine. On-demand dosing with SSRIs have been tried (3–6 hours before intercourse); however, the delay is inferior when compared to daily therapy [23].

Daily Vs. on-Demand Treatment of SSRIs

1. Daily treatment significantly delays ejaculation.
2. Patient adherence to treatment is better with daily dosing.
3. Daily treatment requires 1–3 weeks for onset of significant effect.
4. Associated with increased side effects and possible drug dependance.
5. More suitable for patients with higher sexual frequency.
6. Higher chances of tachyphylaxis.

Clomipramine

Clomipramine hydrochloride is a tricyclic antidepressant with serotonin uptake inhibitory activity and is one of the oldest drugs still being used in the management of PME. This is also a cheaper alternative to the other off-label SSRIs. The efficacy in delaying ejaculation is inferior to paroxetine but equivalent to sertraline/fluoxetine. It was used both for daily and on-demand treatments 2–6 h before sexual intercourse, but obviously the efficacy was higher with daily use (5-fold vs 3–4-fold respectively) [24]. Clomipramine can be started at a low dose of 10 mg and can be increased gradually every 2–3 weeks till the desired effect is achieved to a maximum of 50 mg beyond which there is increased risk of TEAE [25].

Topical Anesthetic Agents

Bearing the concept that penile hypersensitivity is a reason for PME, topical anesthetic agents have been used since ages to reduce the sensitivity of glans and there by prolonging ejaculation without significantly affecting the sensation of ejaculation [26]. It was reported as the efficacy of the topical agents was much higher in comparison to the oral pharmacotherapeutic agents prescribed for PME [27]. Topical anesthetic agents are available as a combination of prilocaine and lidocaine in both cream and sprays (lidocaine: prilocaine—1:1 and 3:1 respectively) and also as plain lignocaine preparations. The cream has to be applied 10–15 min before sexual intercourse and ideally washed off or use a condom before intercourse. Creams have to be avoided in patients who are allergic to the ingredients and couples actively trying to conceive due to the cytotoxic effects on sperms [28].

The eutectic spray is available as a metered dose spray and is the only second pharmaceutical agent approved by EMA for use in PME. It is recommended to apply three sprays (one dose) on the most sensitive area of glans 5–10 mins before sexual intercourse. When compared to creams, metered dose spray delivery systems deposit the drug in a dose-controlled manner, ensure a concentrated film covers the glans penis, maximize the neural blockade, and minimalize the onset of numbness without significant absorption into the penile skin [29].

Although various studies have reported a significant delay in the ejaculatory time (6–seven fold) and also a progressive month by month improvement, patient discontuation rate is close to 70% due to loss of spontaneity and some patients find it difficult to cumbersome to use it for a long term [30].

The reported complications are genital hypoesthesia in both partners, vulvovaginal burning sensation, and ED (in patients who stimulate the penis to achieve an erection). Lidocaine only (5% & 10%) sprays have also been reported to have similar efficacy and similar side effect profiles.

Tramadol

Tramadol is a centrally acting analgesic with mild agonistic activity at μ opioid receptors and antagonistic activity towards serotonin and nor-adrenaline transportation. It has a half-life of 5–6 h and peaks serum concentration in 2 h. EAU guidelines consider on-demand tramadol as an alternative to patients who have failed the first-line medications. On-demand 50 mg tramadol causes a 2–2.5fold delay in ejaculation [31].

It has been studied that daily paroxetine (20 mg) is superior and on-demand paroxetine (20 mg) is inferior to on-demand tramadol (50 mg). The TAEA are sedation, constipation, dry mouth, and a potential for abuse. It can also cause serotonin syndrome either when used alone or in combination with SSRIs. Hence, tramadol has to be used with caution [32].

Phosphodiesterase 5 Inhibitors (PDE5I)

It is hypothesized that PDE5Is cross the blood-brain barrier, by increased cGMP and NO activity in the medial preoptic nuclei in the hypothalamus; it reduces the central sympathetic drive and cause delay in ejaculation. It also causes relaxation of the smooth muscles in the organs involved in ejaculation (seminal vesicles, vas deferens, prostate, and urethra). But various studies have reported that PDE5Is, especially tadalafil (5 mg daily), may cause a delay in ejaculation, and by improving the quality of erection it causes improvement in confidence, perception of control in ejaculation, and a shorter refractory time to a second erection. Thereby it increases the overall sexual satisfaction [33].

A recent Bayesian network meta-analysis has confirmed that a combination of PDE5Is and SSRIs is superior to SSRIs alone and to other monotherapies (topical agents, tramadol, PDE5Is). The routinely used PDE5Is are sildenafil (25–50 mg) and tadalafil (2.5–10 mg) in combination with paroxetine (10–20 mg), sertraline (25 mg) and dopoxetine (30–60 mg) [27].

Alpha Blockers

Selective alpha blockers cause inhibition of alpha 1 receptor in the bladder neck and prostate, and it is theorized that by interfering with the emission phase, it causes delay in ejaculation. Silodosin (4 mg) is reported to be the most effective and widely used alpha blocker in management of PME. When compared to other drugs of the same group, it is reposted to cause a delay in ejaculation upto eightfold when used on-demand 2 h before intercourse [34]. The reported complications were reduction in the semen volume and anejaculation. Hence it has to be avoided in couples trying to conceive. In fact, Silodosin 8 mg was studied as a successful contraception as well [35].

Emerging Drugs under Trial and Future Concepts

Oxytocin Receptor Antagonists

Based on rat studies, it is perceived that blockage of the peripheral and central oxytocin receptors may have a role in the management of PME. Two oxytocin receptor antagonists, Epilsiban (only peripherally acting) and Cligosiban (both centrally and peripherally acting), have been studied, but the reported results are not promising as yet [36].

Modafinil

Modafinil is a wake-promoting agent used in the management of nacrolepsy. By increasing the intracerebral serotonin and interfering with the dopaminergic pathway, it causes a delay in the ejaculation. Few studies have tried modafinil 100 mg on-demand 2–3 h before intercourse and have reported a modest increase (2–2.5 fold) in the IELT with satisfactory control over ejaculation. The TEAE were minimal and transient, dyspepsia and insomnia. Based on the studies, modafinil can be added to the PME armamentarium; however, more RCTs with larger cohorts are required [37].

GSK958108

The GSK958108 molecule is a serotonin $5HT_{1A}$ receptor antagonist which was tried on-demand (3 mg and 7 mg). After 3.5 h of administration, the MELT increased in both the groups when compared to the placebo and a favorable TEAE profile. This drug appears to be promising; however, more trials evaluating the IELT are necessary [38].

Plant Extract Supplements

There is increasing evidence in favor of plant extracts like *Satureja montana*, *Tribulus terrestris*, *Phyllanthus emblica*, *Ecklonia bicyclis*, and *Rhodiola rosea*, in combination with other vitamins and amino acids for use in PME. However, there is limited evidence on their mechanism of action and the long-term effects [13].

Neurobiological Agents

A new class of ion channels termed as PIEZO channels have been identified to play a role in the tactile mechanisms of penile sensitivity. Blockage of these channels specifically has been hypothesized to improve the ejaculation time.

In the rat models, a relationship between the Brain Derived Natriuretic Peptide (BDNP), expressed in the pre-frontal cortex, hippocampus and the central nervous and the ejaculation was observed. The levels of (BDNP) were found to be low in rapidly ejaculating rats. This opens up a new avenue for further research in expanding the armamentarium of PME management [39].

Practical Tips

1. When paroxetine is prescribed more than 20 mg daily, patients develop dullness, lethargy, and gastric discomfort and hence it is associated with poor compliance.
2. Clomipramine can be started from as low as 5 mg once daily, be increased gradually by 5 mg every 3 weeks till the desired effect is achieved. This titration can be done by the patient himself till his desired effect is achieved. This is the most affordable drug for long-term use. Unfortunately, patients develop excessive yawning when the daily dose exceeds 25 mg.

3. In patients who do not respond to paroxetine, it can be substituted with sertraline which has better patient tolerance and overall sexual satisfaction.
4. Always add a low-dose PDE5I as these drugs themselves may cause some degree of erectile dysfunction.
5. Patients of life-long PME may have to take life-long medications.
6. Severe PME (ejaculation even before penetration) will not respond satisfactorily to pharmacotherapeutic drugs alone.

An algorithmic approach to early ejaculation patients (both life-long and acquired) is described in Fig. 9.5. The treatment needs to be customized according to the patient's need.

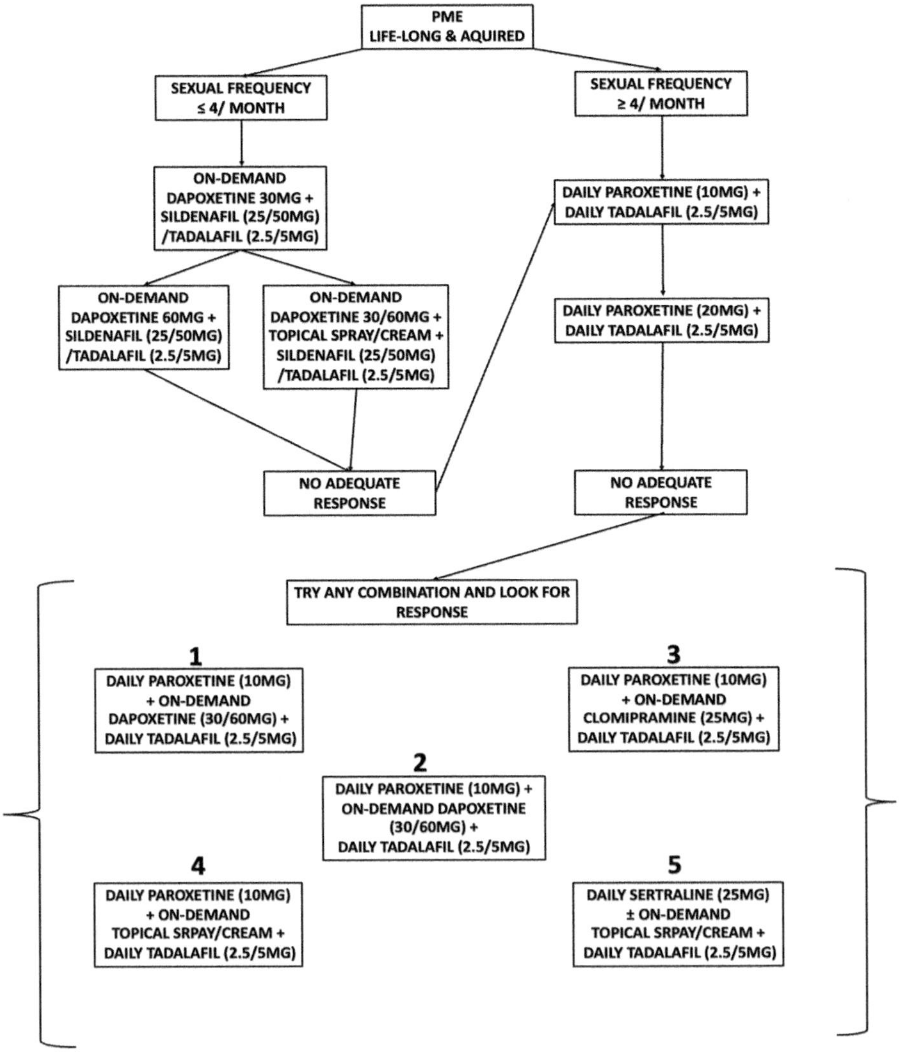

Fig. 9.5 Algorithmic approach to pharmacotherapy in PME

Surgery

Although the standard guidelines weakly recommend surgery as a treatment for PME, it can be considered in men who are unresponsive to pharmacological treatment. The reported results are encouraging. The lack of strong supporting evidence and its technical difficulties seem to be the main barriers in widespread adoption of these procedures [40].

Frenuloplasty and Circumcision

A high frenulum has been described to cause PME as it causes bothersome traction-like sensation during intercourse, encouraging to end coitus soon. Moreover, along with glans penis, frenulum is equally sensitive containing multiple nerve endings [41]. Frenuloplasty for correction of short frenulum, had mixed opinion regarding its efficacy in delaying ejaculation. Few studies have demonstrated a 2.5-fold delay in ejaculation, whereas others have reported no difference in ejaculation time compared to the control group [42].

Circumcision clearly does not improve ejaculation latency [12].

Selective Dorsal Nerve Neurotomy (SDN)

The pathological basis for selective dorsal nerve neurotomy (SDN) is that the number of dorsal nerve branches in patients with PME, especially lifelong PME correlates positively with the penile sensitivity. According to Zhang et al., patients with life-long premature ejaculation had more terminal branches of penile dorsal nerves than the average male (average 7.16 branches vs. average 3.55 branches). SDN suppresses central excitability and penile hypersensitivity, blocks the hypersensitive signals by peripheral sexual stimulation and hence improve IELT and ejaculatory threshold [8].

There is no standard technique or consensus regarding the number of nerve branches that has to be severed [43]. The Korean doctors severe the lateral branches more proximally (at the mid-distal shaft level) whereas the Chinese doctors resect the dorsal nerves more distally (near the coronal sulcus). It has been reported that the IELT significantly improved after SDN in patients with LPE (0.86 ± 0.32 min vs. 6.65 ± 3.90 min). Similar observations have been reported in studies from China and Korea [44, 45].

The Korean study reported a satisfaction rate of 70% with a durable response upto 2 years. Complications were hypoesthesia in 8.1% cases and a recurrence rate of 10%. There are chances of anejaculation, pain due to neuroma formation, Peyronnie's disease and very rarely erectile dysfunction as well. Hence patient selection is very important. However, this is an unpopular procedure in the West [46]. A brief description of the procedure is illustrated in Fig. 9.6.

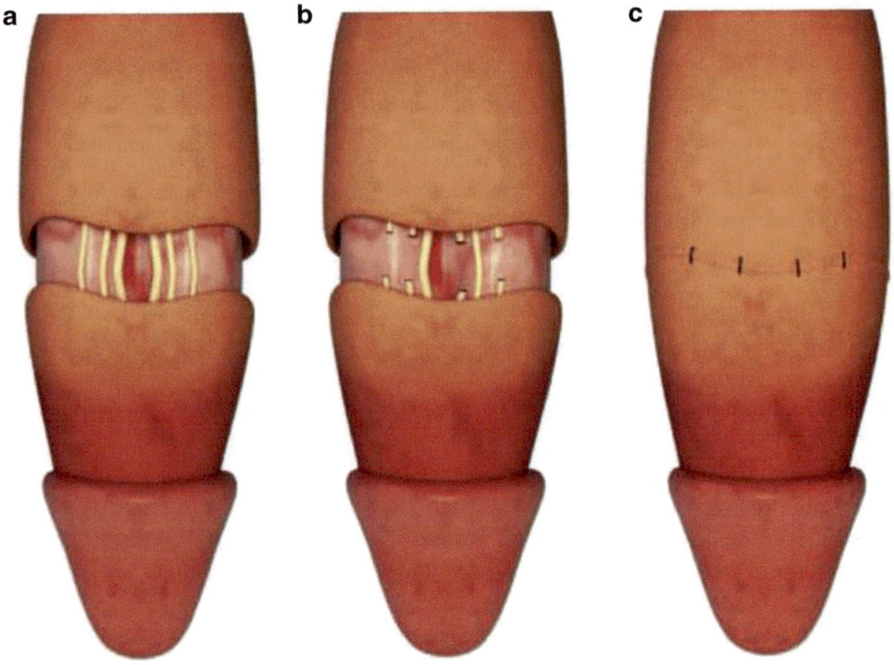

Fig. 9.6 Brief illustration of the SDN procedure. (Adopted from You, H.S. (2000). The Partial Neurectomy of the Dorsal Nerve of the Penis for Patient with Premature Ejaculation.)

Glans Penis Augmentation with Hyaluronic Acid Gel Injection

In this procedure, hyaluronic acid gel is injected deep dermally into the glans to create an artificial barrier (bulking agent) between the branches of dorsal nerve of penis and its receptors and subsequently inhibiting the tactile stimuli. Hyaluronic Acid (HA) has been widely used due to its hygroscopic nature (99% water) and form high viscosity hydrated polymers. HA fills the extracellular space and serves as a structure stabilizing and cellular protective molecule with surprising malleability and superior biocompatibility. HA undergoes slow digestion and isovolumetric degradation, hence has extensive tissue longevity [47].

Studies have used HA at concentrations between 16 mg/ml and 24 mg/ml in prefilled syringes mixed with local anesthetic injections using fine needles (27G and 30G). Different studies have adopted multiple techniques with no clear demonstration of superiority of one over another. It was preferred to use HA with medium molecular weight and viscosity. A large molecular weight and more viscous HA will be difficult to inject considering the small space and will require larger sized needles (18G) which will cause glandular bleeding [48]. The techniques implemented in various studies are depicted in Fig. 9.7.

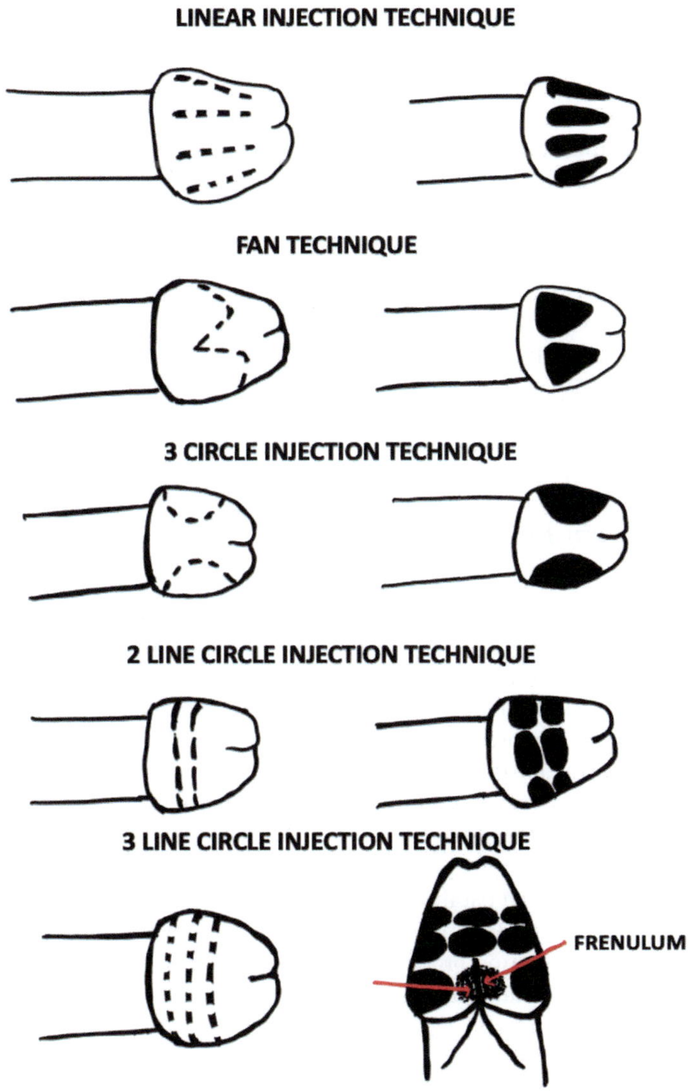

Fig. 9.7 Different techniques of Hyaluronic acid gel injection

This procedure can be performed safe using topical anesthetic cream (mixture of lidocaine and prilocaine) as an outpatient procedure. The starting point of injection is at one-third distance between coronal sulcus and the tip of the glans. The distal third and tip of the glans penis is generally avoided to maintain the conical shape of the penis. To avoid overloading, the recommended volume was 2 ml. The plane of injection is very important. An ideal injection should create a bulge proportional to the volume of injection. Apart from undulations with minimal morphological changes, a too superficial injection may lead to pressure necrosis with ulceration and a too deep injection may not serve the purpose and may rarely enter the vasculature leading to thrombus formation with immediate discoloration of the glans penis [49].

Studies have shown a significant improvement in IELT between 2.43 and 4.46-fold and that lasting upto 5 years. This is significantly high when compared with dopoxetine usage (both 30 mg and 60 mg). The reported patient satisfaction rate is nearly 70%.

The main challenges with the procedure are:

1. absence of a precise measure of the volume required to achieve satisfactory results as the size of the glans penis is not uniform among all men.
2. the technical difficulties involved with regards to the depth of injection.
3. the choice of HA gel.
4. number and distribution of injection sites [50].

Botulinum Toxin Injection

Botulinum toxin (BoNT) is produced by the Clostridium bacteria and seven serotypes exist (A, B, C, D, E, F, G). BoNT-A is the most potent and commercially available for therapeutic purposes (as Botox, Dysport, Xeomin), with each brand having its own preparation, dosage, and potency. In humans, BoNT blocks acetylcholine release from the presynaptic neurons at the neuromuscular junction resulting in interruption of postsynaptic transmission and temporary muscle paralysis. However, this effect reverses with time due to formation of new synaptic connections and recovery of the original nerve terminals as well. The effect lasts for 3–6 months [51].

It was hypothesized that paralyzing the bulbospongiosus muscle by giving BoNT injection into the muscle directly would block the neural transmission and subsequently delay the ejaculation process. It was applied with good success in rats by Serefoglu et al., and Ongün et al., where the IELT increased significantly compared to the pretreatment IELT.

Although human studies are very limited, all have demonstrated 2–3 times improvement in the IELT when compared to the placebo groups. The data on side effect profile is also limited and a theoretical probability of anejaculation [13, 52].

At this moment, this therapy should be considered as only experimental. There is no consensus regarding the dose, the exact location of injection, and safety profile. However, this can evolve as potential treatment for PME, considering its effectiveness in other fields of medicine especially for men with more sensitivity at the base of the penis.

CYROABLATION and *PULSED RADIOFREQUENCY NEUROMODULATION* of the dorsal penile nerve have been tried with acceptable success, but the data available is limited and be considered only experimental.

Retrograde Ejaculation

While treating a patient with retrograde ejaculation (RGE), it is important to understand the necessity to treat him. The usual concern of patients who approach for treatment of RGE is to have a child. In such patients the management should be focused on obtaining sperms without compromising on its quality. Another unusual reason that we encountered in our clinical practice is that wives of patients (from rural background) feel that their husbands have a satisfactory sexual intercourse with them only if he ejaculates inside them. Otherwise, they have the fear of their husband's dissatisfaction and that they would be forbidden. The middle-aged or the elderly patients would be satisfied with reassurance and follow-ups and they do not require aggressive treatments.

Pharmacotherapy

Alpha 1 Sympathomimetics

The alpha 1 receptor agonists cause closure of the bladder neck with contraction of the vas deferens and seminal vesicles, hence antegrade ejaculation. However, these drugs will be helpful only in the neurogenic causes like diabetic neuropathy where there is a progressive dysfunction. The efficacy of these drugs is only 28% in causing antegrade ejaculation and also it reverses with time, so patients become unresponsive to the treatment. Considering the TEAE (headache, tachycardia, insomnia, excess sweating, difficulty in urination) and reversing response, these drugs are better administered for short terms, like 1 week before the ovulation period/planned IUI and discontinued for rest of the cycle [53]. The various drugs used with their doses are enlisted in Fig. 9.8.

Tricyclic Antidepressants

The tricyclic antidepressants (TCA), by inhibiting serotonin and noradrenaline transports, inhibit adrenaline reuptake and hence potentiate sympathomimetic activity leading to contraction of bladder neck. The TEAE are secondary to its anti-muscarinic and anti-histaminic properties, which are dry mouth, constipation, dysuria, and drowsiness. TCAs are contraindicated in glaucoma, post-acute coronary event, and concomitant use of monoamine oxidase inhibitors. The overall efficacy is only 22% in causing antegrade ejaculation. But when combined with sympathomimetics, the efficacy increases to 39%. However, when using a combination therapy, the side effect profile and patient's tolerability should be taken into consideration. The list of various drugs used with their doses are enlisted in the Fig. 9.8. In men desiring fertility, sperm can be retrieved from the bladder for IUI/ICSI. There are different methods of retrieval, which are beyond the interest of this chapter [54].

Fig. 9.8 Drugs used in the treatment of retrograde ejaculation

ALPHA 1 SYMPATHOMIMETICS (Daily)	Dose (Maximum)
Ephedrine Phenylpropanolamine Pseudoephedrine Midodrine	30mg QID 75mg QID 30mg QID 7.5mg QID
(on-demand) Pseudoephedrine	60-120mg, 1-2 hours before intercourse/masturbation
TRICYCLIC ANTIDEPRESSANTS (Daily)	
Imipramine (1st gen) Amoxapine (2nd gen)	25-50mg QID 25-75mg HS ± 25-50mg 1 hour before intercourse/masturbation
Older drugs (uncommonly used) Brompheniramine, Chlorpheniramine, Dextroamphetamine, Synephrine	

Bladder Neck Reconstruction/Augmentation

Bladder neck reconstruction for incompetent bladder neck is a cumbersome procedure associated with complications and poor results. Hence it is not a routinely recommended procedure. However, bladder neck augmentation with collagen and deflux have been reported to cause antegrade ejaculation and the effect lasted between 6 and 22 months. But the pregnancy rates by natural conception is variable, number of studies are also limited, the study population is also less and the complications associated are unclear. Hence it cannot be recommended as a standard procedure; however, once standardized it can be offered in patients who insist on natural conception [55].

Practical Points

1. Patients of neuropathic etiology will only respond to medications.
2. The response to medications depends upon the severity of the etiology.
3. Imipramine is the commonly used drug as the sympathomimetic drugs are not available in all parts of the world.
4. Start with a low dose and gradually titrate the dose every week depending on the patient's response and keeping a watch on the side effects.
5. If adequate response is not achieved, a sympathomimetic drug can be added.

An algorithmic approach to patient with RGE is illustrated in Fig. 9.9.

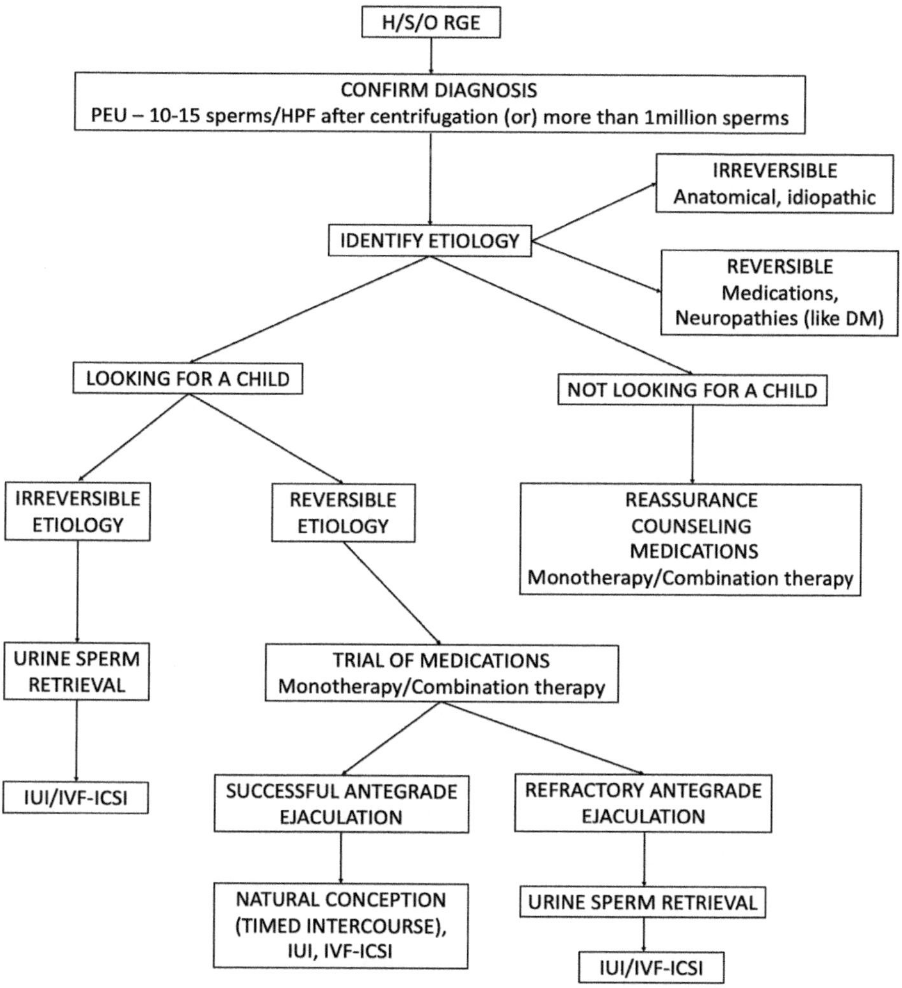

Fig. 9.9 Algorithmic approach to Retrograde Ejaculation

Delayed Ejaculation/Anejaculation

Management of Delayed ejaculation/Anejaculation is quite difficult as the number of unknown factors overtake the treatable factors. And the response to the various treatment modalities are not uniform among all patients. However, a combination of behavioral modification with psychotherapy and pharmacotherapy have been successful in a certain subset of patients. It is important to differentiate between the types of delayed ejaculation / anejaculation to ensure what treatment suits which patient, for counselling about the success and for discussion of infertility management. Figure 9.10 depicts a simplistic way of differentiating between the types of

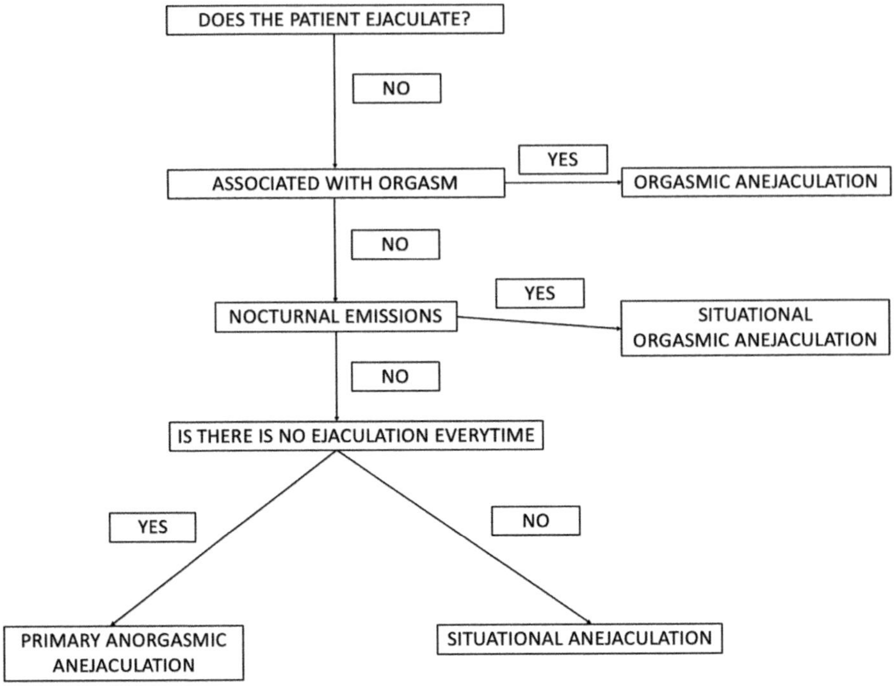

Fig. 9.10 Simple schematic approach to differentiate the types of Delayed/Anejaculation

delayed ejaculation /anejaculation. This section discusses about the practical approach to the treatment modalities and the author's guide to certain gray areas in the management.

Behavioral Therapy and Psychotherapy

This group of patients have a high threshold to achieve orgasm and ejaculation. Some show a strong desire to prolong intercourse, so don't let go and ejaculate. Here are some practices that need to be adopted in an attempt to achieve orgasm and ejaculation.

1. Sex education and a basic understanding of the sexual cycle to evaluate their sexual practices.
2. Try different sexual positions to understand in which position maximum stimulation is achieved and to have sex when not tired.
3. To try alternate sexual practices like oral sex before a penetrative sex.
4. Try to understand the mismatch between fantasies and reality.
5. Retrain masturbation practice with appropriate sexual content and fantasy, correct technique and solo or partnered practice.

6. Spending more time in foreplay to achieve intimacy and arousal.
7. Use of appropriate sex toys after specialist counselling.
8. Partner education and counseling to help patients discover new fantasies.
9. Reducing alcohol consumption and refraining from drugs of abuse [3].

Pharmacotherapy

There are currently no FDA/EMA-approved drugs for treatment of delayed ejaculation / anejaculation. The most commonly used drugs are cabergoline are bupropion to some success. The endocrine causes like hypogonadism and hypothyroidism should be identified and treated before commencing other drugs [56]. The drugs tried in the management of delayed ejaculation /anejaculation are enlisted in Fig. 9.11.

Cabergoline

It is a dopaminergic drug which increases the central level of dopamine and causes increased sexual desire with a pro-ejaculatory effect. It also has agonistic activity at the $5HT_{2B}$ and thus a pro-ejaculatory effect. It has been studied that, elevated levels of serum prolactin results in prolonged ejaculatory time and cabergoline induced hypoprolactinemia caused significant improvement in sexual function as well the ejaculatory time. Cabergoline has been tried at a dose of 0.5 mg twice a week in patient with high normal or mildly elevated prolactin levels. Upto 70% patients reported an improvement in ejaculation time during a period of 8–9 months. The TEAE are nausea, drowsiness, and cardiac valvular regurgitation and cardiac failure [57].

Bupropion

It is a selective reuptake inhibitor of dopamine and noradrenaline. In addition to the dopaminergic effects, it potentiates the sympathetic ejaculatory effect and causes contraction of the epididymal duct. It the only antidepressant that has pro-sexual effects. Upto 70% men were able to achieve ejaculation and orgasm at a dose of 150-300 mg/day during a treatment period of 3–8 weeks. Bupropion requires daily administration and is a relatively safer drug when compared to the other antidepressants. The TEAE are insomnia, headache, irritability, palpitations, blurred vision, and occasionally chest pain and psychosis [58].

<table>
<tr><th>NAME</th><th>MECHANISM OF ACTION</th><th>DOSE</th><th>DURATION</th></tr>
<tr><td colspan="4">COMMONLY USED DRUGS</td></tr>
<tr><td>CABERGOLINE</td><td>Dopamine Agonist, $5HT_{2B}$ activation</td><td>0.5mg twice a week at bedtime</td><td>Long-term</td></tr>
<tr><td>BUPROPION</td><td>Dopamine & Noradrenaline reuptake inhibition</td><td>150-300mg daily in the morning</td><td>Long-term</td></tr>
<tr><td colspan="4">PROMISING DRUG NEEDING FURTHER STUDIES</td></tr>
<tr><td>YOHIMBINE</td><td>$5HT_1$ agonist, central $\alpha 2$ antagonist</td><td>20-50mg daily 1 hour before intercourse</td><td>Long-term/On-demand</td></tr>
<tr><td>OXYTOCIN</td><td>Peripheral oxytocin receptors, Vasopressin receptor stimulation</td><td>16U-24U before intercourse</td><td>On-demand</td></tr>
<tr><td colspan="4">COMMONLY USED DRUGS WITH LIMITED BENEFIT</td></tr>
<tr><td>Pseudoephedrine
Ephedrine
Midodrine
Imipramine</td><td>$\alpha 1$ agonists</td><td>60-120mg
15-60mg
7.5-30mg
25-75mg</td><td>Long-term/On-demand</td></tr>
<tr><td colspan="4">DRUGS TRIED WITH NO EFFECTIVE CONCLUSION</td></tr>
<tr><td>AMANTADINE</td><td>Dopamine release, reuptake inhibition</td><td>-</td><td>Long-term/On-demand</td></tr>
<tr><td>CYPROHEPTADINE</td><td>Anti-serotonergic activity</td><td>-</td><td>Long-term/On-demand</td></tr>
<tr><td>BUSPIRON</td><td>$5HT_1$ agonist, $\alpha 2$ antagonist</td><td>-</td><td>Long-term</td></tr>
<tr><td>BETHANECOL</td><td>Muscarinic receptor activation</td><td>-</td><td>Long-term/On-demand</td></tr>
<tr><td colspan="4">DRUGS UNDER TRIAL</td></tr>
<tr><td colspan="2">Apomorphine, Quinelorane</td><td colspan="2">Dopaminergic activity</td></tr>
<tr><td colspan="2">Anandamide,
Reboxetine</td><td colspan="2">Cannabinoid receptor agonist,
Noradrenaline reuptake inhibitor</td></tr>
<tr><td colspan="4">HERBAL PREPARATIONS</td></tr>
<tr><td colspan="2">Ferula hermonis, Chinese herbal extract, Ginkgo biloba extract, Mucuna pruriens Linn seed, Eurycoma longifolia, Pedalium murex Linn Fruits, Maca root</td><td colspan="2">Unknown effect</td></tr>
</table>

Fig. 9.11 Drugs used in the treatment of delayed/anejaculation

Penile Vibratory Stimulation (PVS)

The first vibrator device was patented in 1880 for use in female sexual dysfunction. Since then, may vibrators have reached the market. But only two medical penile vibrators are approved by FDA for treatment in ejaculatory disorders. One is Ferticare personal (Denmark) and another Viberect X3 (USA) (Fig. 9.12). Penile vibratory devices work on the principle that the ejaculatory threshold of patients is high and by applying prolonged high amplitude vibration to the glans penis it causes orgasm and ejaculation via the spinal reflex. Using these devices, it was determined that vibrations given at a amplitude of 25 and frequency of 100 Hz is optimal to induce ejaculation in men with SCI. This is a simple outpatient procedure [59].

Procedure

1. Patient is made to rest in his comfortable position—supine/reclined/sitting.
2. The applicator of the device is placed on the glans at the region of the frenulum (6 o'clock position) or on both sides when the device with two applicators used (sandwich technique).
3. The settings are appropriately adjusted.
4. As per the standard literature, the vibration is given for 2 min, followed by a rest period of 1 min and it is recommended to continue this cycle upto five times.
5. It has been observed that ejaculation occurs within five cycles.
6. Inspect the contact points during the rest period.
7. If no ejaculate comes despite a bulbocavernous reflex and hip flexor response, urine should be examined for sperms.

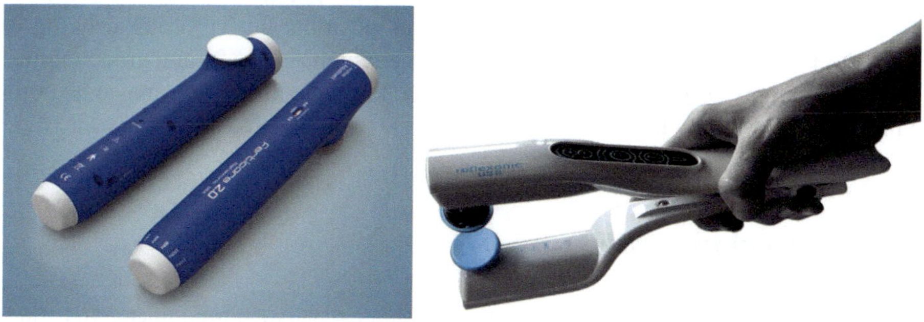

Fig. 9.12 Ferticare Personal and Viberect 3 Penile Vibration Devices

Prerequisites and Precautions While Using PVS

1. The patient has to be in a good mindset for the procedure; hence he should be counselled well to come prepared and also that it may take about an hour for the procedure.
2. A PDE5I may be necessary before starting the procedure.
3. Local penile and glans skin should be inspected for swelling, inflammation, or skin eruptions, where the procedure should be deferred.
4. In patients with spinal cord injury (SCI) where autonomic dysreflexia (Spinal cord injury above T6, incomplete spinal cord transection) characterized by elevation of blood pressure is expected, patients have to be pretreated with oral/sublingual Nifedipine 10-20 mg and should be on continuous BP monitoring.
5. At least two people should be available while the procedure is performed, one for holding the device and another for collection of the sample. The patient may be asked to watch something erotic to maintain the mood which may augment the process.
6. The bulbocavernous reflex and hip flexor response are considered to be good predictors of ejaculation. Hence in men with SCI, the reflexes have to be checked before starting the procedure [60].

The success rate in achieving antegrade ejaculation in SCI men with injury above T10 is 86%, whereas it is 15% in SCI men with injury distal to T11. The success rates in other groups of anejaculators is unavailable. The TEAE are autonomic dysreflexia and erythema of penile skin [59].

Prostatic Massage

Prostatic massage can be used as an alternative for semen collection where the facilities of PVS/EEJ are not available, in patients who failed PVS but unwilling for EEJ. The patient is placed in lateral decubitus position and vigorous stroking of both the prostate and seminal vesicles are done which results in antegrade expression of semen by activation of the spinal reflex. Prostatic massage can also be combined with PVS at the height of orgasm.

Electroejaculation (EEJ)

Electroejaculation devices were initially designed for use in animal husbandry. First human application was done in 1938 with good success. Later in the 1980s, the first FDA-approved EEJ device was introduced by Dr. Seager. This device comes with a main unit and multiple transrectal probes (Fig. 9.13). This is a procedure primarily

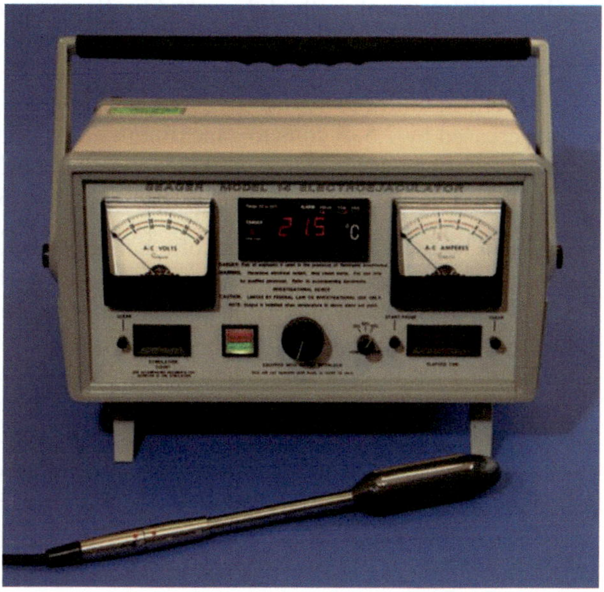

Fig. 9.13 Seager's Electroejaculator with probe

used in men with SCI with nearly 100% success, involves transrectal electrical stimulation of prostate, seminal vesicles with AC current of 5–25 V/100–500 mAmp [59].

Prerequisites for the Procedure

1. A digital rectal examination and proctoscopy is performed to rule out any preexisting lesion.
2. Bladder preparation for sperm retrieval.
3. At least two people are required for the procedure, one person to deliver the current and another to collect the semen.
4. General anesthesia backup in SCI men and mandatory in all others.
5. Patients prone to develop autonomic dysreflexia should be pretreated with nifedipine [60].

Procedure

1. Patient is placed in lateral decubitus position with knees drawn upto the abdomen.
2. The rectal probe is inserted with one electrode towards the prostate and two towards the seminal vesicles.
3. Continuous rectal temperature monitoring via a built-in sensor.
4. Two methods of delivery of current.

5. One is the original method described by Seager, where current is applied continuously and gradually increased till ejaculation occurs.
6. Other method is the start-stop method, where initial current, at 5 volts, is delivered for 5 s, followed by rest for 20 seconds and restarted. Every time the current is increased by 2.5–5 volts to a maximum of 20–30 volts.
7. After completion, bladder should be drained and evaluated for sperms.
8. At the end of procedure, a repeat proctoscopy has to be done [59].

EEJ can be used in anejaculators of other etiology too, but the literature regarding success rate and pregnancy rates is scarce. Although the procedure sounds simple, it is a painful procedure with serious complications like rectal burns, blood in stools, painful defecation, pelvic muscle pain, which many patients may not tolerate. The other major concern is about the quality of the sperms retrieved. Even if a good volume is achieved, the sperm quality and viability were reported to be poor. There are much simpler techniques of sperm retrieval by which good quality sperms can be obtained and used with higher pregnancy rates through IVF-ICSI. Hence this procedure is falling out of favor in the present times [53].

Practical Tips

1. A combination of behavioral modification, psychotherapy, and drug therapy may be effective only in 50–60% of patients.
2. Long-term usage of pharmacotherapeutic drugs may be associated with complications and tachyphylaxis. Hence, these drugs can be used intermittently providing drug free intervals during the course of treatment.
3. Partner cooperation is very important for this group of patients. Hence, they should be counselled adequately well.
4. All patients do not respond equally to PVS, as all patients do not have sensitivity at the tip of penis. Patients should be allowed to evaluate at which point from the root of penis to the tip they feel maximum stimulation with PVS. The intensity of vibration has to be gradually increased. Patient should not be tired and be in a good mindset avoiding anxiety.
5. Before PVS, a PDE5I may be given to achieve good erection. Patient should be adequately erotized (visual/imaginary). He should be instructed to inform when he is achieving maximum pleasure with a sense of letting go. At that point, providing a prostatic massage may be successful in achieving both an orgasm and ejaculation.
6. If PVS is successful, patients can be advised to buy their personal vibrator devices.

7. Primary anorgasmic anejaculators are the difficult group to treat and may not respond to any mode of treatment. In this subset, if fertility is the issue, then they should be advised to proceed with surgical sperm retrieval and IVF-ICSI.
8. EEJ is a morbid procedure associated with poor quality sperms and significant complications. If fertility is the issue, then the patient should be advised to proceed with surgical sperm retrieval and IVF-ICSI.

An algorithmic approach to patient with RGE is illustrated in Fig. 9.14.

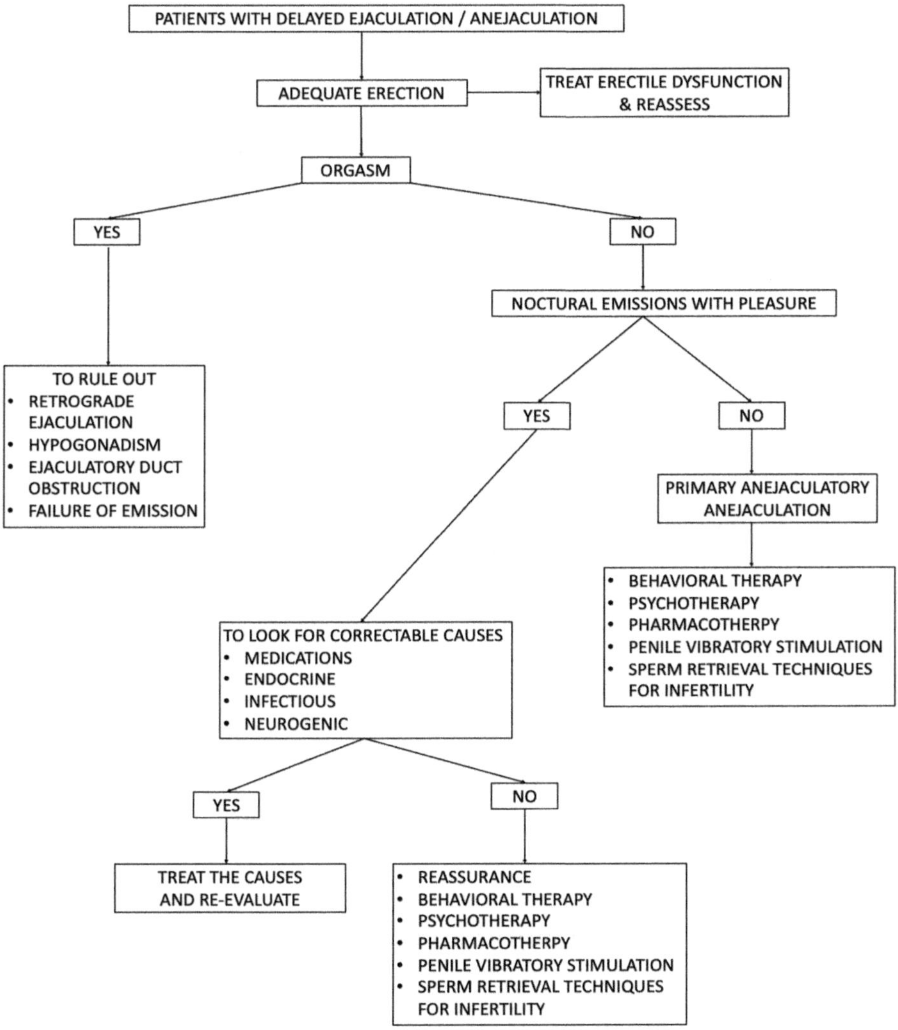

Fig. 9.14 Algorithmic approach to Delayed/Anejaculation

ETIOLOGY	MANAGEMENT
INFECTION / INFLAMMATION (prostatitis, urethritis, orchitis, epididymitis)	Antibiotics, Anti-inflammatory, α-blockers, scrotal nerve denervation
EJACULATORY DUCT OBSTRUCTION	Transurethral resection of ejaculatory duct
SEMINAL VESICLE STONES	Seminal vesiculoscopy with laser lithotripsy and antibiotic wash
BENIGN PROSTATIC ENLAREMENT	Medical/Surgical management
NEUROPATHIC (post radical prostatectomy, post-vasectomy, post-radiotherapy)	Reassurance, Pudendal nerve block
PROSTATIC CANCER	Specific Management
STIs (sexually transmitted infections)	Antibiotics, Antivirals, Anti-inflammatory drugs
MEDICATIONS (antidepressants, muscle relaxants)	Withdrawal of specific medications
CPPS (Chronic Pelvic Pain Syndrome)	Antibiotics, Anti-inflammatory, α-blockers, perineal shockwave therapy
POST INGUINAL HERNIOPLASTY (due to vas entrapment)	Release of vas and ilioinguinal neurectomy
PSYCHOLOGICAL	Reassurance, Counseling, Psychotherapy

Fig. 9.15 Etiologies of painful ejaculation and their respective managements

Painful Ejaculation

Painful ejaculation, also known as dysorgasmia or dysejaculation or orgasmalgia, is a poorly understood phenomenon where the patient experiences mild discomfort to severe pain in the penis, perineum, scrotum, and testis during or shortly after ejaculation. It is usually associated with an orgasm. The reported incidence is from 1.9% to 25%. Painful ejaculation is a highly underrated and ignored symptom which interferes with the quality of sexual life. There no specific guidelines available for its management [61]. The various possible causes with its management discussed in the literature are enlisted in the Fig. 9.15.

Post-Orgasmic Illness Syndrome (POIS)

POIS is yet another rare disorder caused by poorly understood mechanisms and is characterized by a symptom complex that occurs following ejaculation. The symptoms may occur within seconds or minutes or a few hours of ejaculation and may persist for 2–7 days. There are no recommended FDA therapeutic agents available for its management and no specific guidelines too. It has also been discussed that a

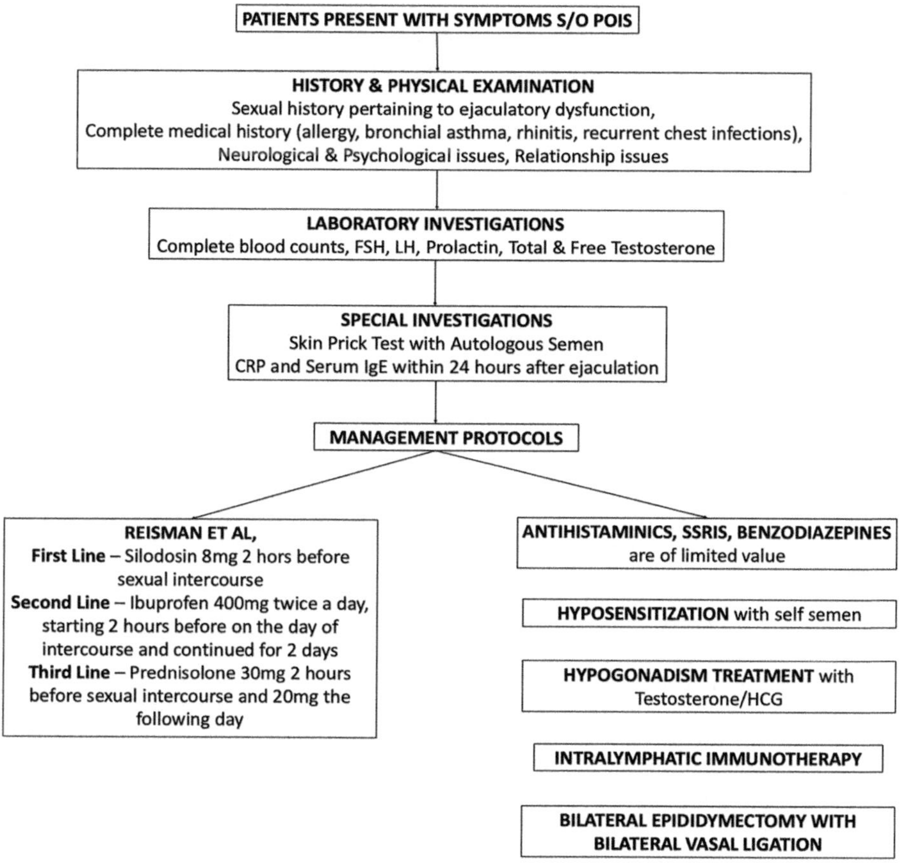

Fig. 9.16 Algorithmic management of Post Orgasmic Illness Syndrome

single drug treatment will not control all the symptoms unless any etiology is identified and treated specifically. Figure 9.16 describes the algorithmic approach to PCOS and the various treatment modalities tried. Unfortunately, the evidence and sample size of the studies are limited and no RCTs are available. Further researches are required to identify a definitive therapy [62].

Conclusion

Ejaculatory disorders encompasses a wide range of symptomatology and severity, which varies from individual to individual. Hence the treatment strategies should be customised according to the patients requirements. Better understanding of patients and analyzing from their pain points will be effective in deciding a strategy for them. A multimodal treatment approach could be effective for this subset of patients.

With better understanding of the disease process and emergence of newer modalities of treatment, the future of management strategies of ejaculatory disorders looks bright, and more bonafide studies are required to cement these strategies.

References

1. Rowland DL, Dabbs CR, Medina MC. Sex differences in attributions to positive and negative sexual scenarios in men and women with and without sexual problems: reconsidering stereotypes. Arch Sex Behav. 2019 Apr 6;48(3):855–66.
2. Gao P, Gao J, Wang Y, Peng D, Zhang Y, Li H, et al. Temperament-character traits and attitudes toward premature ejaculation in 4 types of premature ejaculation. J Sex Med. 2021 Jan;18(1):72–82.
3. Althof SE. Psychological interventions for delayed ejaculation/orgasm. Int J Impot Res [Internet]. 2012;24(4):131–6. [cited 2023 Jul 23]. Available from: https://pubmed.ncbi.nlm.nih.gov/22378496/
4. Sridharan K, Sivaramakrishnan G, Sequeira RP, Al-Khaja KA. Pharmacological interventions for premature ejaculation: a mixed-treatment comparison network meta-analysis of randomized clinical trials. Int J Impot Res [Internet]. 2018;30(5):215–23. [cited 2023 Jun 19]. Available from: https://pubmed.ncbi.nlm.nih.gov/29921893/
5. Semans JH. Premature ejaculation: a new approach. South Med J [Internet]. 1956;49(4):353–8. [cited 2023 Jul 13]. Available from: https://pubmed.ncbi.nlm.nih.gov/13311629/
6. McMahon CG. Premature ejaculation. Indian J Urol [Internet]. 2007;23(2):97. [cited 2023 Jul 13]. Available from: /pmc/articles/PMC2721550/
7. Raveendran AV, Agarwal A. Premature ejaculation-current concepts in the management: a narrative review. Int J Reprod BioMed Research and Clinical Center for Infertitlity. 2021;19:5–22.
8. Hu QB, Zhang D, Ma L, Ng DM, Haleem M, Ma Q. Progresses in pharmaceutical and surgical management of premature ejaculation. Chin Med J (Engl) [Internet]. 2019 Oct 10 [cited 2023 Jun 19];132(19):2362. Available from: /pmc/articles/PMC6819047/.
9. Cormio L, Massenio P, La Rocca R, Verze P, Mirone V, Carrieri G. The combination of dapoxetine and behavioral treatment provides better results than dapoxetine alone in the management of patients with lifelong premature ejaculation. J Sex Med [Internet]. 2015;12(7):1609–15. [cited 2023 Jun 19]. Available from: https://pubmed.ncbi.nlm.nih.gov/26077706/
10. Bronner G, Kitrey ND, Uziel N, Eli I, Raviv G, Ramon J, et al. Correlation between premature ejaculation and female vaginal penetration difficulties. Int J Impot Res [Internet]. 2015;27(4):152–6. [cited 2023 Jul 16]. Available from: https://pubmed.ncbi.nlm.nih.gov/25716748/
11. Salonia A, Bettocchi C, Boeri L, Capogrosso P, Carvalho J, Cilesiz NC, et al. European Association of Urology Guidelines on sexual and reproductive Health-2021 update: male sexual dysfunction. Eur Urol [Internet]. 2021;80(3):333–57. [cited 2023 Jun 29]. Available from: https://pubmed.ncbi.nlm.nih.gov/34183196/
12. Shindel AW, Althof SE, Carrier S, Chou R, McMahon CG, Mulhall JP, et al. Disorders of ejaculation: an AUA/SMSNA guideline. J Urol [Internet]. 2022;207(3):504–12. [cited 2023 Jul 15]. Available from: https://pubmed.ncbi.nlm.nih.gov/34961344/
13. Gul M, Bocu K, Serefoglu EC. Current and emerging treatment options for premature ejaculation. Nat Rev Urol [Internet]. 2022;19(11):659–80. [cited 2023 Jun 29]. Available from: https://www.nature.com/articles/s41585-022-00639-5

14. Andersson KE, Mulhall JP, Wyllie MG. Pharmacokinetic and pharmacodynamic features of dapoxetine, a novel drug for "on-demand" treatment of premature ejaculation. BJU Int [Internet]. 2006;97(2):311–5. [cited 2023 Jun 29]. Available from: https://pubmed.ncbi.nlm.nih.gov/16430636/
15. Porst H, McMahon CG, Althof SE, Sharlip I, Bull S, Aquilina JW, et al. Baseline characteristics and treatment outcomes for men with acquired or lifelong premature ejaculation with mild or no erectile dysfunction: integrated analyses of two phase 3 dapoxetine trials. J Sex Med [Internet]. 2010;7(6):2231–42. [cited 2023 Jun 29]. Available from: https://pubmed.ncbi.nlm.nih.gov/20412423/
16. Peng J, Yang L, Liu L, Zhou R, Liu J, Li N, et al. Safety and effectiveness of Dapoxetine on demand in Chinese men with premature ejaculation: results of a multicenter, prospective, open-label phase IV study. Sex Med [Internet]. 202;9(2) [cited 2023 Jul 5]. Available from: https://pubmed.ncbi.nlm.nih.gov/33529810/
17. Park HJ, Park NC, Kim TN, Baek SR, Lee KM, Choe S. Discontinuation of Dapoxetine treatment in patients with premature ejaculation: a 2-year prospective observational study. Sex Med [Internet]. 2017;5(2):e99–105. [cited 2023 Aug 20]. Available from: https://pubmed.ncbi.nlm.nih.gov/28395997/
18. Olivier B, Van Oorschot R, Waldinger MD. Serotonin, serotonergic receptors, selective serotonin reuptake inhibitors and sexual behaviour. Int Clin Psychopharmacol [Internet]. 1998;13(SUPPL. 6) [cited 2023 Jun 29]. Available from: https://pubmed.ncbi.nlm.nih.gov/9728669/
19. Waldinger MD, Hengeveld MW, Zwinderman AH, Olivier B. Effect of SSRI antidepressants on ejaculation: a double-blind, randomized, placebo-controlled study with fluoxetine, fluvoxamine, paroxetine, and sertraline. J Clin Psychopharmacol [Internet]. 1998;18(4):274–81. [cited 2023 Jun 29]. Available from: https://pubmed.ncbi.nlm.nih.gov/9690692/
20. Fallon B. "Off-label" drug use in sexual medicine treatment. Int J Impot Res [Internet]. 2008;20(2):127–34. [cited 2023 Jul 5]. Available from: https://pubmed.ncbi.nlm.nih.gov/17851582/
21. Machado M, Iskedjian M, Ruiz I, Einarson TR. Remission, dropouts, and adverse drug reaction rates in major depressive disorder: a meta-analysis of head-to-head trials. Curr Med Res Opin [Internet]. 2006;22(9):1825–37. [cited 2023 Jul 5]. Available from: https://pubmed.ncbi.nlm.nih.gov/16968586/
22. Koyuncu H, Serefoglu EC, Ozdemir AT, Hellstrom WJ. Deleterious effects of selective serotonin reuptake inhibitor treatment on semen parameters in patients with lifelong premature ejaculation. Int J Impot Res [Internet] 2012 ;24(5):171–173. [cited 2023 Jul 5]. Available from: https://pubmed.ncbi.nlm.nih.gov/22573230/
23. Jern P, Johansson A, Piha J, Westberg L, Santtila P. Antidepressant treatment of premature ejaculation: discontinuation rates and prevalence of side effects for dapoxetine and paroxetine in a naturalistic setting. Int J Impot Res [Internet]. 2015;27(2):75–80. [cited 2023 Jul 5]. Available from: https://pubmed.ncbi.nlm.nih.gov/25410962/
24. Waldinger MD, Zwinderman AH, Olivier B. On-demand treatment of premature ejaculation with clomipramine and paroxetine: a randomized, double-blind fixed-dose study with stopwatch assessment. Eur Urol [Internet]. 2004;46(4):510–6. [cited 2023 Jul 6]. Available from: https://pubmed.ncbi.nlm.nih.gov/15363569/
25. Eaton H. Clomipramine (Anafranil) in the treatment of premature ejaculation. J Int Med Res [Internet]. 1973;1(5):432–4. [cited 2023 Jul 6]. Available from: https://journals.sagepub.com/doi/10.1177/030006057300100531
26. Wyllie MG, Hellstrom WJG. The link between penile hypersensitivity and premature ejaculation. BJU Int [Internet]. 2011;107(3):452–7. [cited 2023 Jul 6]. Available from: https://pubmed.ncbi.nlm.nih.gov/20553259/

27. Liu H, Zhang M, Huang M, Cai H, Zhang Y, Liu G, et al. Comparative efficacy and safety of drug treatment for premature ejaculation: a systemic review and Bayesian network meta-analysis. Andrologia [Internet]. 2020;52(11) [cited 2023 Jul 9]. Available from: https://pubmed.ncbi.nlm.nih.gov/32892379/
28. Sutton M, Hunn C, Summers-Colquitt RB, Chen SH, Kavoussi SK, Kavoussi KM, et al. Promescent has a cytotoxic impact on fresh human sperm in vitro. Urology [Internet]. 2018;114:95–8. [cited 2023 Jul 6]. Available from: https://pubmed.ncbi.nlm.nih.gov/29307732/
29. Dinsmore WW, Hackett G, Goldmeier D, Waldinger M, Dean J, Wright P, et al. Topical eutectic mixture for premature ejaculation (TEMPE): a novel aerosol-delivery form of lidocaine-prilocaine for treating premature ejaculation. BJU Int [Internet]. 2007;99(2):369–75. [cited 2023 Jul 6]. Available from: https://pubmed.ncbi.nlm.nih.gov/17129234/
30. Morales A. Evolving therapeutic strategies for premature ejaculation: the search for on-demand treatment—topical versus systemic. Can Urol Assoc J [Internet]. 2012;6(5):380–5. [cited 2023 Jul 7]. Available from: https://pubmed.ncbi.nlm.nih.gov/23093633/
31. Bar-Or D, Salottolo KM, Orlando A, Winkler JV. A randomized double-blind, placebo-controlled multicenter study to evaluate the efficacy and safety of two doses of the tramadol orally disintegrating tablet for the treatment of premature ejaculation within less than 2 minutes. Eur Urol [Internet]. 2012;61(4):736–43. [cited 2023 Jul 9]. Available from: https://pubmed.ncbi.nlm.nih.gov/21889833/
32. Kirby EW, Carson CC, Coward RM. Tramadol for the management of premature ejaculation: a timely systematic review. Int J Impot Res [Internet]. 2015;27(4):121–7. [cited 2023 Jul 9]. Available from: https://pubmed.ncbi.nlm.nih.gov/25971856/
33. Chen J, Keren-Paz G, Bar-Yosef Y, Matzkin H. The role of phosphodiesterase type 5 inhibitors in the management of premature ejaculation: a critical analysis of basic science and clinical data. Eur Urol [Internet]. 2007;52(5):1331–9. [cited 2023 Jul 9]. Available from: https://pubmed.ncbi.nlm.nih.gov/17728050/
34. Bhat GS, Shastry A. Effectiveness of "on demand" silodosin in the treatment of premature ejaculation in patients dissatisfied with dapoxetine: a randomized control study. Cent European J Urol [Internet]. 2016;69(3):280–4. [cited 2023 Jul 11]. Available from: https://pubmed.ncbi.nlm.nih.gov/27729995/
35. Bhat GS, Shastry A. A prospective double-blind, randomized, placebo-controlled study to evaluate the efficacy of silodosin 8 mg as an on-demand, reversible, nonhormonal oral contraceptive for males: a pilot study. World J Urol [Internet]. 2020;38(3):747–51. [cited 2023 Jul 11]. Available from: https://pubmed.ncbi.nlm.nih.gov/31076850/
36. Gul M, Serefoglu EC. Oxytocin antagonists: the next frontier in PE treatment. Nat Rev Urol [Internet]. 2019;16(12):696–7. [cited 2023 Jul 11]. Available from: https://pubmed.ncbi.nlm.nih.gov/31551585/
37. Tuken M, Kiremit MC, Serefoglu EC. On-demand Modafinil improves ejaculation time and patient-reported outcomes in men with lifelong premature ejaculation. Urology [Internet]. 2016;94:139–42. [cited 2023 Jul 12]. Available from: https://pubmed.ncbi.nlm.nih.gov/27151339/
38. Migliorini F, Tafuri A, Bettica P, Ziviani L, Lund J, Poggesi I, et al. A double-blind, Placebo-Controlled Parallel Group study to evaluate the effect of a single oral dose of 5-HT1A Antagonist GSK958108 on ejaculation latency time in male patients suffering from premature ejaculation. J Sex Med [Internet]. 2021;18(1):63–71. [cited 2023 Jul 12]. Available from: https://pubmed.ncbi.nlm.nih.gov/33223426/
39. Miranda M, Morici JF, Zanoni MB, Bekinschtein P. Brain-derived neurotrophic factor: a key molecule for memory in the healthy and the pathological brain. Front Cell Neurosci [Internet]. 2019;13. [cited 2023 Jul 13]. Available from: /pmc/articles/PMC6692714/
40. Serefoglu C, E, Saitz TR. New insights on premature ejaculation: a review of definition, classification, prevalence and treatment. Asian J Androl. 2012 Nov 15;14(6):822–9.

41. Song B, Cai ZM. Possible function of the frenulum of prepuce in penile erection. Andrologia [Internet]. 2012;44(1):23–5. [cited 2023 Jul 15]. Available from: https://pubmed.ncbi.nlm.nih.gov/22126255/
42. Gallo L, Perdonà S, Gallo A. The role of short frenulum and the effects of frenulectomy on premature ejaculation. J Sex Med [Internet]. 2010;7(3):1269–76. [cited 2023 Jul 15]. Available from: https://pubmed.ncbi.nlm.nih.gov/20074312/
43. Althof SE, Abdo CHN, Dean J, Hackett G, McCabe M, McMahon CG, et al. International Society for Sexual Medicine's guidelines for the diagnosis and treatment of premature ejaculation. J Sex Med [Internet]. 2010;7(9):2947–69. [cited 2023 Jun 19]. Available from: https://pubmed.ncbi.nlm.nih.gov/21050394/
44. Liu Q, Li S, Zhang Y, Cheng Y, Fan J, Jiang L, et al. Anatomic basis and clinical effect of selective dorsal neurectomy for patients with lifelong premature ejaculation: a randomized controlled trial. J Sex Med. 2019 Apr 1;16(4):522–30.
45. You HS. The partial neurectomy of the dorsal nerve of the penis for patient with premature ejaculation. Korean J Androl [Internet]. 2014;18(2):143–8. [cited 2023 Jun 19]. Available from: http://www.koreamed.org/SearchBasic.php?RID=1573716
46. Zhang GX, Yu LP, Bai WJ, Wang XF. Selective resection of dorsal nerves of penis for premature ejaculation. Int J Androl [Internet]. 2012;35(6):873–9. [cited 2023 Jun 21]. Available from: https://onlinelibrary.wiley.com/doi/full/10.1111/j.1365-2605.2012.01296.x
47. Gibbs DA, Merrill EW, Smith KA, Balazs EA. Rheology of hyaluronic acid. Biopolymers. 1968 Jun;6(6):777–91.
48. Califano G, Arcaniolo D, Ruvolo CC, Manfredi C, Smarrazzo F, Cilio S, et al. Glans penis augmentation: when, how, and why? Int J Impoten Res [Internet]. 2021;34(4):343–6. [cited 2023 Jun 23]. Available from: https://www.nature.com/articles/s41443-021-00464-1
49. Moon DG. Is there a place for surgical treatment of premature ejaculation? Transl Androl Urol [Internet]. 2016 Aug 1 [cited 2023 Jun 23];5(4):502. Available from: /pmc/articles/PMC5002006/.
50. Kosseifi F, Chebbi A, Raad N, Ndayra A, El Samad R, Achkar K, et al. Glans penis augmentation using hyaluronic acid for the treatment of premature ejaculation: a narrative review. Transl Androl Urol. 2020 Dec;9(6):2814–20.
51. Reddy AG, Dick BP, Natale C, Akula KP, Yousif A, Hellstrom WJG. Application of Botulinum Neurotoxin in male sexual dysfunction: where are we now? Sex Med Rev [Internet]. 2021;9(2):320–30. [cited 2023 Jun 24]. Available from: https://pubmed.ncbi.nlm.nih.gov/32641225/
52. Serefoglu EC, Silay MS. Botulinum toxin-A injection may be beneficial in the treatment of life-long premature ejaculation. Med Hypotheses [Internet]. 2010;74(1):83–4. [cited 2023 Jun 24]. Available from: https://pubmed.ncbi.nlm.nih.gov/19683401/
53. Otani T. Clinical review of ejaculatory dysfunction. Reprod Med Biol [Internet]. 2019 Oct 1 [cited 2023 Jul 21];18(4):331. Available from: /pmc/articles/PMC6780042/.
54. Jefferys A, Siassakos D, Wardle P. The management of retrograde ejaculation: a systematic review and update. Fertil Steril [Internet]. 2012;97(2):306–312.e6. [cited 2023 Jul 19]. Available from: https://pubmed.ncbi.nlm.nih.gov/22177462/
55. Han H, Liu S, Liang X, Lei H, Li G, Zhang J, et al. Restoration of antegrade ejaculation after transurethral bladder neck injection of Deflux for retrograde ejaculation: a case report of natural conception. Transl Androl Urol [Internet]. 2020;9(5):2270–4. [cited 2023 Jul 19]. Available from: https://pubmed.ncbi.nlm.nih.gov/33209692/
56. Gray M, Zillioux J, Khourdaji I, Smith RP. Contemporary management of ejaculatory dysfunction. Transl Androl Urol [Internet]. 2018;7(4):686–702. [cited 2023 Jul 23]. Available from: https://pubmed.ncbi.nlm.nih.gov/30211060/
57. Hollander AB, Pastuszak AW, Hsieh TC, Johnson WG, Scovell JM, Mai CK, et al. Cabergoline in the Treatment of Male Orgasmic Disorder-A Retrospective Pilot Analysis. Sex Med [Internet]. 2016 ;4(1):e28–e33. [cited 2023 Jul 23]. Available from: https://pubmed.ncbi.nlm.nih.gov/26944776/

58. Abdel-Hamid IA, Elsaied MA, Mostafa T. The drug treatment of delayed ejaculation. Transl Androl Urol [Internet]. 2016 Aug 1 [cited 2023 Jul 23];5(4):576. Available from: /pmc/articles/PMC5001980/.
59. Ibrahim E, Brackett NL, Lynne CM. Advances in the management of infertility in men with spinal cord injury. Asian J Androl [Internet]. 2016;18(3):382–90. [cited 2023 Jul 20]. Available from: https://pubmed.ncbi.nlm.nih.gov/27048781/
60. Ohl DA, Quallich SA, Sønksen J, Brackett NL, Lynne CM. Anejaculation and retrograde ejaculation. Urol Clin North Am [Internet]. 2008;35(2):211–20. [cited 2023 Jul 20]. Available from: https://pubmed.ncbi.nlm.nih.gov/18423241/
61. Waqar M, Omar K, Moubasher A, Brunckhorst O, Ahmed K. Painful ejaculation—an ignored symptom. Cureus [Internet]. 2020, 12(10) [cited 2023 Jul 24]. Available from: /pmc/articles/PMC7707127/
62. Reisman Y. Clinical experience with post-orgasmic illness syndrome (POIS) patients-characteristics and possible treatment modality. Int J Impot Res [Internet]. 2021;33(5):556–62. [cited 2023 Aug 20]. Available from: https://pubmed.ncbi.nlm.nih.gov/32472106/

Chapter 10
Initial Management of the Newly Diagnosed PE Patient

Peter Huat Chye Lim

Introduction

The initial management of the patient with PE can be conveniently done by first dividing the condition as to whether it is primary or secondary PE. Decision-making regarding management strategy follows and is heavily predicated on what is derived from a detailed history taking.

History

The history should determine whether premature ejaculation is lifelong (i.e. primary) or acquired (i.e. secondary) and assess the severity of the problem (Fig. 10.1).

For completeness screen for other medical conditions that might be relevant, e.g. if the patient has angina with subsequent fear of myocardial infarction (MI) during sexual activity, he might present with PE when the actual underlying problem is his cardiac disease and his worry regarding MI Resolution of the heart problem usually solves the PE.

P. H. C. Lim (✉)
Department of Andrology, Urology Continence Center, Gleneagles Hospital, Singapore, Singapore

H.T. Naval Medical School, Surabaya, Indonesia

Edith Cowan University, Joondalup, WA, Australia

Society for Men's Health Singapore, Midview City, Singapore

Singapore Gleneagles Medical Centre, Singapore, Singapore

Department of Urology, Changi General Hospital, Singapore, Singapore
e-mail: tphphcl@pacific.net.sg

Vasan S S et al. (eds.), *Men's Health*,
https://doi.org/10.1007/978-3-031-76898-9_10

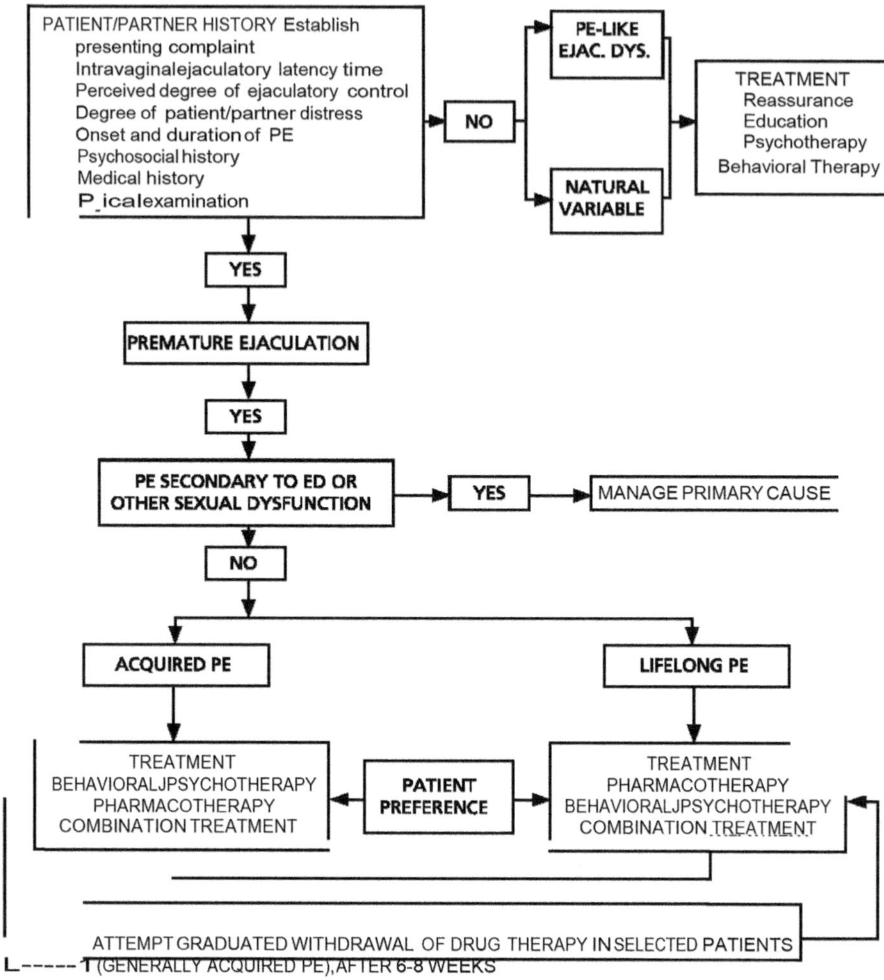

Fig. 10.1 Algorithmfor the management of premature ejaculation PE. (With permission of D. Rowland [1])

If the patient has always had PE from the time he began coitus, then he has primary PE. If he had successful coitus in the past and developed PE with the current relationship, then he has secondary premature ejaculation. In most cases, secondary PE is easier to treat and has a better prognosis.

Primary Premature Ejaculation [6]

- *Prior psychological difficulties*, as psychiatric conditions are more common in males with primary PE in the general population.
- *Patient's early sexual experiences*. Any traumatic sexual episode as a child or teenager? For example, parental discovery of masturbation, with guilt feelings or punishment/threats for masturbation.
- *Family relationships* whilst growing up. What was the relationship with mother, father, brother(s), sister(s)? Any history of incest or sexual assault? Males can be sexually assaulted by other males and, in rare instances, by females, including siblings.
- *Peer relationships*. Male friends, female friends? *Self-regard* with respect to peers (e.g. inferior, superior, athletic, frail, more intelligent, less intelligent)?
- *Difficulties at work* (or school, if still a student)?
- *General attitude toward sex* (i.e. regarded as dirty etc.), and what is the patient's sexual preference, fantasy, and arousal pattern?
- *Strict religious upbringing*? If so, what was he taught about sex?
- *Guilt feelings* when PE began with earlier nonmarital relationship
- If PE started from first coital marital relationship, ask about *premarital, noncoital sexual play* between the partners.
- Sexual attitude and *response of the female partner*; Any dyspareunia which could relate to the male's problem or may have preceded it.
- *Nonsexual part of the relationship*—fights, power struggles?
- If sexual partner is not present, ask why (i.e. *partner not supportive* or blaming him).
- Clues from these and similar questions usually point toward causation factors.

Secondary Premature Ejaculation [6]

- Prior relationships when PE was not present and any prior relationships in which transient episodes of PE occurred.
- In the current relationship, *was PE always a problem* or did it start after an initial time frame when coitus was OK to both partners?
- Quality of the relationship vis-a-vis *nonsexual factors*. Partners get along mostly or conflict present? Who is dominant and is the relationship equal?
- If *female sexual partner accompany him* did not come with him, ask why. She may regard the problem as only his rather than a couple's issue.
- Does he have *impotence*? If he has erectile dysfunction (ED), did it begin after the PE or before? If no ED, what is the general timing for PE for the male-intromission or what stage later.
- Was actual *coitus achieved or prevented by PE*?

- Is PE present at self-stimulation (i.e. masturbation), with non- intercourse stimulation by the partner, or *just with coitus*?
- *Time required for the female partner to reach climax*? Climax with intercourse, or require direct clitoral stimulation (oral or manual) to be able to climax?
- If *ED began after the PE*, then treatment of both conditions may be required; ED may resolve when confidence in controlling ejaculation is restored. If ED is started initially, PE may be a secondary sexual dysfunction, which resolves upon successful treatment of ED.

Physical Examination

Usually the physical examination is normal in males whose only presenting condition is premature ejaculation. However, chronic preputial infection or inflammation/ balanitis or an uncorrected phimosis may be found and correction of the latter may help resolve PE. Abnormal penile curvatures and thin and atrophic skin of the prepuce and glans penis can contribute to the condition if left unresolved.

Causes of Premature Ejaculation

The cause of premature ejaculation is mainly considered psychological, although this has not been definitively confirmed. Recent reports [7] have located the ejaculatory center in the lower lumbar spinal cord and disorders of this center may be causative.

Primary Premature Ejaculation

- In *Primary PE and no prior sexual experiences, a deep-seated emotional disturbance* may be present and the causes may be multiple.
- Behavior may be a *conditioned response* resulting from teen masturbatory practice or there is *deep anxiety* about sex connected to past traumatic experiences, e.g., family incest, sexual assault, conflict with one or both parents etc.
- *Consultation* with a psychiatrist, psychologist may be needed.

Secondary Premature Ejaculation

- Some type of *performance anxiety* is often present.
- Performance pressure (i.e., fear of failure to satisfy the partner) can arise from *various precipitating events, e.g., ED.*
- Careful history is needed because the situation may be *complex.*

- If ED is not the problem, the *partner may have difficulty achieving climax* through intercourse and may require direct clitoral stimulation to reach a climax and this is not communicated to him.
- Most doctors are not trained sex therapists, *sorting out conflicts* in the relationship may need referral if simple counseling and/or medication unsuccessful.

Differential Diagnoses and Other Problems [6]

- In *anorgasmia* or severely delayed orgasm in the female partner, nearly all men would be considered to have PE.
- Adverse effect from a psychotropic drug: If PE occurred after starting the drug but ceases when the drug is withdrawn,
- Pre-ejaculate: This may be confused as PE. Pre-ejaculate is the lubricating fluid produced by Cowper glands and other glands during the excitement phase of sexual stimulation. Reassurance of the male is needed.
- Erectile dysfunction (ED): This may occur in some men who are actually having premature ejaculation. Differentiating between the two problems is important.

Workup and Laboratory Studies [6]

- In males with PE and no other medical problems, no specific lab tests aid or affect treatment.
- Checking serum testosterone (free, total or bioavailable) level and prolactin level is useful if PE presents together with impotence.
- If depression or other conditions coexist, lab studies specific to depression or to other medical or psychological problems are appropriate.
- Occasionally, vibrational threshold testing or nerve conduction time, somatosensory latency testing, or both are useful in a research setting.

Medical Care

Medical treatment for PE includes several options and must also include treatment of any concomitant erection problem. Include the female partner as much as possible in the treatment and counseling sessions in order to achieve the optimal response.

Treatment of Premature Ejaculation

The principles of therapy are essentially the following:

- Lifelong PE—pharmacotherapy
- Acquired or situational PE—Pharmacotherapy and/or behavioral therapy in particular men with significant contributing psychogenic or relationship factors may benefit from concomitant behavioral therapy

Counseling/Behavioral Therapy

- Stop/Start.
- Squeeze Technique.
- Post-Coital Masturbation.
- Sensate Focus Relationship Counseling (best done by trained professional).

Withdrawal of Pharmacotherapy

- Attempt gradual withdrawal of drugs once condition stabilizes.

Behavioral Therapy—Strategy [6]

Performance Anxiety

Treat Performance Anxiety/Relieve underlying performance pressure on the male.

- If PE occurs at intercourse, the couple should be instructed that intercourse should not be attempted until PE is treated. The male may use manual stimulation, oral sex, or other means to satisfy the female partner meantime.
- If the male always experiences ejaculation with initial sexual excitement or early foreplay, this probably indicates primary PE.

Sexual Therapy

Treat couple with the stop-start or squeeze-pause technique (Masters and Johnson) [1].

The "Stop and Start" Method

- This technique involves sexually stimulating the man until he feels like he is about to reach orgasm. Stop the stimulation for about 30 seconds and then start it again. Repeat this pattern until the man wants to ejaculate. The last time continue stimulation until the man reaches orgasm.

The "Squeeze" Method (Masters and Johnson).

- This technique involves sexually stimulating the man until he recognizes that he is about to ejaculate. At that point, the man or his partner gently squeezes the end of the penis (where the glans meets the shaft) for several seconds. Stop sexual stimulation for about 30 seconds, and then start it again. The person or couple may repeat this pattern until the man wants to ejaculate. The last time continue stimulation until the man reaches orgasm.

Pre-coital Masturbation

If the male is relatively young and can achieve another erection in a few minutes following an episode of premature ejaculation, he may find that his control is much better the second time.

- Advise young men to masturbate (or have their partner stimulate them rapidly to climax) 1–2 h before sexual relations are planned.
- The interval for achieving a second climax often includes a much longer period of latency, and the male can usually exert better control in this setting.
- In an older man, such a strategy may be less effective because the older man may have difficulty achieving a second erection after his first rapid sexual release. If this occurs, it can damage his confidence and may result in secondary impotence.

Pharmacological Treatment of PE

- Selective serotonin reuptake inhibitors (SSRIs).
- PDE-5 inhibitors.
- Topical local anesthetics.

NB: For SSRI's only Dapoxetine has regulatory approval for treatment of PE

The most effective pharmacologic modality found to aid men with premature ejaculation is the selective serotonin reuptake inhibitors (SSRIs) class drugs, which are used normally as antidepressants in the clinical setting.

- Some tricyclic antidepressants with SSRI-like activity yield the same result.
- As a side effect, many of these agents have been found to cause a significant delay in reaching orgasm in both male and female patients.
- For this reason, medications with SSRI side effects have been used in men who experience premature ejaculation.

Medical Therapy Options for the Treatment of Premature Ejaculation

Nonselective Serotonin Reuptake Inhibitor

- Clomipramine.
- Anafranil 25 mg to 50 mg/day or 25 mg 4–24 h pre-intercourse.

Selective Serotonin Reuptake Inhibitors

- Anafranil, Fluxetine (Prozac) (Sarafern), Paroxetine(Paxil).
- Sertraline (Zoloft): 5 mg to 20 mg/day, 10, 20, 40 mg/day, or 20 mg, or 3–4 h pre-intercourse, 25 mg to 200 mg/day or 50 mg 4–8 h pre-intercourse.

Dapoxetine [9–11]

Dapoxetine is an SSRI developed specifically for the treatment of premature ejaculation. Dapoxetine is an approved SSRI for PE in seven European Union countries, South Korea, Australia, New Zealand, Philippines, Malaysia, and Singapore. It is rapidly absorbed (Tmax-1.5h) following oral administration. Dapoxetine acts by decreasing brain concentrations of 5HT metabolites (5-HIAA). Dapoxetine may be effective at first dose (i.e. on-demand) for premature ejaculation when given 1–3 h prior to sexual intercourse, with an adverse-effect profile comparable to those of other SSRIs [17–19]. Dapoxetine is now approved for use in Singapore by the HAS and will be available for use soon.

Topical Therapies

- Lidocaine 2.5% cream.
- EMLA* cream.
- Prilocaine 2.5% 20–30 min pre-intercourse.

  Use of desensitizing creams for the male.

- In Korea and other areas of the Far East, SS cream (a combination of nine ingredients, mainly herbal; SS stands for Super Secret) has been shown to desensitize the penis, decrease the vibratory threshold, and help men with premature ejaculation to significantly delay their ejaculatory response [2, 3].
- Unfortunately, SS Cream is not yet approved by the US Food and Drug Administration (FDA), but simple combinations of lidocaine cream or related

topical anesthetic agents can be used with similar effects and they are safe as long as the patient has no history of allergy to the substance [4, 5].

PDE-5 Inhibitors in the Treatment of PE

- Can be used in older patients with PE or in those who have concomitant ED.
- PDE-5 Inhibitors can be employed alone or in combination with SSRIs when SSRIs alone fail to treat PE.
- Behavioral therapy should be used to prevent the recurrence of PE following withdrawal of PDE-5 Inhibitors.
- For the PE patient with a definite etiological cause, the etiology should be cured first; if PE still exists, then PDE-5Is should be prescribed.

Concomitant ED and PE

ED and PE frequently overlap. When both are present, erectile dysfunction should be treated first. In the PE patient with a definite etiological cause, the etiology should be cured first.

The Choice of Therapeutic Approach Should Be

- PDE-5 inhibitors.
- PDE-5 inhibitors + SSRIs or *topical anesthetics*.
- Pharmaceuticals + Sex therapy (Behavioral therapy).

Surgical Care

No recommended surgical treatment per se exists for premature ejaculation. However, chronic preputial infection or inflammation/balanitis or an uncorrected phimosis may occasionally be found and correction of the latter may help resolve PE. Abnormal penile curvatures can contribute to the condition if left uncorrected. A urological opinion under these circumstances is mandated. Denervation techniques are still largely experimental and not currently deemed appropriate.

Consultations

- Consultation with a sex therapist, psychologist, or psychiatrist may prove helpful if the primary care physician or urologist cannot provide successful treatment or does not have the time to explore psychological issues and implement behavioral techniques (e.g. squeeze-pause). Some doctors are comfortable implementing medication therapy but not behavioral therapy. The patient should be offered all treatment options.
- For men who may be experiencing a severe emotional disturbance that is an underlying factor for PE, referral to a mental health professional is appropriate.

Prevention

- The incidence of PE in young men may possibly be decreased by better sex education during adolescence. Early successful treatment of ED in like fashion possibly prevent secondary PE in older men.

Complications

- Severe premature ejaculation can cause stress within a marriage or other relationship, which might contribute to conflicts and separation or divorce.
- Conception is also difficult in cases of premature ejaculation before vaginal intromission.

Prognosis

- Masters and Johnson state that the great majority of men with PE (>85%) can be treated successfully with the squeeze-pause technique alone within 3 months of therapy. Others have observed much poorer success [8].
- With a combination of methods including use of SSRI type medications, improvement or cure is possible provided that the couple (not just the man) is committed.
- Counseling and medical therapy can help achieve success rates as high as 85%.
- The problem with all treatments for PE is that the relapse rate is 20–50%. Hence a long-term commitment to periodically repeating the behavioral techniques is needed. Some who succeed with medical therapy, i.e., SSRIs may need to use the medication for the rest of their lives.

Patient Education

- Patients with premature ejaculation may be referred to a sex therapist, psychologist, psychiatrist, or marital counselor for additional help.
- Numerous books and articles in the lay press are available.
- Many can also find information on the Internet regarding this subject.

References

1. Masters WH, Johnson VE. Premature ejaculation. In: Human sexual inadequacy. Boston: Little Brown & Company; 1970. p. 92–115.
2. Choi HK, Jung GW, Moon KH, et al. Clinical study of SS-cream in patients with lifelong premature ejaculation. Urology. 2000;55(2):257–61.
3. Xin ZC, Choi YD, Seong DH, Choi HK. Sensory evoked potential and effect of SS- cream in premature ejaculation. Yonsei Med J. 1995;36(5):397–401.
4. Busato W, Galindo CC. Topical anaesthetic use for treating premature ejaculation: a double-blind, randomized, placebo-controlled study. BJU Int. 2004;93(7):1018–5.
5. Henry R, Morales A. Topical lidocaine-prilocaine spray for the treatment of premature ejaculation: a proof of concept study. Int J Impot Res. 2003;15(4):277–81.
6. Benson A, Ost LB, Noble M, Lakin M at http://emedicine.medscape.com/article/435884-overview
7. Personal communication: Spinal Reflex Centre for Ejaculation Guiliano, 2010.
8. Patrick DL, Althof SE, Pryor JL, Rosen R, Rowland DL, Ho KF, et al. Premature ejaculation: an observational study of men and their partners. J Sex Med. 2005;2(3):358–67.
9. Pryor JL, Althof SE, Steidle C, Rosen RC, Hellstrom WJ, Shabsigh R, et al. Efficacy and tolerability of dapoxetine in treatment of premature ejaculation: an integrated analysis of two double-blind, randomised controlled trials. Lancet. 2006;368(9539):929–37.
10. Safarinejad MR. Comparison of dapoxetine versus paroxetine in patients with premature ejaculation: a double-blind, placebo-controlled, fixed-dose, randomized study. Clin Neuropharmacol. 2006;29(5):243–52.
11. Safarinejad MR. Safety and efficacy of dapoxetine in the treatment of premature ejaculation: a double-blind, placebo-controlled, fixed-dose, randomized study. Neuropsychopharmacology. 2008;33(6):1259–65.

Chapter 11
Choice of Drugs in Ejaculatory Dysfunction

Onuralp Ergun and Ege Can Serefoglu

Introduction

Ejaculatory dysfunction (EjD) is recognized as the most prevalent disorder among male sexual disorders [124]. This condition encompasses a range of issues, including but not limited to premature ejaculation (PE), delayed ejaculation (DE), anejaculation (complete inability to ejaculate), retrograde ejaculation (RE), painful ejaculation, ejaculatory anhedonia, and post-orgasmic illness syndrome (POIS) [198, 270]. In this chapter, we focus on these issues and explain the epidemiology, pathophysiology, evaluation & approach strategies, and treatment modalities in detail for each type of disease under this spectrum.

Physiology of Ejaculatory Response

The sexual response cycle, consists of four stages: desire, arousal, orgasm, and resolution [143]. During sexual activity, as sexual arousal levels increase, a threshold is reached that triggers the ejaculatory response. Typically, this marks the end of the sexual episode for males. The perception of the contractions of the striated muscles and the expulsion of semen during ejaculation, mediated by sensory neurons in the pelvic region, contribute to the experience of orgasm, which is a distinct cortical event with cognitive and emotional dimensions [53]. Ejaculatory latency, the duration between the initiation of penile stimulation and the moment of ejaculation,

O. Ergun
Department of Urology, University of Minnesota, Minneapolis, MN, USA
e-mail: oergun@umn.edu

E. C. Serefoglu (✉)
Department of Urology, Biruni University School of Medicine, Istanbul, Turkey

Vasan S S et al. (eds.), *Men's Health*,
https://doi.org/10.1007/978-3-031-76898-9_11

varies across individuals and situations, forming a continuum of time [269]. While the majority of men achieve ejaculation and orgasm after several minutes of penile-vaginal stimulation and are satisfied with their ejaculatory latency, some individuals report dissatisfaction. Specifically, certain men ejaculate very quickly after, or even before, penetration with minimal stimulation. On the other hand, some may experience difficulty ejaculating or may not ejaculate at all, even after prolonged stimulation [154]. Additionally, various pharmacological, anatomical, and neurological factors can disrupt the ejaculation reflex by inhibiting bladder neck contraction, leading to RE . Painful ejaculation (also known as dysejaculation, odynorgasmia, post-orgasmic pain, dysorgasmia, or orgasmalgia) is another common sexual complaint, often misdiagnosed and mistreated [175].

The ejaculatory response is governed by a complex network involving sensory receptors, afferent and efferent pathways, as well as various cerebral and spinal centers [53]. This reflex is part of a broader brain circuitry that regulates multiple aspects of the sexual response. Neurochemically, the ejaculatory process entails an intricate interplay between central serotonergic and dopaminergic neurons, the involvement of cholinergic, adrenergic, oxytocinergic, and gamma-aminobutyric acid (GABA) neurons. At the peripheral level, autonomic (sympathetic and parasympathetic) and somatic divisions of the nervous system synergistically control the events leading to ejaculation [53].

The autonomic and somatic motor efferents originate from specific spinal nuclei located in the thoracolumbar and lumbosacral segments. Coordinated activation of these efferents is governed by a group of lumbar spinal interneurons known as the spinal generator of ejaculation, along with autonomic and somatic spinal nuclei. This spinal network is heavily influenced by sensory input from the genitals and supraspinal inputs that can either stimulate or inhibit the ejaculatory process [53].

Within the brain, several interconnected groups of neurons located in different sensory/integrative, excitatory, and inhibitory areas form a dedicated neural network for ejaculatory control. Notably, the posteromedial division of the bed nucleus of the stria terminalis, the posterodorsal area of the medial amygdala, the posterodorsal pre-optic nucleus, and the parvicellular part of the subparafascicular thalamus harbor neurons that are activated during ejaculation [262].

Based on functional and anatomical considerations, the ejaculatory process can be divided into three synchronized phases: emission, ejection (or penile expulsion), and orgasm [53]. Emission involves contractions of the vas deferens, seminal vesicles, and prostate, leading to the release of sperm and seminal fluid into the posterior urethra. This phase is mediated by the combined activation of sympathetic and parasympathetic pathways (T10-L2) and may also involve cholinergic mechanisms.

Ejection, on the other hand, is mediated by somatic nerves (S2 to S4) within the pudendal nerve. It encompasses pulsatile contractions of the bulbospongiosus, ischiocavernosus, and levator ani muscles, as well as relaxation of the internal urinary sphincter. Ejection also entails a sympathetic spinal cord reflex that is subject to limited voluntary control. During this phase, the bladder neck (internal urinary sphincter) closes to prevent retrograde flow, while the bulbocavernosus, bulbospongiosus, and other pelvic floor muscles contract rhythmically, and the external urinary sphincter relaxes. The external urinary sphincter exhibits intense contractions interrupted by silent periods during semen ejection [53].

Finally, orgasm is the result of cerebral processing of sensory stimuli from the pudendal nerve, arising from increased pressure in the posterior urethra, sensory stimuli from the verumontanum, and contraction of the urethral bulb and accessory sexual organs [53].

Numerous neurotransmitters play a role in the control of ejaculation, including dopamine, norepinephrine, serotonin, acetylcholine, oxytocin, GABA, and nitric oxide (NO) [152]. Among these, dopamine and serotonin have emerged as crucial neurochemical factors in the regulation of sexual functioning. Dopamine, through its D2 receptors, promotes seminal emission and ejaculation, while serotonin exerts inhibitory effects. Serotonergic neurons are widely distributed in the brain and spinal cord, with significant concentrations found in the brainstem, raphe nuclei, and reticular formation. Stimulation of the 5-HT2C receptor with 5-HT2C agonists leads to DE in male rats, whereas stimulation of postsynaptic 5-HT1A receptors results in shortened ejaculation latency. This has led to the hypothesis that individuals with PE may exhibit hyposensitivity of 5-HT2C and/or hypersensitivity of the 5-HT1A receptor [159, 265, 268].

Premature Ejaculation (PE)

Classification and Prevalence

The classification of PE has evolved over time, with various attempts to specify subtypes [174]. In 1943, Schapiro [225] proposed a classification into two types, B and A, which were later renamed lifelong (primary) and acquired (secondary) PE by Godpodinoff [81]. Subsequent classifications have considered factors such as global vs. situational nature of the disease and the influence of substances [174].

Lifelong PE is characterized by core symptoms, including early ejaculation within 30–60 s in the majority of cases (80%) or between 1–2 m (20%), occurring consistently with nearly every sexual partner and from the first sexual encounters onwards. On the other hand, acquired PE manifests as early ejaculation that develops at some point in a person's life, often in specific situations, following previously normal ejaculation experiences. The key distinguishing features between these two syndromes are the onset of symptoms and the reduction in previously normal ejaculatory latency observed in acquired PE [219]. Research on intravaginal ejaculatory latency time (IELT) in the general population and observational studies of men with PE have shown that while IELTs of less than 1 min are rare (around 2.5% prevalence), a higher percentage of men with normal IELTs report experiencing PE [80, 177, 216, 222, 223]. In order to account for this diversity, Waldinger and Schweitzer proposed a new classification of PE, which includes lifelong PE, acquired PE, variable PE, and subjective PE [271, 272]. Variable PE refers to occasional instances of early ejaculation, considered a natural variation in ejaculation time. On the other hand, subjective PE involves complaints of PE despite normal or extended ejaculation time [82]. The prevalence rates of these four PE subtypes have been confirmed in various studies, with the frequency of PE complaints ranging from 19.8% to 25.8% among sexually active males, and the prevalence of each subtype ranging from 2.3% to 6.4% [77, 222]. The prevalence varies widely depending on the study methodology and definitions used. Epidemiological studies relying on patient self-report and inconsistent definitions have reported prevalence rates ranging from 4% to 39% in the general community [84, 124, 165, 185, 191, 240, 242]. PE is often regarded as the most commonly self-reported male sexual disorder [98]. However, there is a notable disparity between prevalence estimates based on patient self-report and those utilizing the more conservative International Society for Sexual Medicine (ISSM) definition of PE [204, 205].

Regarding global prevalence estimates, data from the Global Study of Sexual Attitudes and Behaviours (GSSAB), which surveyed 27,500 men and women aged 40–80 years, reported a global prevalence of PE (based on self-report) of approximately 30% across all age groups [123, 168]. However, a limitation of the GSSAB survey is that participants were aged 40 years and older, potentially affecting the incidence of PE compared to younger males [98]. In contrast, the Premature Ejaculation Prevalence and Attitude (PEPA) Survey found the prevalence of PE among men aged 18 to 70 to be 22.7% [185].

Taking into account the various subtypes, the overall prevalence of PE has been estimated to be around 19.8%, comprising lifelong PE (2.3%), acquired PE (3.9%), variable PE (8.5%), and subjective PE (5.1%) [222]. Similar prevalence rates have been reported in a Chinese population, with 25.8% of men complaining of PE, including lifelong PE (3.18%), acquired PE (4.84%), variable PE (11.38%), and subjective PE (6.4%) [78]. It is worth noting that men with acquired PE are more likely to seek medical treatment compared to those with lifelong PE [77, 222].

Evaluation of PE

When evaluating men who complain of PE, a comprehensive medical and sexual history should be taken, along with a focused physical examination and an assessment of erectile function [16, 220]. It is beneficial to involve the partner in the management process. A cooperative partner can provide support, enhance the man's self-confidence and skills, and contribute to improving the couple's sexual and overall relationship. Including a focus on interpersonal factors has been shown to be critical for treatment success in sexual disorders.

Patients may be hesitant to discuss their sexual concerns, and it is important for clinicians to initiate discussions about sexual health. Inquiring about sexual health not only gives patients permission to discuss their concerns but also helps screen for associated health risks. Table 11.1 summarizes recommended questions for evaluating PE.

Table 11.1 Recommended questions for premature ejaculation (PE) evaluation (Adopted from [16])

Questions for evaluating PE	
Severity	What is the duration between penetration and ejaculation? Are you able to delay ejaculation? Are you bothered, annoyed or frustrated by your PE?
Lifelong vs. acquired	When did you first experience PE? Have you experienced PE since your first sexual experience on every/almost every attempt and with every partner?
Erectile function	Is your erection hard enough to penetrate? Do you have difficulty in maintaining your erection until you ejaculate during intercourse? Do you ever rush intercourse to prevent loss of your erection?
Impact on relationship	How upset is your partner with your PE? Does your partner avoid sexual intercourse? Is your PE affecting your overall relationship?
Previous treatment	Have you received any treatment for your PE before?
Impact on quality of life	Do you avoid sexual intercourse because of embarrassment? Do you feel anxious, depressed, or embarrassed because of your PE?

Diagnosis Criteria

The ISSM unified definition of lifelong and acquired PE should be used as the basis for diagnosing PE [219]. However, a significant portion of men with self-reported PE may not meet the criteria of the ISSM definition [204]. This led to the categorization of these individuals as having either variable PE or subjective PE [100, 273]. Variable PE refers to occasional early ejaculation, which can be considered a normal variation in sexual response. Subjective PE involves a complaint of PE despite having a normal ejaculatory latency, often accompanied by reduced ejaculatory control [220].

Intravaginal Ejaculatory Latency Time (IELT)

In clinical practice, self-estimation by the patient and partner of ejaculatory latency should be used to determine IELT [16, 208, 232]. Stopwatch measurements of IELT are commonly used in research studies, but they are not recommended for routine clinical management of PE due to their potential intrusiveness and disruption of sexual pleasure or spontaneity [217]. Studies have shown that patient or partner self-report of ejaculatory latency correlates relatively well with objective stopwatch measurements and can serve as a proxy measure of IELT [197]. Therefore, self-estimation by the patient and partner is recommended as the method for determining IELT in clinical practice [16, 208, 232].

Patient-Reported Outcomes (PRO)

Standardized assessment measures, such as validated questionnaires and PRO measures, can be used as adjuncts to the medical history and self-estimation of ejaculatory latency [217, 223]. These measures can provide valuable information for clinical screening and assessment. Several PE measures and questionnaires have been developed, but only a few have undergone extensive psychometric testing and validation. The Premature Ejaculation Profile (PEP) and the Index of Premature Ejaculation (IPE) are two questionnaires with extensive databases and good psychometric properties [14, 178]. The premature ejaculation diagnostic tool (PEDT) [248] is a brief diagnostic measure with a modest database that is available for clinical use. Other measures have limited validation or clinical trial data and are not recommended for clinical use.

Physical Examination

The diagnosis of lifelong PE is based purely on medical/sexual history as there are no predictive physical findings or confirmatory investigations [16, 207, 232]. However, a physical examination is highly desirable and represents an opportunity for screening for cardiovascular or gender-specific diseases, especially in young men or those with limited sexual experience [16, 207, 232]. In men with acquired PE, a physical examination is mandatory in an effort to identify the etiology of the PE and alleviate its possible cause [61]. The presence of erectile dysfunction (ED) should be evaluated either by medical history or with a validated instrument, and laboratory or imaging investigations may be required based on the patient's medical history [49]. A digital prostate examination, routine in an andrological setting for all men over 40, is helpful in identifying possible evidence of prostatic inflammation or infection [16].

Treatment

There are various psychosexual and pharmacological treatments available for PE. For men with lifelong PE, the recommended approach is PE pharmacotherapy either alone or in combination with graded levels of patient and couple psychosexual therapy [16, 208, 232]. On the other hand, men with acquired PE should receive etiology-specific treatment, such as psychosexual counseling or ED pharmacotherapy, either alone or in combination with PE pharmacotherapy [16, 208, 232]. Variable or subjective PE should primarily be treated with psychosexual education and graded patient and couple psychotherapy. It is important for physicians to recognize the association between PE and comorbid conditions such as ED, metabolic syndrome, sedentary lifestyle, obesity, alcohol consumption, and drug addiction. Patients should be counseled to improve their overall lifestyle by exercising more

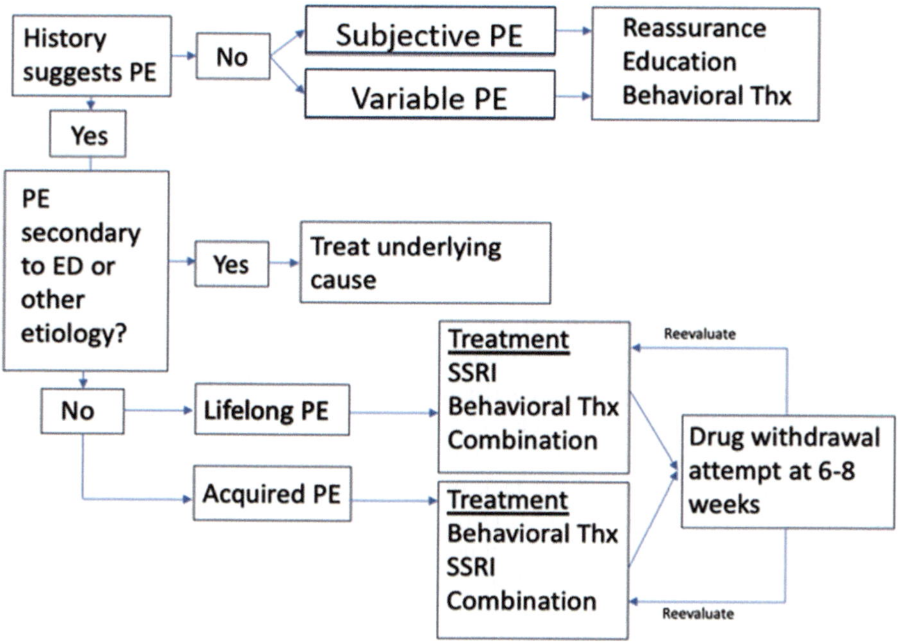

Fig. 11.1 Management of premature ejaculation (PE). *PE* premature ejaculation, *Thx* therapy, *ED* erectile dysfunction, *SSRI* selective serotonin reuptake inhibitor

and adopting healthier habits [111, 263]. Figure 11.1 is a flowchart demonstrating the management of PE.

Conventional Treatments

Psychosexual Therapy

All men seeking treatment for PE may benefit from basic psychosexual education or coaching [16, 208, 232]. This includes providing information on the prevalence of PE and the typical IELT in the general population to dismiss myths and misconceptions about PE. Education may also involve discussing enjoyable sexual activities to expand the man and his partner's sexual repertoire and addressing any avoidance of sexual activity or reluctance to discuss sex with the partner. These educational strategies aim to build the man's confidence, reduce performance anxiety, and modify maladaptive sexual patterns [11, 12, 180, 182]. However, it is important to acknowledge that the psychological-behavioral approach to treating PE has certain drawbacks. It can be time-consuming and may require significant resources in terms of both time and money. Additionally, the effects of psychosexual therapy may not be immediate, and it relies on the active cooperation of the partner. Lastly, there is a lack of long-term data to support the sustained efficacy of psychological interventions for PE.

Selective Serotonin Reuptake Inhibitors (SSRIs) and Tricyclic Antidepressants (TCAs)

Pharmacological treatment typically involves the use of selective serotonin reuptake inhibitors (SSRIs)[87]. Dapoxetine is a specific SSRI that has been approved for the treatment of PE in many countries, although it has not received FDA approval in the United States [211]. Dapoxetine is an on-demand medication with a rapid onset of action and a short half-life. Clinical studies have shown its effectiveness in increasing ejaculatory control, prolonging IELT, and improving satisfaction in men with both lifelong and acquired PE. Side effects are generally mild and dose-dependent, including nausea, diarrhea, headache, and dizziness. However, discontinuation rates can be high due to cost and the lack of spontaneity associated with on-demand administration [103, 153, 161, 172, 184, 187].

In addition to dapoxetine, off-label use of SSRIs such as paroxetine (20–40 mg) [267], clomipramine (15–30 mg) [114], sertraline (50–200 mg) [157, 238], fluoxetine (20–40 mg daily/90 mg per week) [138], and citalopram (20–40 mg) [203] has been found to be effective in delaying ejaculation and improving PE symptoms. These medications are usually taken daily and may take 2–3 weeks to achieve the full therapeutic effect. Adverse effects are generally minor and transient, including fatigue, nausea, diarrhea, and sweating [251]. Other rare adverse effects of SSRIs include priapism [213] and potential impact on fertility [118, 119]. It is important to monitor patients for any signs of suicidal ideation, particularly in younger individuals or those with comorbid depressive disorders [150]. Treatment with SSRIs should be avoided in men with a history of bipolar depression [139].

On-demand administration of clomipramine, paroxetine, sertraline, and fluoxetine a few hours before sexual activity is another treatment option, although it generally provides less ejaculatory delay compared to daily dosing [87]. Patients may have reservations about starting or continuing treatment with SSRIs due to concerns about side effects, taking an antidepressant, or the cost [150, 161, 210, 288].

Topical Local Anesthetics

The use of topical local anesthetics, such as lidocaine and/or prilocaine, in the form of creams, gels, or sprays, is an established approach for delaying ejaculation in men with PE [6, 33, 37]. These anesthetics work by reducing the sensitivity of the glans penis, which can help inhibit the spinal reflex arc responsible for ejaculation [87, 277]. However, it is important to note that topical anesthetics may cause penile hypo-anesthesia, leading to reduced penile sensitivity. There is also a risk of transvaginal absorption, potentially resulting in vaginal numbness and anorgasmia in female partners unless a condom is used [36].

PSD502, an aerosolized eutectic mixture of lidocaine–prilocaine delivered as a metered spray, has been promising in clinical studies. It is designed to optimize tissue penetration and provide a rapid onset of effect. In placebo-controlled trials, treatment with PSD502 applied to the penis at least 5 min before intercourse resulted in a significant increase in IELT and improvements in patient-reported outcome measures [40, 67]. The use of PSD502 was associated with minimal reports of penile hypo-anesthesia and transfer to the partner. It received approval by the European Medicines Agency in 2014 for the treatment of PE in the European Union and was supported for the treatment of lifelong PE by the ISSM guidelines [16].

While topical anesthetics have shown effectiveness in delaying ejaculation, there are drawbacks to their use. Loss of spontaneity and the need for application before intercourse can be a barrier for many patients, leading to discontinuation of treatment. There is limited data available on the long-term safety and efficacy of topical anesthetics for PE [31, 142]. Further research is warranted to better understand their use and address these limitations.

Phosphodiesterase-5 (PDE5) Inhibitors

Off-label use of PDE5 inhibitors, such as sildenafil, tadalafil, and vardenafil, has shown promise in the treatment of PE, both in men with and without comorbid ED [88]. While the primary indication for PDE5 inhibitors is ED, several studies have reported their effectiveness in improving PE symptoms [3, 23, 25, 46, 47, 70, 99, 104, 127, 130, 133, 144–146, 151, 209, 239, 245, 246, 250, 255, 285, 286].

The mechanism of action of PDE5 inhibitors in treating PE is speculative, but it is believed to involve the NO/cGMP transduction system, which plays a role in inhibitory nitrergic neurotransmission in the urogenital system [137]. While early systematic reviews did not provide strong empirical evidence for the use of PDE5 inhibitors in PE, more recent well-designed studies and meta-analyses have shown promising results, indicating a potential role for these agents [25, 104, 142, 246, 285]. These findings have led to recent guidelines recommending the use of PDE5 inhibitors in the treatment of PE, either alone or in combination with SSRIs, for men with or without ED [207].

Tramadol

Tramadol, a centrally acting synthetic opioid analgesic, has been explored as a potential treatment for PE [115]. Its exact mode of action is not fully understood, but it is believed to involve binding to μ-opioid receptors and weak inhibition of the reuptake of GABA, norepinephrine, and serotonin [75].

Studies evaluating the efficacy of on-demand tramadol in the treatment of PE have shown controversial results [10, 28, 68, 90, 108, 134, 141, 206, 226, 250, 278–280].

Tramadol is associated with adverse effects such as nausea, vomiting, dizziness, somnolence, tiredness, and headache [43]. There have also been reports of serotonin syndrome when tramadol is used alone or in combination with SSRIs [79, 160, 249]. Dependence may occur, although it appears to be minimal in clinical practice [148]. The risk of addiction and side effects should be considered, and tramadol should not be combined with SSRIs due to the risk of serotonin syndrome [16].

Alpha-Blockers

α1-adrenoceptor antagonists, commonly used for the treatment of lower urinary tract symptoms (LUTS) associated with or without benign prostatic hyperplasia (BPH), have been explored for their potential in treating PE. These drugs, including alfuzosin, terazosin, and silodosin, are approved primarily for the treatment of LUTS in men with obstructive BPH [126].

Their mechanism of action in the treatment of PE may involve the relaxation of the bladder neck, prostate, and urethra due to the inhibition of α1A-adrenergic receptors by these drugs [158]. Additionally, these antagonists can inhibit semen emission, leading to abnormal ejaculation [92, 116].

Several studies have reported on the use of selective α1-adrenergic blockers, such as alfuzosin (10 mg), terazosin (5 mg), tamsulosin (0.4 mg), and silodosin (4 mg), in the treatment of PE [8, 30, 42, 48, 212]. Silodosin (4 mg daily) has shown promising results in improving IELT, patient-reported outcomes, and quality of life in patients with PE [105, 212].

However, these studies have limitations, including the use of subjective endpoints and the lack of evaluation of IELT.

Common adverse effects of α1-adrenoceptor antagonists include postural hypotension, dizziness, somnolence, and nasal congestion. However, overall, the safety profile of α1-adrenoceptor antagonists in men with PE is comparable to that observed in men with hypertension or BPH [105].

The use of α1-adrenoceptor antagonists, particularly silodosin, as treatment options for PE shows potential, but further placebo-controlled studies are needed to assess their clinical usefulness.

Experimental Treatments

DA-8031

DA-8031, a potent SSRI, shows promise as a potential therapeutic agent for the treatment of PE, based on preclinical studies [102]. It exhibits high affinity and selectivity for the serotonin transporter and low selectivity for dopamine and norepinephrine transporters. In preclinical studies using rat models, DA-8031 demonstrated significant inhibition of ejaculation when administered orally or intravenously [102]. It modulates the bulbospongiosus muscle activity, inhibits the expulsion phase of ejaculation, and blocks the seminal vesicular pressure rise [173]. Currently, a human clinical trial is underway to evaluate the efficacy and safety of DA-8031 but results have not yet been reported (NCT01798667, Dong-A ST, Seoul, South Korea). There is also a recently published human study on healthy males for the pharmacokinetics, tolerability, and pharmacogenetics of the drug that reports well-tolerability but does not evaluate effectiveness [96, 231].

Oxytocin Antagonists

Oxytocin is a peptide hormone of nine amino acids, which facilitates sexual reproduction in mammals [41]. Oxytocin affects male sexual behavior through both central and peripheral pathways [63, 65, 89].

In human males, plasma oxytocin levels are elevated during penile erection and orgasm [39, 258]. Systemic administration of oxytocin reduces the number of intromissions required for ejaculation in young adult rats and shortens ejaculation latencies and post-ejaculation intervals in older sexually sluggish rats which prompted the potential use of antagonists in the treatment of PE [19, 20, 243]. In male rats, administration of an oxytocin receptor antagonist inhibits ejaculation [18, 54].

Epelsiban, formerly known as GSK557296, was used to treat PE in clinical trials after showing promise in animal experiments [18, 52, 54]. Epelsiban (50 mg and 150 mg) therapy did not, however, improve IELT in comparison to placebo [233]. This failure was primarily caused by epelsiban's capacity to operate on peripheral but not central oxytocin receptors. The investigation of another oxytocin antagonist, IX-01 (now known as cligosiban), resulted from the persistence of interest in examining the effects of inhibiting both central and peripheral oxytocin receptors in the treatment of PE. The Phase IIA trial of cligosiban demonstrated clinically and statistically significant treatment-related effects in favor of cligosiban for IELT and PRO measures related to ejaculation control and distress [155]. Cligosiban was well tolerated and exhibited a safety profile similar to placebo.

Contradictory results were obtained in two Phase II trials of cligosiban (PEPIX and PEDRIX). PEPIX showed significant improvements in IELT and PRO measures with cligosiban compared to placebo [149]. However, PEDRIX did not find significant changes in efficacy endpoints between any of the cligosiban groups and placebo [13].

It is important to note that the contradictory results in these trials may be attributed to differences in drug administration methods, the degree of placebo response, and potential biases in the study design [86]. Further research is needed to confirm the efficacy of oxytocin receptor antagonists in the treatment of PE.

Modafinil

Modafinil, a wake-promoting agent used for the treatment of narcolepsy, has shown potential effects on male sexual behavior in animal studies. Acute oral administration of d-modafinil in rats resulted in a significant delay in ejaculation and an increase in the number of intromissions [140].

The mechanism of modafinil's effect on ejaculation is not fully understood but may involve changes in serotonin and dopamine systems. Although animal studies have shown promising results, caution is necessary when applying these findings to humans [214]. A pilot study by Tuken et al. men with lifelong PE reported modest changes in self-reported IELT and PROs with on-demand modafinil treatment [256]. The authors attributed the modest increase in IELT to the pharmacokinetic properties of modafinil, with patients instructed to take the medication before noon to avoid sleep disturbances. Human trials with careful consideration of safety, side effect profile, and optimal dosing are needed before modafinil can be considered as a potential treatment for PE.

Botulinum-A Toxin

The *Clostridium botulinum* bacteria produce botulinum toxin, which prevents acetylcholine from being released from presynaptic receptors in the neuromuscular junction [95]. The bulbospongiosus and ischiocavernosus muscles, both of which play a significant part in the expulsion phase of the ejaculation reflex, have been postulated to be inhibited by botulinum toxin [221]. The efficacy of botulinum toxin A injection into the bulbospongiosus muscle in delaying ejaculation have been demonstrated in animal studies [169, 218]. A study conducted in China investigated the injection of botulinum toxin A into the bulbospongiosus muscle in individuals with lifelong PE [128]. Seventy patients with lifelong PE were randomly assigned to receive either 100 units of botulinum toxin A (10 U/ml) or an equal amount of saline into the bulbospongiosus muscles. After 4 weeks of treatment, the mean IELT of patients in the botulinum group showed a significant improvement compared to both baseline and saline-treated patients.

Specifically, the mean IELT of patients in the botulinum group was considerably better (2.35 ± 1.83 min) than at baseline (0.79 ± 0.21 min, $p < 0.001$) and compared to patients receiving saline (0.74 ± 0.27 min, $p < 0.001$). This indicates that the injection of botulinum toxin A into the bulbospongiosus muscle resulted in a significant increase in IELT compared to both baseline and saline treatment.

Furthermore, patients treated with botulinum toxin showed a statistically significant improvement in the PEP scores of the ejaculation control domain (1.21 ± 1.04) compared to both baseline and saline-treated patients (0.47 ± 0.51 and 0.49 ± 0.56, respectively, $p < 0.05$). This suggests that botulinum toxin treatment had a positive impact on patients' perceived control over ejaculation.

These findings indicate that the injection of botulinum toxin A into the bulbospongiosus muscle may be a safe and effective means to prolong ejaculatory latency without affecting other aspects of sexual behavior.

Hyaluronic Acid

Penile enlargement with hyaluronic acid is thought to act as a bulky barrier that inhibits the sensation from the glans penis' sensory receptors [44]. Thus, many clinical trials have evaluated bulking agent (hyaluronic acid) injections into the glans penis for the treatment of PE [1, 9, 38, 112, 113, 121, 163, 164, 227]. In 2019, a randomized, controlled, cross-over study randomized 30 patients with PE to receive glans penis injections of hyaluronic acid or saline [9]. The Arabic Index of PE (AIPE) scores and IELT values were obtained at various intervals following the injections. After 1 month, the mean IELT in the hyaluronic acid group was significantly higher than the saline group (two-way repeated ANOVA, $p = 0.001$). Additionally, the total AIPE scores obtained at 1 month were significantly higher in hyaluronic acid group compared to baseline ($p = 0.003$) and compared to scores from the saline group ($p = 0.002$). Mean IELTs decreased proportionally with time in the hyaluronic acid group, especially after the first month, on the other hand, even after 9 months, IELTs were still higher than pretreatment values, indicating a lasting improvement.

No severe adverse events were encountered. Local soreness at the injection site, penile ecchymosis, and papule formation in the injection site were the most common mild side effects [9]. That being said, glans penis augmentation is not entirely safe, especially if done with irreversible fillers. Unnatural cosmetics, granuloma formation, anaphylaxis, and glans necrosis have previously been documented post-penile enhancement procedures [7, 282].

Surgical Treatment

Various studies have suggested selective resection of the dorsal penile nerves (SRDN) as a potential treatment for PE [132, 230, 284, 287]. In Korea, SRDN is reported to be the second most commonly used treatment option after SSRIs, showing higher effectiveness in PE patients aged between 22–30 years [280, 281]. Instead of resection, several authors have proposed neuromodulation of the dorsal penile nerves using pulsed radiofrequency [29]. In a randomized, placebo-controlled trial conducted in China, 101 patients with PE were assigned to either circumcision alone (control group, $n = 61$) or circumcision combined with SRDN (treatment group, $n = 40$) [283]. The postoperative IELT in the SRDN group significantly increased compared to baseline (1.1 ± 0.9 min vs. 3.8 ± 3.1 min, $p < 0.01$), while the postoperative IELT in the control group did not show significant differences from baseline (1.2 ± 0.7 min vs. 1.5 ± 1.1 min, $p > 0.05$). Assessment of erectile function using the Brief Male Sexual Function Inventory questionnaire showed no significant differences between the treatment and control groups ($p = 0.59$).

In a study involving 24 patients with PE, the efficacy and safety of computed tomography-guided interventional cryoablation of the dorsal penile nerve were evaluated. The study revealed a significant increase in IELT values at 6 months (54.7 ± 7.8 s vs. 182.5 ± 27.6 s, $p < 0.0001$) and 1 year after the surgery (54.7 ± 7.8 s vs. 140.9 ± 83.6 s, $p < 0.001$) [62]. Moreover, PEP scores improved, with 83% of participants expressing that they would undergo the surgery again.

Despite the positive results observed with SRDN, current guidelines [16, 207, 232] do not recommend it as a standard treatment for PE due to its invasive and irreversible nature. Further well-designed clinical trials are needed before considering this therapy as a recommended option for PE patients.

Neuromuscular Electrical Stimulation

In 2017, a novel approach known as perineal transcutaneous electrical nerve stimulation (TENS) was introduced as a potential treatment for PE [85]. The underlying principle of this treatment is to inhibit the rhythmic contractions during the expulsion phase by inducing a plateau action potential in the bulbospongiosus and ischiocavernosus muscles. Sustained stimulation of these muscles through TENS maintains a state of sub-tetanic persistent contraction, potentially leading to DE [50, 85].

To investigate this concept, a study was conducted involving 23 individuals with lifelong PE who were divided into two groups: an active TENS treatment group and a sham treatment group. Masturbation ejaculation latency time (MELT) during self-stimulation was measured as an outcome [229]. The results showed that the active TENS group had significantly higher mean MELT values compared to the sham group ($p = 0.0009$; 311.4 ± 237.14 s vs. 124.6 ± 107.02 s; a four-fold increase in MELT). It is important to note that this study did not establish specific threshold values for MELT and assumed a correlation between MELT and IELT in PE patients. No severe adverse effects or ED were reported, although some participants experienced minor side effects such as unpleasant sensations during stimulation and a burning sensation during urination afterwards.

A more recent prospective bi-center international study by Shechter et al. [228] further examined the efficacy and safety of a miniaturized on-demand perineal TENS device (vPatch) for treating PE. The study included 59 patients with lifelong PE, and the group treated with the vPatch device showed a significant increase in the geometric mean IELT (from 67 to 123 s, $p < 0.01$), whereas the sham treatment group had a nonsignificant increase (from 63 to 81 s, $p = 0.17$).

To determine the comparative efficacy of on-demand neuromuscular TENS therapy in delaying ejaculation for individuals with PE, future head-to-head trials are warranted, particularly in comparison to pharmacological treatments. Furthermore, the development of user-friendly TENS devices that minimize sexual discomfort should be a focus of future research.

Transcutaneous Posterior Tibial Nerve Stimulation (TPTNS)

The rationale for employing TPTNS in the management of PE is based on the intricate sensory role of the posterior tibial nerve, which is rooted in the T4-S3 region. The emission phase of ejaculation is primarily governed by stimuli originating from the T12-L1 area, while the expulsion phase is predominantly controlled at the S2-S4 level. By stimulating the posterior tibial nerve, it is hypothesized that both the sympathetic-mediated emission phase and the parasympathetic-somatic expulsion phase of ejaculation can be inhibited.

To explore the potential therapeutic efficacy of TPTNS for PE, a phase II study was conducted involving 11 patients [259]. These patients underwent 30-min TPTNS sessions three times per week over a span of 12 weeks. Among the patients who completed the full 12-week therapy period, 54% exhibited a threefold increase in IELT compared to baseline ($p = 0.037$). Adverse effects were reported by two patients, including constipation ($n = 1$) and a sensation of heat in the leg ($n = 1$), but these side effects did not impact treatment adherence. It is important to note that this study is limited by the small sample size and the absence of both a control group and randomization. Further randomized controlled trials with larger sample sizes are warranted to confirm the therapeutic efficacy of TPTNS for PE.

Acupuncture

In a randomized placebo-controlled clinical study conducted by Sunay et al. [247], the efficacy of acupuncture therapy administered twice a week was compared to paroxetine (20 mg/day) and sham acupuncture (placebo) for the treatment of PE. The study involved 90 patients and revealed that acupuncture had a significantly greater ejaculation-delaying effect than placebo (65.7 vs. 33.1 s), although it was less effective than daily paroxetine (82.7 s, $p = 0.001$). PRO measures also indicated improvement in both the acupuncture and paroxetine groups.

In another recent study, electroacupuncture was evaluated in 50 PE patients, with the control group receiving Long Dan Xie Gan herbal medicine [135]. The researchers observed a significant increase in IELT in both groups ($p < 0.05$). However, after 4 weeks of treatment, the electroacupuncture group demonstrated a significantly higher IELT compared to the control group. Interestingly, a significant decrease in testosterone levels was observed in both groups compared to baseline ($p < 0.05$), with the electroacupuncture group showing a greater decline ($p < 0.05$).

These findings suggest that acupuncture and electroacupuncture may have a positive impact on delaying ejaculation and improving symptoms of PE. However, it is important to emphasize that further well-designed clinical trials are necessary to validate these results and explore the underlying mechanisms, particularly with regard to metabolic effects.

Delayed Ejaculation, Anejaculation, and Anorgasmia

Classification and Prevalence

DE, also known as retarded ejaculation or inhibited ejaculation, is a male sexual dysfunction that is less common, less studied, less reported, and less understood compared to other sexual dysfunctions [202]. It refers to difficulties or delays in achieving ejaculation during sexual activity, resulting in a lack of sexual fulfillment for both the man and his partner. In some cases, a complete inability to ejaculate, known as anejaculation, may occur. Additionally, reductions in the volume, force, and sensation of ejaculation can be experienced. [45].

Anorgasmia is another related disorder, which refers to the perceived absence of the orgasm experience or sexual anhedonia, irrespective of whether the physiological components of ejaculation have occurred [101].

Historically, the reported rates of DE have been low, rarely exceeding 3% [124, 237, 241]. However, a multinational survey conducted in 2003 in the United States and Europe revealed that approximately 40% of men aged 50–79 experienced some form of DE, with a prevalence similar to ED [196].

Age has been moderately and positively associated with the prevalence of DE, as ejaculatory function tends to diminish with increasing age. For example, one study reported DE prevalence of 16.2%, 22.7%, and 33.2% in men aged 57–65, 65–74, and 75–85 years, respectively [129]. The prevalence of DE and anejaculation has also been found to differ among different racial groups, and it has been associated with ED, LUTS, hyperlipidemia, and low serum testosterone [55, 56, 171, 196]. However, there is limited research on the demographic and clinical correlates of DE/ anejaculation in community-dwelling populations, and few studies have differentiated between different types of DE or used validated scales to assess it.

DE can be either a lifelong problem or an acquired problem [183]. It can occur in every sexual encounter (global) or be intermittent or situational [201]. While coital anejaculation often drives the treatment-seeking behavior of individuals referred for fertility problems, men may also seek treatment when distressed by their inability to achieve orgasm in response to various types of sexual stimulation by their partner. Some men with acquired DE may still be able to achieve orgasm through masturbation, while others may have lost the capacity to do so due to emotional or physical trauma [166]. Just like PE, men with DE often experience high levels of relationship distress, sexual dissatisfaction, anxiety about sexual performance, and general health issues compared to sexually functional men [4]. They also tend to have lower frequencies of sexual intercourse and higher frequencies of masturbation [2]. Notably, men with DE may exhibit normal erectile function but report lower levels of subjective sexual arousal compared to sexually functional men [15, 56, 200].

Further research is needed to better understand the prevalence, etiology, causes, mechanisms, and optimal treatment approaches for DE and anorgasmia in various populations. Psychometrically validated scales and comprehensive assessments are necessary to differentiate between different ejaculatory disorders and improve diagnostic accuracy and treatment outcomes.

Etiology

DE or anorgasmia can be either lifelong or acquired, and it may manifest as a global issue or be situational in nature [232]. The pathophysiology of DE is multifactorial, and various underlying factors have been associated with it [2]. These factors can include congenital disorders, psychological factors, surgical or radiotherapeutic treatment for male pelvic cancers, neurological diseases such as multiple sclerosis and Parkinson's disease, hypogonadism, hypothyroidism, infections, and the use of medications for conditions such as schizophrenia or mood disorders (e.g., major tranquilizers or SSRI antidepressants) [45].

Psychological factors can play a significant role in DE and include performance anxiety, relationship conflicts, poor sexual communication, hypoactive sexual desire, and psychological conflicts related to fears of fathering a child, harm to oneself or the partner, or shame induced by religious beliefs [15, 199]. Some men develop idiosyncratic patterns of solitary masturbation that cannot be replicated during intercourse, leading to conditioned DE or anejaculation [181].

In clinical practice, the most common causes of DE are psychogenic inhibited ejaculation, degeneration of penile afferent nerves and Pacinian corpuscles associated with aging, hypogonadism, diabetic autonomic neuropathy, treatment with SSRI antidepressants and major tranquilizers, and radical prostatectomy or other major pelvic surgeries and/or radiotherapy [166].

Evaluation

When evaluating men presenting with DE or anejaculation, a comprehensive assessment is necessary to determine the underlying cause and potential contributing factors [166, 232]. The evaluation process involves obtaining a detailed medical and sexual history, conducting a focused physical examination, and performing additional investigations as warranted by the findings.

The assessment begins by distinguishing between lifelong or acquired DE and determining whether it is a global issue or situational. Important aspects to consider include the frequency of ejaculation during intercourse, the IELT, and the ability to achieve ejaculation through post-coital self or partner-assisted masturbation. Table 11.2 reviews questions to ask for evaluating DE.

The evaluation should also assess the negative psychological consequences experienced by the patient, partner, or in the interpersonal relationship, such as bother, distress, frustration, or avoidance of sexual contact. The frequency of intercourse and the dynamics of initiation can serve as indicators of these psychological consequences. Additionally, the quality of the nonsexual relationship should be explored as it can have an impact on sexual function.

For men with acquired DE, a review of previous illnesses, surgeries, medications, or life events/circumstances is essential. Identifying any psychological factors or stressors that may contribute to the ejaculatory difficulties is important, such as fears or concerns related to a partner's health or societal and religious attitudes towards sexuality [166].

A focused physical and genital examination is necessary to assess the testes, epididymes, and vas deferentia for any abnormalities. A screening morning total testosterone level may be obtained, and further hormonal or imaging investigations

Table 11.2 Recommended Questions for Delayed Ejaculation (DE) Evaluation [166]

Questions for evaluating DE	
Severity	How often can you ejaculate during sexual intercourse? During intercourse, how long after penetration does it take for you to either ejaculate or stop intercourse?
	When you cannot ejaculate during sexual intercourse, how often do you feel that you are close to ejaculation? If you cannot ejaculate, why do you stop intercourse?
	Do you ever feel that you have ejaculated but fail to release semen? Do you feel bothered, annoyed, and/or frustrated by your DE?
	How often can you ejaculate during masturbation by yourself or with your partner?
Lifelong vs. acquired	When did you first experience DE? Have you experienced DE since your first sexual experience on every/almost every attempt and with every partner?
Erectile function	Is your erection hard enough to penetrate? Do you have difficulty in maintaining your erection during intercourse?
Impact on relationship	How upset is your partner with your DE? Do you or your partner avoid sexual intercourse? Is your DE affecting your overall relationship?
Previous treatment	Have you received any treatment for you DE previously?
Impact on quality of life	Do you feel anxious, depressed, or embarrassed because of your DE?

may be indicated based on the history and physical examination findings. Digital rectal examination can help assess prostate size, anal sphincter tone, and the quality of the bulbo-cavernous reflex. In cases where neuropathy is suspected, electrophysiological evaluations of the neural pathways controlling ejaculation, such as pudendal somatosensory and motor evoked potentials, sacral reflex arc testing, and sympathetic skin responses, may be considered.

In cases where DE is accompanied by absent or low-volume prograde ejaculation, further differentiation between RE and ejaculatory duct obstruction is necessary. The presence of spermatozoa in post-masturbation first void urine suggests RE, while low viscosity, low fructose, and low pH semen on semen analysis suggest ejaculatory duct obstruction. In cases where the etiology of DE remains unclear, additional investigations such as culture of expressed prostatic secretion and urine, urine cytology, and serum prostate-specific antigen may be performed to exclude prostatitis, bladder, and prostatic cancer. Perineal and/or transrectal ultrasound may be utilized to identify pelvic function and local diseases [71]. Overall, a thorough evaluation of men with DE or anejaculation is necessary to identify the underlying causes and guide appropriate management strategies.

Management of DE/Anejaculation

Treatment for DE or anejaculation should be tailored to the underlying cause and address the specific needs of the patient and his partner. The treatment options include patient/couple psychoeducation and/or psychosexual therapy, pharmacotherapy, or integrated treatment approaches [166, 232].

Lifestyle changes and psychotherapy can be beneficial for some individuals. Lifestyle modifications may involve spending more time together to enhance intimacy, minimizing alcohol consumption, and optimizing arousal through techniques like pelvic floor training. Psychotherapy, particularly psychosexual therapy, can help address the psychological and behavioral factors contributing to DE. It may involve sex education, reducing performance anxiety, increasing genital-focused stimulation, masturbatory retraining, and realigning sexual fantasies with arousal strategies.

Therapeutic interventions should aim to facilitate the bond between partners while maintaining a therapeutic alliance and optimizing the man's response to various forms of sexual stimulation.

The effectiveness of treatments for DE is difficult to assess due to limited evidence, and success rates vary among individuals [156]. Pharmacotherapy options have shown limited success, and no drugs are approved specifically for DE. Medications such as cabergoline (0.5–3 mg every 3 days) [94], a central D2 agonist, and alpha-1 adrenergic receptor agonists like pseudoephedrine (120 mg 1–2 h pre-coitus) [106] or serotonin-norepinephrine reuptake inhibitors (SNRI) antidepressant reboxetine (4–8 mg daily) [51, 106] have been used but may have limited efficacy and side effects. Other medications like cyproheptadine (2–16 mg) [21, 195] and loratadine [22, 24, 147] have been reported anecdotally to reverse anorgasmia induced by SSRI antidepressants, but controlled studies are lacking. Several other pharmacological agents have been suggested as potential treatments, but robust randomized controlled trials are needed to evaluate their efficacy.

Intra-coital administration of intranasal oxytocin has shown some promise in case reports, but there is a lack of robust evidence from randomized controlled trials to support its effectiveness [35, 97, 136, 264]. Further research is needed to determine its efficacy and optimal dosage.

In cases where DE is irreversible, alternative methods to achieve sexual satisfaction with the partner should be explored. Overall, treatment for DE should be individualized, bearing in mind the specific etiology, psychological factors, and needs of the patient and his partner. Collaborative efforts between healthcare providers, psychosexual therapists, and couples are essential to achieve satisfactory outcomes.

Retrograde Ejaculation

Definition and Prevalence

The closure of the bladder neck and proximal urethra is necessary for antegrade ejaculation [175]. Surgical procedures that compromise the closure mechanism of the bladder neck can lead to RE. Transurethral incision of the prostate (TUIP) has been associated with RE in 5–45% of patients, depending on factors such as the number of incisions made and the extent of the incision [91, 110]. The contraction of the urethral smooth muscle at the level of the verumontanum has also been suggested to play a role in preventing RE [192].

Transurethral resection of the prostate (TURP) has a higher incidence of RE compared to TUIP. Reported incidences of RE following TURP range from 42% to 100% [69, 188]. While men who undergo TURP may still experience some antegrade ejaculation and orgasmic sensation, these events may be reduced due to age-related changes in the male sexual response. Modified-TURP and modified-prostate photo-vaporization techniques have been developed to preserve ejaculatory function in patients with BPH, with antegrade ejaculation rates reported as 66–91% and 87–96%, respectively [125]. More recent procedures like prostatic urethral lift and aquablation have demonstrated superiority over TURP in terms of ejaculatory disorders in prospective randomized-controlled trials [125].

RE is more common in individuals with diabetes mellitus (DM) compared to age-matched controls, with a reported incidence of 30% in men with DM. However, it is not statistically associated with waist circumference, the body mass index (BMI), HbA1c levels, or testosterone levels [66, 275].

Differentiating between RE and failure of emission can be done by examining a post-masturbatory urine specimen for the presence of spermatozoa and fructose. The presence of more than 5–10 sperm per high-power field confirms the diagnosis of RE. In cases of low-volume ejaculate, finding more sperm in the urine than in the ejaculate suggests RE [235].

Management of RE

Bladder neck reconstruction is a surgical option for the treatment of RE, but the results have been poor [5, 131]. Drug treatment is currently considered the most promising approach. Sympathomimetic amine agents have been used with mixed results to stimulate the release of noradrenaline from nerve axon terminals and facilitate ejaculation. These agents include pseudoephedrine, ephedrine, midodrine, and phenylpropanolamine [109, 186]. Pseudoephedrine, administered at a dose of 120 mg every 6 h on the day prior to coitus and twice on the day of coitus, resulted in prograde ejaculation in 58% of predominantly diabetic men [234].

The tricyclic antidepressant imipramine, which blocks the reuptake of noradrenaline, has also been used for the treatment of RE with some success [234]. The usual dose is 25 mg twice daily, and long-term treatment with imipramine is considered more effective. Preliminary data suggest a potential role for endourethral injection of collagen type 2 in the treatment of RE [120]. However, further research is needed to evaluate the effectiveness and safety of these treatment options for RE.

Anhedonia

Sexual anhedonia, also known as ejaculatory anhedonia or Pleasure Dissociative Orgasm Disorder (PDOD), is a condition where individuals experience little or no pleasure despite being aware of orgasm and ejaculation [83]. It is an uncommon disorder. Sexual anhedonia can occur in both males and females and may be associated with various factors such as depression, fatigue, physical illness, hypoactive sexual desire disorder (HSDD), hypogonadism, hyperprolactinemia, spinal cord injury, multiple sclerosis, or the use of SSRI antidepressants or antipsychotic medications [59, 72].

The pathophysiology of PDOD is not clearly understood, but it is believed to involve a central neurochemical dysfunction, particularly involving dopamine [257]. Dopaminergic neurons in the mesolimbic pathway, which project into the nucleus accumbens (NAc), play a role in the release of dopamine in response to rewarding stimuli, including sexual arousal and orgasm. PDOD may result from a defect in dopamine release or the interaction between dopamine and GABAergic neurons in the NAc. Chronic depression is often associated with this disorder, and there may be a bidirectional relationship between sexual anhedonia and depression [252]. The frustration and negativity resulting from the underlying neurochemical disorder contribute to the psychogenic component of the condition [59]. When evaluating individuals with sexual anhedonia, androgen studies including total and free testosterone, pituitary gonadotropins, and prolactin levels should be conducted. If there is evidence of hyperprolactinemia or secondary hypogonadism, a pituitary MRI may be necessary. Other potential causes of sexual disorders, such as HSDD, opiate addiction, the use of psychotropic medications, or genital sensory neuropathy, should be ruled out. It is important to acknowledge that individuals with sexual anhedonia are often resistant to the idea that their condition has a psychogenic cause or contribution, and they may be correct in their assessment [59].

The management of sexual anhedonia typically involves an integrated approach with both pharmacotherapy and psychotherapy. Central dopamine agonists, such as cabergoline at a dose of 0.5–3 mg every 3 days, may be considered as part of the pharmacological treatment [59]. Psychotherapy can help address the psychogenic component of the disorder and provide support to individuals coping with the frustration and negative emotions associated with sexual anhedonia.

Post-SSRI Sexual Dysfunction (PSSD)

Post-SSRI Sexual Dysfunction (PSSD) is a condition that can occur after the abrupt cessation, interruption, or dose reduction of antidepressant drugs, particularly SSRIs or SNRIs. While antidepressant withdrawal syndrome is a transient and mild condition, PSSD is a debilitating condition that can persist for months to years and adversely affect the quality of life of individuals [59]. The exact prevalence of persistent sexual side effects after discontinuing SSRIs is unknown, although one study reported an incidence of PSSD ranging from 5% to 15% [26]. Symptoms may include genital anesthesia, HSDD, ED, PE, and ejaculatory anhedonia [274].

The etiology of PSSD remains unknown, but several theories have been proposed. One theory suggests that there may be interactions between dopamine and serotonin, serotonin neurotoxicity, or downregulation of 5-HT-IA receptors [27]. Serotonin-receptor downregulation theory suggests that high concentrations of serotonin in the hypothalamus can lead to downregulation of the hypothalamic-pituitary-testicular axis, resulting in decreased testosterone levels [58, 60, 193].

Diagnosing PSSD can be challenging and requires a thorough review of the patient's drug history, onset and type of symptoms, and the patient's premorbid sexual function. It is important to distinguish PSSD symptoms from those of the actual mental illness.

Currently, there is no definitive treatment for PSSD, and management is limited to treating specific symptoms with pharmacotherapy, such as using PDE5 inhibitors for ED or pharmacotherapy for SSRI-induced sexual dysfunction, either alone or in combination with individual and couple psychotherapy [64]. Some anecdotal reports have suggested potential treatment options such as low-power laser irradiation, serotonergic antagonists, dopaminergic agonists, or switching SSRIs to dopaminergic antidepressants [93, 162, 274]. However, these strategies lack definitive evidence, and their efficacy is limited. Spontaneous recovery of symptoms has been reported in some patients over time, ranging from a few days to decades, indicating that these symptoms may not arise from permanent damage [193]. Nonetheless, PSSD is underdiagnosed and can significantly impact patients' quality of life, so a multidisciplinary approach involving urology, psychology, and endocrinology is necessary for managing patients with suspected PSSD. Patients should also be well-informed about the potential side effects of SSRIs, and their sexual function should be assessed before starting treatment, during medication use, and after discontinuation [32].

Orgasmic Headache

There have been numerous reports of a headache that occurs during sexual activity, specifically at or around the time of orgasm. Lance et al. identified two variants of sexual headache, one characterized by muscle contraction headache and the other by severe throbbing vascular headache [122]. Structural lesions are not typically found in the majority of patients, although the possibility of intracranial vascular or other lesions should be considered. The population prevalence of orgasmic headache is estimated to be between 1% and 1.6% [190, 254]. Risk factors for orgasmic headache include male gender, a history of migraine, familial occurrence, stress, and fatigue [17, 74, 122, 170, 176, 179, 189, 236]. There is no definitive treatment for orgasmic headache, but migraine treatments such as triptans, indomethacin, and beta-blockers have been reported to alleviate symptoms [74, 176, 179]. Medications such as rizatriptan, almotriptan, and sumatriptan taken 30 min before planned sexual activity have also shown potential benefits in the treatment of orgasmic headaches [74].

Painful Ejaculation

Painful ejaculation, also known as odynorgasmia, is a syndrome that is not well-characterized [175]. It can be associated with various conditions such as urethritis, BPH, acute or chronic prostatitis, chronic pelvic pain syndrome, seminal vesiculitis, seminal vesicular calculi, or ejaculatory duct obstruction [57, 117, 167, 276]. However, in many cases, no clear underlying cause can be identified.

Painful ejaculation is reported in 17–23% of men with BPH&LUTS [34, 73, 253, 260]. It is worth noting that treatment with alpha-blocking drugs for LUTS may be associated with painful ejaculation [76], although the incidence of pain appears to be lower with uroselective alpha-1 blockers such as alfuzosin [261].

Management of painful ejaculation should primarily focus on addressing and treating the underlying cause. This may involve targeted therapies for conditions such as prostatitis, BPH, or other associated factors. Consulting with a healthcare professional, such as a urologist, is recommended for appropriate evaluation and treatment.

Post-Orgasmic Illness Syndrome

Post-Orgasmic Illness Syndrome (POIS) is a rare and poorly understood condition characterized by a collection of symptoms that occur shortly after orgasm [244]. The symptoms of POIS typically include severe fatigue, myalgia (muscle pain), and flu-like symptoms such as fever, chills, headache, nasal congestion, and cognitive difficulties. These symptoms typically arise within 30 min of orgasm and can last for hours to days [270].

The exact cause of POIS is unknown, and the pathophysiology of the syndrome remains poorly understood [215]. Some theories suggest that it may be an autoimmune response triggered by the release of certain substances during orgasm, while others propose a potential allergic or hypersensitivity reaction [107]. Diagnosing

POIS can be challenging, as there are no specific diagnostic tests available. It is typically based on a thorough evaluation of the patient's symptoms and medical history, with a focus on the temporal relationship between orgasm and the onset of symptoms. Keeping a detailed diary of symptoms and their association with sexual activity can aid in the diagnostic process. Currently, there is no definitive treatment for POIS. Management strategies focus on symptom relief and improving the patient's quality of life. Some treatment approaches that have shown variable success include antihistamines [224], nonsteroidal anti-inflammatory drugs (NSAIDs), corticosteroids, alpha-blockers [194], and desensitization therapy [266]. Due to the rarity and lack of awareness surrounding POIS, many individuals with the condition may face challenges in obtaining an accurate diagnosis and appropriate care. Seeking the expertise of healthcare professionals who are knowledgeable about the syndrome, such as urologists or sexual medicine specialists, can be beneficial for individuals experiencing POIS symptoms.

Conclusion

EjDs can significantly impact the sexual health and well-being of individuals. Whether it is PE, DE, or RE, these conditions can cause distress, frustration, and strain on relationships. However, it is important to remember that most of EjDs are treatable, and seeking medical advice can lead to effective solutions. With the help of healthcare professionals, individuals can explore various treatment options, including medications, psychotherapy and lifestyle changes, to improve their ejaculatory function and regain control over their sexual experiences. Additionally, open communication, understanding, and support from partners can play a crucial role in managing EjD and promoting overall sexual satisfaction. By addressing EjD proactively and seeking appropriate care, individuals can reclaim their sexual confidence and enhance their overall quality of life.

References

1. Abdallah H, Abdelnasser T, Hosny H, Selim O, Al-Ahwany A, Shamloul R. Treatment of premature ejaculation by glans penis augmentation using hyaluronic acid gel: a pilot study. Andrologia. 2012;44(Suppl 1):650–3.
2. Abdel-Hamid IA, Ali OI. Delayed ejaculation: pathophysiology, diagnosis, and treatment. World J Mens Health. 2018;36:22–40.
3. Abdel-Hamid IA, El Naggar EA, El Gilany AH. Assessment of as needed use of pharmacotherapy and the pause-squeeze technique in premature ejaculation. Int J Impot Res. 2001;13:41–5.
4. Abdo CH. The impact of ejaculatory dysfunction upon the sufferer and his partner. Transl Androl Urol. 2016;5:460–9.
5. Abrahams JI, Solish GI, Boorjian P, Waterhouse RK. The surgical correction of retrograde ejaculation. J Urol. 1975;114:888–90.

6. Abu El-Hamd M. Effectiveness and tolerability of lidocaine 5% spray in the treatment of lifelong premature ejaculation patients: a randomized single-blind placebo-controlled clinical trial. Int J Impot Res. 2021;33:96–101.
7. Ahn ST, Il Kwak T, Park KS, Kim JJ, Moon DG. Complications of glans penis augmentation. Int J Impot Res. 2019;31:245–55.
8. Akin Y, Gulmez H, Ates M, Bozkurt A, Nuhoglu B. Comparison of alpha blockers in treatment of premature ejaculation: a pilot clinical trial. Iran Red Crescent Med J. 2013;15:e13805.
9. Alahwany A, Ragab MW, Zaghloul A, Abdallah H, Mostafa T. Hyaluronic acid injection in glans penis for treatment of premature ejaculation: a randomized controlled cross-over study. Int J Impot Res. 2019;31:348–55.
10. Alghobary M, El-Bayoumy Y, Mostafa Y, Mahmoud El H, M. & Amr, M. Evaluation of tramadol on demand vs. daily paroxetine as a long-term treatment of lifelong premature ejaculation. J Sex Med. 2010;7:2860–7.
11. Althof S. Sex therapy in the age of pharmacotherapy. Annu Rev Sex Res. 2006;17:116–32.
12. Althof S. Treatment of rapid ejaculation: psychotherapy, pharmacotherapy, and combined therapy. In: Leiblum S, editor. Principles and practice of sex therapy. 4th ed. New York: Guilford Press; 2007.
13. Althof S, Osterloh IH, Muirhead GJ, George K, Girard N. The oxytocin antagonist cligosiban fails to prolong intravaginal ejaculatory latency in men with lifelong premature ejaculation: results of a randomized, double-blind, placebo-controlled phase IIb trial (PEDRIX). J Sex Med. 2019;16:1188–98.
14. Althof S, Rosen R, Symonds T, Mundayat R, May K, Abraham L. Development and validation of a new questionnaire to assess sexual satisfaction, control and distress associated with premature ejaculation. J Sex Med. 2006;3:465–75.
15. Althof SE. Psychological interventions for delayed ejaculation/orgasm. Int J Impot Res. 2012;24:131–6.
16. Althof SE, Mcmahon CG, Waldinger MD, Serefoglu EC, Shindel AW, Adaikan PG, Becher E, Dean J, Giuliano F, Hellstrom WJ, Giraldi A, Glina S, Incrocci L, Jannini E, Mccabe M, Parish S, Rowland D, Segraves RT, Sharlip I, Torres LO. An update of the International Society of Sexual Medicine's guidelines for the diagnosis and treatment of premature ejaculation (PE). J Sex Med. 2014;11:1392–422.
17. Angus-Leppan H, Caulfield A. Orgasmic migraine aura: report of two cases. Cephalalgia. 2019;39:153–6.
18. Argiolas A, Collu M, D'aquila P, Gessa GL, Melis MR, Serra G. Apomorphine stimulation of male copulatory behavior is prevented by the oxytocin antagonist d(CH2)5 Tyr(Me)-Orn8-vasotocin in rats. Pharmacol Biochem Behav. 1989;33:81–3.
19. Arletti R, Bazzani C, Castelli M, Bertolini A. Oxytocin improves male copulatory performance in rats. Horm Behav. 1985;19:14–20.
20. Arletti R, Benelli A, Bertolini A. Sexual behavior of aging male rats is stimulated by oxytocin. Eur J Pharmacol. 1990;179:377–81.
21. Arnott S, Nutt D. Successful treatment of fluvoxamine-induced anorgasmia by cyproheptadine. Br J Psychiatry. 1994;164:838–9.
22. Ashton K, Hamer R, Rosen R. Serotonin reuptake inhibitor-induced sexual dysfunction and its treatment: a large-scale retrospective study of 596 psychiatric outpatients. J Sex Marital Ther. 1997;23:165–75.
23. Atan A, Basar MM, Tuncel A, Ferhat M, Agras K, Tekdogan U. Comparison of efficacy of sildenafil-only, sildenafil plus topical EMLA cream, and topical EMLA-cream-only in treatment of premature ejaculation. Urology. 2006;67:388–91.
24. Aukst-Margetic B, Margetic B. An open-label series using loratadine for the treatment of sexual dysfunction associated with selective serotonin reuptake inhibitors. Prog Neuro-Psychopharmacol Biol Psychiatry. 2005;29:754–6.
25. Aversa A, Pili M, Francomano D, Bruzziches R, Spera E, La Pera G, Spera G. Effects of vardenafil administration on intravaginal ejaculatory latency time in men with lifelong premature ejaculation. Int J Impot Res. 2009;21:221–7.

26. Bahrick AS. Post SSRI sexual dysfunction. Am Soc Adv Pharmacother Tablet. 2006;7:2–3.
27. Bala A, Nguyen HMT, Hellstrom WJG. Post-SSRI sexual dysfunction: a literature review. Sex Med Rev. 2018;6:29–34.
28. Bar-Or D, Salottolo KM, Orlando A, Winkler JV. A randomized double-blind, placebo-controlled multicenter study to evaluate the efficacy and safety of two doses of the tramadol orally disintegrating tablet for the treatment of premature ejaculation within less than 2 minutes. Eur Urol. 2011;61:736–43.
29. Basal S, Goktas S, Ergin A, Yildirim I, Atim A, Tahmaz L, Dayanc M. A novel treatment modality in patients with premature ejaculation resistant to conventional methods: the neuromodulation of dorsal penile nerves by pulsed radiofrequency. J Androl. 2010;31:126–30.
30. Basar MM, Yilmaz E, Ferhat M, Basar H, Batislam E. Terazosin in the treatment of premature ejaculation: a short-term follow-up. Int Urol Nephrol. 2005;37:773–7.
31. Bebi C, Turetti M, Lievore E, Ripa F, Bilato M, Rocchini L, Gallioli A, Spinelli MG, De Lorenzis E, Albo G, Longo F, Gadda F, Dell'orto PG, Montanari E, Boeri L. Sexual and ejaculatory function after holmium laser enucleation of the prostate and bipolar transurethral enucleation of the prostate: a single-center experience. Int J Impot Res. 2022;34:71–80.
32. Ben-Sheetrit J, Aizenberg D, Csoka AB, Weizman A, Hermesh H. Post-SSRI sexual dysfunction: clinical characterization and preliminary assessment of contributory factors and dose-response relationship. J Clin Psychopharmacol. 2015;35:273–8.
33. Boeri L, Pozzi E, Fallara G, Montorsi F, Salonia A. Real-life use of the eutectic mixture lidocaine/prilocaine spray in men with premature ejaculation. Int J Impot Res. 2022;34:289–94.
34. Brookes ST, Donovan JL, Peters TJ, Abrams P, Neal DE. Sexual dysfunction in men after treatment for lower urinary tract symptoms: evidence from randomised controlled trial. BMJ. 2002;324:1059–61.
35. Burri A, Heinrichs M, Schedlowski M, Kruger TH. The acute effects of intranasal oxytocin administration on endocrine and sexual function in males. Psychoneuroendocrinology. 2008;33:591–600.
36. Busato W, Galindo CC. Topical anaesthetic use for treating premature ejaculation: a double-blind, randomized, placebo-controlled study. Br J Urol Int. 2004;93:1018–21.
37. Cai T, Gallelli L, Verze P, Salonia A, Palmieri A. Prilocaine/lidocaine spray for the treatment of premature ejaculation: a dose- and time-finding study for clinical practice use. Int J Impot Res. 2023;35:378–84.
38. Califano G, Arcaniolo D, Ruvolo CC, Manfredi C, Smarrazzo F, Cilio S, Verze P. Glans penis augmentation: when, how, and why? Int J Impot Res. 2022;34:343–6.
39. Carmichael MS, Humbert R, Dixen J, Palmisano G, Greenleaf W, Davidson JM. Plasma oxytocin increases in the human sexual response. J Clin Endocrinol Metab. 1987;64:27–31.
40. Carson C, Wyllie M. Improved ejaculatory latency, control and sexual satisfaction when PSD502 is applied topically in men with premature ejaculation: results of a phase III, double-blind, placebo-controlled study. J Sex Med. 2010;7:3179–89.
41. Carter CS. Oxytocin and sexual behavior. Neurosci Biobehav Rev. 1992;16:131–44.
42. Cavallini G. Alpha-1 blockade pharmacotherapy in primitive psychogenic premature ejaculation resistant to psychotherapy. Eur Urol. 1995;28:126–30.
43. Cepeda MS, Camargo F, Zea C, Valencia L. Tramadol for osteoarthritis: a systematic review and metaanalysis. J Rheumatol. 2007;34:543–55.
44. Cepeda-Emiliani A, Gándara-Cortés M, Otero-Alén M, García H, Suárez-Quintanilla J, García-Caballero T, Gallego R, García-Caballero L. Immunohistological study of the density and distribution of human penile neural tissue: gradient hypothesis. Int J Impot Res. 2023;35:286–305.
45. Chen J. The pathophysiology of delayed ejaculation. Transl Androl Urol. 2016;5:549–62.
46. Chen J, Mabjeesh NJ, Matzkin H, Greenstein A. Efficacy of sildenafil as adjuvant therapy to selective serotonin reuptake inhibitor in alleviating premature ejaculation. Urology. 2003;61:197–200.

47. Chia, S. 2002. Management of premature ejaculation -- a comparison of treatment outcome in patients with and without erectile dysfunction. Int J Androl, 25, 301–305.
48. Choi JH, Hwa JS, Kam SC, Jeh SU, Hyun JS. Effects of tamsulosin on premature ejaculation in men with benign prostatic hyperplasia. World J Mens Health. 2014;32:99–104.
49. Cilio S, Pozzi E, Fallara G, Belladelli F, Corsini C, D'arma A, Boeri L, Capogrosso P, Imbimbo C, Mirone V, Montorsi F, Salonia A. Premature ejaculation among men with erectile dysfunction—findings from a real-life cross-sectional study. Int J Impot Res. 2022;44:S18.
50. Cizmeci S, Ongun S, Sarac A, Sel E, Tozburun S, Durmus N. Low frequency neuromuscular electrical stimulation applied to the bulbospongiosus muscle prolongs the ejaculation latency in a rat model. Int J Impot Res. 2023;36:261.
51. Clayton AH, Zajecka J, Ferguson JM, Filipiak-Reisner JK, Brown MT, Schwartz GE. Lack of sexual dysfunction with the selective noradrenaline reuptake inhibitor reboxetine during treatment for major depressive disorder. Int Clin Psychopharmacol. 2003;18:151–6.
52. Clement P, Bernabe J, Compagnie S, Alexandre L, Mccallum S, Giuliano F. Inhibition of ejaculation by the non-peptide oxytocin receptor antagonist GSK557296: a multi-level site of action. Br J Pharmacol. 2013;169:1477.
53. Clement P, Giuliano F. Physiology and pharmacology of ejaculation. Basic Clin Pharmacol Toxicol. 2016;119(Suppl 3):18–25.
54. Clement P, Peeters M, Bernabe J, Denys P, Alexandre L, Giuliano F. Brain oxytocin receptors mediate ejaculation elicited by 7-hydroxy-2-(di-N-propylamino) tetralin (7-OH-DPAT) in anaesthetized rats. Br J Pharmacol. 2008;154:1150–9.
55. Corona G, Jannini EA, Mannucci E, Fisher AD, Lotti F, Petrone L, Balercia G, Bandini E, Chiarini V, Forti G, Maggi M. Different testosterone levels are associated with ejaculatory dysfunction. J Sex Med. 2008;5:1991–8.
56. Corona G, Mannucci E, Petrone L, Fisher AD, Balercia G, De Scisciolo G, Pizzocaro A, Giommi R, Chiarini V, Forti G, Maggi M. Psychobiological correlates of delayed ejaculation in male patients with sexual dysfunctions. J Androl. 2006;27:453–8.
57. Corriere JN Jr. Painful ejaculation due to seminal vesicle calculi. J Urol. 1997;157:626.
58. Coskuner ER, Culha MG, Ozkan B, Kaleagasi EO. Post-SSRI sexual dysfunction: preclinical to clinical. Is it fact or fiction? Sex Med Rev. 2018;6:217–23.
59. Csoka AB, Bahrick A, Mehtonen OP. Persistent sexual dysfunction after discontinuation of selective serotonin reuptake inhibitors. J Sex Med. 2008;5:227–33.
60. Csoka AB, Shipko S. Persistent sexual side effects after SSRI discontinuation. Psychother Psychosom. 2006;75:187–8.
61. Culha MG, Tuken M, Gonultas S, Cakir OO, Serefoglu EC. Frequency of etiological factors among patients with acquired premature ejaculation: prospective, observational, single-center study. Int J Impot Res. 2020;32:352–7.
62. David Prologo J, Snyder LL, Cherullo E, Passalacqua M, Pirasteh A, Corn D. Percutaneous CT-guided cryoablation of the dorsal penile nerve for treatment of symptomatic premature ejaculation. J Vasc Interv Radiol. 2013;24:214–9.
63. De Jong TR, Veening JG, Olivier B, Waldinger MD. Oxytocin involvement in SSRI-induced delayed ejaculation: a review of animal studies. J Sex Med. 2007;4:14–28.
64. De Luca R, Bonanno M, Manuli A, Calabrò RS. Cutting the first turf to heal post-SSRI sexual dysfunction: a male retrospective Cohort study. Medicines (Basel). 2022;9
65. De Wied D, Diamant M, Fodor M. Central nervous system effects of the neurohypophyseal hormones and related peptides. Front Neuroendocrinol. 1993;14:251–302.
66. Desai A, Chen R, Cayetano A, Jayasena CN, Minhas S. Understanding and treating ejaculatory dysfunction in men with diabetes mellitus. Andrology. 2022;11:379.
67. Dinsmore WW, Wyllie MG. PSD502 improves ejaculatory latency, control and sexual satisfaction when applied topically 5 min before intercourse in men with premature ejaculation: results of a phase III, multicentre, double-blind, placebo-controlled study. BJU Int. 2009;103:940–9.

68. Eassa BI, El-Shazly MA. Safety and efficacy of tramadol hydrochloride on treatment of premature ejaculation. Asian J Androl. 2013;15:138–42.
69. Edwards L, Powell C. An objective comparison of transurethral resection and bladder neck incision in the treatment of prostatic hypertrophy. J Urol. 1982;128:325–7.
70. Erenpreiss J, Zalkalns J. Premature ejaculation: comparison of patroxetine alone, paroxetine plus local lidocaine and paroxetine plus sildenafil. Int J Imp Res. 2002;14, S33:abstract PS-7-4.
71. Forbes CM, Flannigan R, Paduch DA. Perineal ultrasound: a review in the context of ejaculatory dysfunction. Sex Med Rev. 2018;6:419–28.
72. Fortier P, Mottard JP, Trudel G, Even S. Study of sexuality-related characteristics in young adults with schizophrenia treated with novel neuroleptics and in a comparison group of young adults. Schizophr Bull. 2003;29:559–72.
73. Frankel SJ, Donovan JL, Peters TI, Abrams P, Dabhoiwala NF, Osawa D, Lin AT. Sexual dysfunction in men with lower urinary tract symptoms. J Clin Epidemiol. 1998;51:677–85.
74. Frese A, Eikermann A, Frese K, Schwaag S, Husstedt IW, Evers S. Headache associated with sexual activity: demography, clinical features, and comorbidity. Neurology. 2003;61:796–800.
75. Frink MC, Hennies HH, Englberger W, Haurand M, Wilffert B. Influence of tramadol on neurotransmitter systems of the rat brain. Arzneimittelforschung. 1996;46:1029–36.
76. Gacci M, Ficarra V, Sebastianelli A, Corona G, Serni S, Shariat SF, Maggi M, Zattoni F, Carini M, Novara G. Impact of medical treatments for male lower urinary tract symptoms due to benign prostatic hyperplasia on ejaculatory function: a systematic review and meta-analysis. J Sex Med. 2014;11:1554–66.
77. Gao J, Zhang X, Su P, Liu J, Xia L, Yang J, Shi K, Tang D, Hao Z, Zhou J, Liang C. Prevalence and factors associated with the complaint of premature ejaculation and the four premature ejaculation syndromes: a large observational study in China. J Sex Med. 2013a;10:1874.
78. Gao J, Zhang X, Su P, Liu J, Xia L, Yang J, Shi K, Tang D, Hao Z, Zhou J, Liang C. Prevalence and factors associated with the complaint of premature ejaculation and the four premature ejaculation syndromes: a large observational study in China. J Sex Med. 2013b;10:1874–81.
79. Garrett PM. Tramadol overdose and serotonin syndrome manifesting as acute right heart dysfunction. Anaesth Intensive Care. 2004;32:575–7.
80. Giuliano F, Patrick DL, Porst H, La Pera G, Kokoszka A, Merchant S, Rothman M, Gagnon DD, Polverejan E. Premature ejaculation: results from a five-country European observational study. Eur Urol. 2008;53:1048–57.
81. Godpodinoff ML. Premature ejaculation: clinical subgroups and etiology. J Sex Marital Ther. 1989;15:130–4.
82. Gopalakrishna A, Bole R, Alom M, Meng Y, Jimbo M, Trost L, Helo S, Kohler T, Ziegelmann M. Characteristics of men who are bothered by rapid ejaculation: results from clinical intake surveys. Int J Impot Res. 2021;33:369–75.
83. Gray M, Zillioux J, Khourdaji I, Smith RP. Contemporary management of ejaculatory dysfunction. Transl Androl Urol. 2018;7:686–702.
84. Grenier G, Byers ES. The relationships among ejaculatory control, ejaculatory latency, and attempts to prolong heterosexual intercourse. Arch Sex Behav. 1997;26:27–47.
85. Gruenwald I, Serefoglu EC, Gollan T, Springer S, Meiry G, Appel B, Shechter A. Transcutaneous neuromuscular electrical stimulation may be beneficial in the treatment of premature ejaculation. Med Hypotheses. 2017;109:181–3.
86. Gul A, Pastuszak A, Kabasakal L, Bates J, Altinay S, Celik DS, Semercioz A, Serefoglu EC. Tadalafil preserves penile nitric oxide synthase from detrimental effect of paroxetine in rats. Eurasian J Med. 2019;51:60–3.
87. Gul M, Bocu K, Serefoglu EC. Current and emerging treatment options for premature ejaculation. Nat Rev Urol. 2022;19:659–80.
88. Gur S, Kadowitz PJ, Serefoglu EC, Hellstrom WJ. PDE5 inhibitor treatment options for urologic and non-urologic indications: 2012 update. Curr Pharm Des. 2012;18:5590–606.
89. Hallbeck M, Larhammar D, Blomqvist A. Neuropeptide expression in rat paraventricular hypothalamic neurons that project to the spinal cord. J Comp Neurol. 2001;433:222–38.

90. Hamidi-Madani A, Motiee R, Mokhtari G, Nasseh H, Esmaeili S, Kazemnezhad E. The efficacy and safety of on-demand tramadol and paroxetine use in treatment of life long premature ejaculation: a randomized double-blind placebo-controlled clinical trial. J Reprod Infertil. 2018;19:10–5.
91. Hedlund H, Ek A. Ejaculation and sexual function after endoscopic bladder neck incision. Br J Urol. 1985;57:164–7.
92. Hisasue S, Furuya R, Itoh N, Kobayashi K, Furuya S, Tsukamoto T. Ejaculatory disorder caused by alpha-1 adrenoceptor antagonists is not retrograde ejaculation but a loss of seminal emission. Int J Urol. 2006;13:1311–6.
93. Hogan C, Le Noury J, Healy D, Mangin D. One hundred and twenty cases of enduring sexual dysfunction following treatment. Int J Risk Saf Med. 2014;26:109–16.
94. Hsieh T-C, Hollander AB, Walters RC, Lipshultz LI. 1495 Cabergoline for the treatment of male anorgasmia. J Urol. 2012;187:e605.
95. Huang W, Foster JA, Rogachefsky AS. Pharmacology of botulinum toxin. J Am Acad Dermatol. 2000;43:249–59.
96. Hwang S, Lee DY, Cho JY, Chung JY, Jang IJ, Yu KS, Lee S. Pharmacokinetics, tolerability and pharmacogenetics of DA-8031 after multiple ascending doses in healthy male subjects. Drug Des Devel Ther. 2021;15:2375–84.
97. Ishak WW, Berman DS, Peters A. Male anorgasmia treated with oxytocin. J Sex Med. 2007;5:1022.
98. Jannini E, Lenzi A. Epidemiology of premature ejaculation. Curr Opin Urol. 2005;15:399–403.
99. Jannini EA, Mcmahon C, Chen J, Aversa A, Perelman M. The controversial role of phosphodiesterase type 5 inhibitors in the treatment of premature ejaculation. J Sex Med. 2011;8:2135–43.
100. Janssen PKC, Waldinger MD. Men with subjective premature ejaculation have a similar lognormal IELT distribution as men in the general male population and differ mathematically from males with lifelong premature ejaculation after an IELT of 1.5 minutes (part 2). Int J Impot Res. 2019;31:341–7.
101. Jenkins LC, Mulhall JP. Delayed orgasm and anorgasmia. Fertil Steril. 2015;104:1082–8.
102. Jeon HJ, Kim HS, Lee CH, Lee YG, Choi SM, Sohn YS, Shin CY, Kim J, Shim HJ, Kang KK, Ahn BO, Kim SH. Candidate molecule for premature ejaculation, DA-8031: in vivo and in vitro characterization of DA-8031. Urology. 2011;77(1006):e17–21.
103. Jiann BP, Huang YJ. Assessing satisfaction in men with premature ejaculation after dapoxetine treatment in real-world practice. Int J Clin Pract. 2015;69:1326–33.
104. Jin K, Deng L, Qiu S, Tu X, Li J, Bao Y, Yang L, Wei Q. Comparative efficacy and safety of phosphodiesterase-5 inhibitors with selective serotonin reuptake inhibitors in men with premature ejaculation: a systematic review and Bayesian network meta-analysis. Medicine (Baltimore). 2018;97:e13342.
105. Jindan L, Xiao W, Liping X. Evolving role of silodosin for the treatment of urological disorders—a narrative review. Drug Des Devel Ther. 2022;16:2861–84.
106. Kamischke A, Nieschlag E. Update on medical treatment of ejaculatory disorders 1. Int J Androl. 2002;25:333–44.
107. Kawamura H, Watanabe T, Yamamura H, Sano S, Kanaoka M, Watanabe Y, Ohta M, Yamaguchi Y. Post-orgasmic illness syndrome with positive intradermal test for autologous semen. J Dermatol. 2023;50:951–5.
108. Kaynar M, Kilic O, Yurdakul T. On-demand tramadol hydrochloride use in premature ejaculation treatment. Urology. 2011;79:145–9.
109. Kedia K, Markland C. The effect of pharmacological agents on ejaculation. J Urol. 1975;114:569–73.
110. Kelly MJ, Roskamp D, Leach GE. Transurethral incision of the prostate: a preoperative and postoperative analysis of symptoms and urodynamic findings. J Urol. 1989;142:1507–9.
111. Kilinc MF, Aydogmus Y, Yildiz Y, Doluoglu OG. Impact of physical activity on patient self-reported outcomes of lifelong premature ejaculation patients: results of a prospective, randomised, sham-controlled trial. Andrologia. 2017;50

112. Kim JJ, Kwak TI, Jeon BG, Cheon J, Moon DG. Effects of glans penis augmentation using hyaluronic acid gel for premature ejaculation. Int J Impot Res. 2004;16:547–51.
113. Kim NN. Phosphodiesterase type 5 inhibitors: a biochemical and clinical correlation survey. Int J Impot Res. 2003;15(Suppl 5):S13–9.
114. Kim SW, Choi JB, Kim SJ, Kim KS, Kim CM, Lee DH, Choi WS. Tolerability and adequate therapeutic dosage of oral clomipramine for the treatment of premature ejaculation: a randomized, double-blind, placebo-controlled, fixed-dose, parallel-grouped clinical study. Int J Impot Res. 2018;30:65–70.
115. Kirby EW, Carson CC, Coward RM. Tramadol for the management of premature ejaculation: a timely systematic review. Int J Impot Res. 2015;27:121–7.
116. Kobayashi K, Masumori N, Hisasue S, Kato R, Hashimoto K, Itoh N, Tsukamoto T. Inhibition of seminal emission is the main cause of anejaculation induced by a new highly selective alpha1A-blocker in normal volunteers. J Sex Med. 2008;5:2185–90.
117. Kochakarn W, Leenanupunth C, Muangman V, Ratana-Olarn K, Viseshsindh V. Ejaculatory duct obstruction in the infertile male: experience of 7 cases at Ramathibodi Hospital. J Med Assoc Thail. 2001;84:1148–52.
118. Koyuncu H, Serefoglu EC, Ozdemir AT, Hellstrom WJ. Deleterious effects of selective serotonin reuptake inhibitor treatment on semen parameters in patients with lifelong premature ejaculation. Int J Impot Res. 2012;24:171–3.
119. Koyuncu H, Serefoglu EC, Yencilek E, Atalay H, Akbas NB, Sarica K. Escitalopram treatment for premature ejaculation has a negative effect on semen parameters. Int J Impot Res. 2011;23:257–61.
120. Kurbatov D, Russo GI, Galstyan GR, Rozhivanov R, Lepetukhin A, Dubsky S, Shwartz YG, Cimino S, Morgia G, Sansalone S. Correction of retrograde ejaculation in patients with diabetes mellitus using Endourethral collagen injection: preliminary results. J Sex Med. 2015;12:2126–9.
121. Kwak TI, Jin MH, Kim JJ, Moon DG. Long-term effects of glans penis augmentation using injectable hyaluronic acid gel for premature ejaculation. Int J Impot Res. 2008;20:425–8.
122. Lance JW. Headaches related to sexual activity. J Neurol Neurosurg Psychiatry. 1976;39:1226–30.
123. Laumann EO, Nicolosi A, Glasser DB, Paik A, Gingell C, Moreira E, Wang T. Sexual problems among women and men aged 40-80 y: prevalence and correlates identified in the global study of sexual attitudes and behaviors. Int J Impot Res. 2005;17:39–57.
124. Laumann EO, Paik A, Rosen RC. Sexual dysfunction in the United States: prevalence and predictors. JAMA. 1999;281:537–44.
125. Lebdai S, Chevrot A, Doizi S, Pradere B, Delongchamps NB, Benchikh A, Cornu JN, Della Negra E, Fourmarier M, Misrai V, Theveniaud PE, Descazeaud A, Robert G, CTMH-AFU group. Do patients have to choose between ejaculation and miction? A systematic review about ejaculation preservation technics for benign prostatic obstruction surgical treatment. World J Urol. 2019;37:299–308.
126. Lepor H. The evolution of alpha-blockers for the treatment of benign prostatic hyperplasia. Rev Urol. 2006;8(Suppl 4):S3–9.
127. Li X, Zhang SX, Cheng HM, Zhang WD. Clinical study of sildenafil in the treatment of premature ejaculation complicated by erectile dysfunction. Zhonghua Nan Ke Xue. 2003;9:266–9.
128. Li ZT, Li YF, Zhang Y, Luo Y, Zhu T, Li K, Feng QX, Jiang J. Injection of botulinum-A toxin into bulbospongiosus muscle for primary premature ejaculation: A preliminary clinical study. Zhonghua Nan Ke Xue. 2018;24:713–8.
129. Lindau ST, Schumm LP, Laumann EO, Levinson W, O'muircheartaigh CA, Waite LJ. A study of sexuality and health among older adults in the United States. N Engl J Med. 2007;357:762–74.
130. Linn R, Ginesin Y, Hardak S, Mertyk S. Treatment of sildenfil as part of the treatment in premature ejaculation. Int J Imp Res. 2002;14, S39. abstract P-168

131. Lipshultz LI, Mcconnell J, Benson GS. Current concepts of the mechanisms of ejaculation. Normal and abnormal states. J Reprod Med. 1981;26:499–507.
132. Liu L, Xu H, Ding S, Wang D, Song G, Huang X. Phosphodiesterase 5 inhibitors as novel agents for the treatment of Alzheimer's disease. Brain Res Bull. 2019;153:223–31.
133. Lozano AF. Premature ejaculation. Pharmacological treatment. Three years after. Int J Imp Res. 2003;15, S11:abstract MP-2-6.
134. Lu GL, Ding YM, Zhang YM, Huang HT, Liang YP, Chen CR. The correlation between mobile phone addiction and coping style among Chinese adolescents: a meta-analysis. Child Adolesc Psychiatry Ment Health. 2021;15:60.
135. Lu X, Han H, Zhang Z, Chen H, Huang X, Zhang R. Study on the efficacy of electric acupuncture in the treatment of premature ejaculation based on testosterone level. J Healthc Eng. 2022;2022:8331688.
136. Macdonald K, Feifel D. Dramatic improvement in sexual function induced by intranasal oxytocin. J Sex Med. 2012;9:1407–10.
137. Mamas MA, Reynard JM, Brading AF. Nitric oxide and the lower urinary tract: current concepts, future prospects. Urology. 2003;61:1079–85.
138. Manasia P, Pomerol J, Ribè N, Gutierrez Del Pozo R, Alcover Garcia J. Comparison of the efficacy and safety of 90 mg versus 20 mg fluoxetine in the treatment of premature ejaculation. J Urol. 2003;170:164–5.
139. Marangell, L., Dennehy, E., Wisniewski, S. & Et Al 2008. Case-control analyses of the impact of pharmacotherapy on prospectively observed suicide attempts and completed suicides in bipolar disorder: findings from STEP-BD J Clin Psych, 69, 916–922.
140. Marson L, Yu G, Farber NM. The effects of oral administration of d-modafinil on male rat ejaculatory behavior. J Sex Med. 2010;7:70–8.
141. Martyn-St James M, Cooper K, Kaltenthaler E, Dickinson K, Cantrell A, Wylie K, Frodsham L, Hood C. Tramadol for premature ejaculation: a systematic review and meta-analysis. BMC Urol. 2015;15:6.
142. Martyn-St James M, Cooper K, Ren S, Kaltenthaler E, Dickinson K, Cantrell A, Wylie K, Frodsham L, Hood C. Phosphodiesterase type 5 inhibitors for premature ejaculation: a systematic review and meta-analysis. Eur Urol Focus. 2017;3:119–29.
143. Masters WH, Johnson VE. Human sexual inadequacy. Boston: Little Brown; 1970.
144. Mathers MJ, Klotz T, Roth S, Lummen G, Sommer F. Safety and efficacy of vardenafil versus sertraline in the treatment of premature ejaculation: a randomised, prospective and crossover study. Andrologia. 2009;41:169–75.
145. Mattos RM, Lucon AM. Tadalafil and slow-release fluoxetine in premature ejaculation—a prospective study. J Urol. 2005;173, 239:abst.880.
146. Mattos RM, Marmo Lucon A, Srougi M. Tadalafil and fluoxetine in premature ejaculation: prospective, randomized, double-blind, placebo-controlled study. Urol Int. 2008;80:162–5.
147. Mccormick S, Olin J, Brotman AW. Reversal of fluoxetine-induced anorgasmia by cyproheptadine in two patients. J Clin Psychiatry. 1990;51:383–4.
148. Mcdiarmid T, Mackler L, Schneider DM. Clinical inquiries. What is the addiction risk associated with tramadol? J Fam Pract. 2005;54:72–3.
149. Mcmahon C, Althof S, Rosen R, Giuliano F, Miner M, Osterloh IH, Muirhead GJ, Harty B, PEPIX Multi-Centre Study Group. The oxytocin antagonist cligosiban prolongs intravaginal ejaculatory latency and improves patient-reported outcomes in men with lifelong premature ejaculation: results of a randomized, double-blind, placebo-controlled proof-of-concept trial (PEPIX). J Sex Med. 2019;16:1178–87.
150. Mcmahon CG. Long term results of treatment of premature ejaculation with selective serotonin re-uptake inhibitors. IntJImpRes. 2002;14:S19.
151. Mcmahon CG. The etiology and management of premature ejaculation. Nat Clin Pract Urol. 2005;2:426–33.
152. Mcmahon CG, Abdo C, Incrocci L, Perelman M, Rowland D, Waldinger M, Xin ZC. Disorders of orgasm and ejaculation in men. J Sex Med. 2004;1:58–65.

153. Mcmahon CG, Giuliano F, Dean J, Hellstrom WJ, Bull S, Tesfaye F, Sharma O, Rivas DA, Aquilina JW. Efficacy and safety of dapoxetine in men with premature ejaculation and concomitant erectile dysfunction treated with a phosphodiesterase type 5 inhibitor: randomized, placebo-controlled, phase III study. J Sex Med. 2013a;10:2312–25.
154. Mcmahon CG, Jannini E, Waldinger M, Rowland D. Standard operating procedures in the disorders of orgasm and ejaculation. J Sex Med. 2013b;10:204–29.
155. Mcmahon CG, Osterloh IH, Rosen R, Althof S, Muirhead GJ, Harty B, Giuliano F, Miner M. A phase IIA study to investigate the efficacy and safety of the selective oxytocin receptor antagonist, IX-01, in men with lifelong premature ejaculation. J Urol. 2017;1997:e1344.
156. Mcmahon CG, Waldinger M, Rowland DL, Assalian P, Chan Kim Y, Bechara A, Riley A. Ejaculatory disorders. In: Porst H, Buvat J, editors. Standard practice in sexual medicine. Oxford: Blackwell Publishing; 2006.
157. Mendels J, Camera A, Sikes C. Sertraline treatment for premature ejaculation. J Clin Psychopharmacol. 1995;15:341–6.
158. Michel MC. Alpha1-adrenoceptors and ejaculatory function. Br J Pharmacol. 2007;152:289–90.
159. Migliorini F, Tafuri A, Bettica P, Ziviani L, Lund J, Poggesi I, Marcer A, Cacciamani GE, Lorenzo-Gomez MF, Porcaro AB, Antonelli A, Milleri S. A double-blind, placebo-controlled parallel group study to evaluate the effect of a single Oral dose of 5-HT1A antagonist GSK958108 on ejaculation latency time in male patients suffering from premature ejaculation. J Sex Med. 2021;18:63–71.
160. Mittino D, Mula M, Monaco F. Serotonin syndrome associated with tramadol-sertraline coadministration. Clin Neuropharmacol. 2004;27:150–1.
161. Mondaini N, Fusco F, Cai T, Benemei S, Mirone V, Bartoletti R. Dapoxetine treatment in patients with lifelong premature ejaculation: the reasons of a “Waterloo”. Urology. 2013;82:620–4.
162. Montejo AL, Llorca G, Izquierdo JA, Carrasco JL, Daniel E, Pérez-Sola V, Vicens E, Bousoño M, Sánchez-Iglesias S, Franco M, Cabezudo A, Rubio V, Ortega MA, Puigdellivol M, Domenech JR, Allué B, Sáez C, Mezquita B, Gálvez I, Pacheco L, De Miguel E. Sexual dysfunction with antidepressive agents. Effect of the change to amineptine in patients with sexual dysfunction secondary to SSRI. Actas Esp Psiquiatr. 1999;27:23–34.
163. Moon DG, Kwak TI, Cho HY, Bae JH, Park HS, Kim JJ. Augmentation of glans penis using injectable hyaluronic acid gel. Int J Impot Res. 2003;15:456–60.
164. Moon Du G, Kwak TI, Kim JJ. Glans penis augmentation using hyaluronic acid gel as an injectable filler. World J Mens Health. 2015;33:50–61.
165. Nathan SG. The epidemiology of the DSM-III psychosexual dysfunctions. J Sex Marital Ther. 1986;12:267–81.
166. Nguyen V, Dolendo I, Uloko M, Hsieh T-C, Patel D. Male delayed orgasm and anorgasmia: a practical guide for sexual medicine providers. Int J Impot Res. 2023;36:186.
167. Nickel JC, Elhilali M, Vallancien G, ALF-ONE Study Group. Benign prostatic hyperplasia (BPH) and prostatitis: prevalence of painful ejaculation in men with clinical BPH. BJU Int. 2005;95:571–4.
168. Nicolosi A, Laumann E, Glaser D, Moreira E, Paik A, Gingell C. Global study of sexual attitudes and behaviors investigator's group. Sexual behavior and sexual dysfunctions after age 40: the global study of sexual attitudes and behaviors. Urology. 2004;64:991–7.
169. Ongün Ş, Acar S, Koca P, Uzut M, Esen AA, Durmus N, Demir O. Can botulinum-A toxin be used to delay ejaculation: results of an ejaculation model in male rats. J Sex Med. 2019;16:1338–43.
170. Ostergaard JR, Kraft M. Benign coital headache. Cephalalgia. 1992;12:353–5.
171. Paduch DA, Bolyakov A, Beardsworth A, Watts SD. Factors associated with ejaculatory and orgasmic dysfunction in men with erectile dysfunction: analysis of clinical trials involving the phosphodiesterase type 5 inhibitor tadalafil. BJU Int. 2012;109:1060–7.

172. Park HJ, Park NC, Kim TN, Baek SR, Lee KM, Choe S. Discontinuation of dapoxetine treatment in patients with premature ejaculation: a 2-year prospective observational study. Sex Med. 2017;5:e99–e105.
173. Park HS, Jung IS, Lim NH, Sung JH, Lee S, Moon BS, Lee BC, Kang KK, Kim SE. Proof of mechanism study of a novel serotonin transporter blocker, DA-8031, using [11C]DASB positron emission tomography and in vivo microdialysis. Urology. 2014;84:245.e1–7.
174. Parnham A, Serefoglu EC. Classification and definition of premature ejaculation. Transl Androl Urol. 2016a;5:416–23.
175. Parnham A, Serefoglu EC. Retrograde ejaculation, painful ejaculation and hematospermia. Transl Androl Urol. 2016b;5:592–601.
176. Pascual J, Iglesias F, Oterino A, Vazquez-Barquero A, Berciano J. Cough, exertional, and sexual headaches: an analysis of 72 benign and symptomatic cases. Neurology. 1996;46:1520–4.
177. Patrick DL, Althof SE, Pryor JL, Rosen R, Rowland DL, Ho KF, Mcnulty P, Rothman M, Jamieson C. Premature ejaculation: an observational study of men and their partners. J Sex Med. 2005;2:358–67.
178. Patrick DL, Giuliano F, Ho KF, Gagnon DD, Mcnulty P, Rothman M. The premature ejaculation profile: validation of self-reported outcome measures for research and practice. Br J Urol Int. 2008;103:358–67.
179. Paulson GW, Klawans HL Jr. Benign orgasmic cephalgia. Headache. 1974;13:181–7.
180. Perelman M. Sex coaching for physicians: combination treatment for patient and partner. Int J Impot Res. 2003;15:S67–74.
181. Perelman M. Idiosyncratic masturbation patterns: a key unexplored variable in the treatment of retarded ejaculation by the practicing urologist. J Urol. 2005;173:S340.
182. Perelman M. A new combination treatment for premature ejaculation. A sex therapist's perspective. J Sex Med. 2006;3:1004–12.
183. Perelman MA. Reexamining the definitions of PE and DE. J Sex Marital Ther. 2017;43:633–44.
184. Porst H, Mcmahon CG, Althof SE, Sharlip I, Bull S, Aquilina JW, Tesfaye F, Rivas DA. Baseline characteristics and treatment outcomes for men with acquired or lifelong premature ejaculation with mild or no erectile dysfunction: integrated analyses of two phase 3 dapoxetine trials. J Sex Med. 2010;7:2231–42.
185. Porst H, Montorsi F, Rosen RC, Gaynor L, Grupe S, Alexander J. The Premature Ejaculation Prevalence and Attitudes (PEPA) survey: prevalence, comorbidities, and professional help-seeking. Eur Urol. 2007;51:816-23; discussion 824.
186. Proctor KG, Howards SS. The effect of sympathomimetic drugs on post-lymphadenectomy aspermia. J Urol. 1983;129:837–8.
187. Pryor JL, Althof SE, Steidle C, Rosen RC, Hellstrom WJ, Shabsigh R, Miloslavsky M, Kell S, for the Dapoxetine Study Group. Efficacy and tolerability of dapoxetine in treatment of premature ejaculation: an integrated analysis of two double-blind, randomised controlled trials. Lancet. 2006;368:929–37.
188. Quinlan DM, Epstein JI, Carter BS, Walsh PC. Sexual function following radical prostatectomy: influence of preservation of neurovascular bundles. J Urol. 1991;145:998–1002.
189. Rabiee B, Mohammadinejad P, Kordi R, Yunesian M. The epidemiology of exertional headache in the general population of Tehran, Iran. Headache. 2015;55:1225–32.
190. Rasmussen BK, Olesen J. Symptomatic and nonsymptomatic headaches in a general population. Neurology. 1992;42:1225–31.
191. Reading A, Wiest W. An analysis of self-reported sexual behavior in a sample of normal males. Arch Sex Behav. 1984;13:69–83.
192. Reiser C. The etiology of retrograde ejaculation and a method for insemination. Fertil Steril. 1961;12:488–92.
193. Reisman Y. Sexual consequences of post-SSRI syndrome. Sex Med Rev. 2017;5:429–33.
194. Reisman Y. Clinical experience with post-orgasmic illness syndrome (POIS) patients—characteristics and possible treatment modality. Int J Impot Res. 2021;33:556–62.

195. Riley AJ, Riley EJ. Cyproheptadine and antidepressant-induced anorgasmia. Br J Psychiatry. 1986;148:217–8.
196. Rosen R, Altwein J, Boyle P, Kirby RS, Lukacs B, Meuleman E, O'leary MP, Puppo P, Robertson C, Giuliano F. Lower urinary tract symptoms and male sexual dysfunction: the multinational survey of the aging male (MSAM-7). Eur Urol. 2003;44:637–49.
197. Rosen RC, Mcmahon CG, Niederberger C, Broderick GA, Jamieson C, Gagnon DD. Correlates to the clinical diagnosis of premature ejaculation: results from a large observational study of men and their partners. J Urol. 2007;177:1059–64. discussion 1064
198. Rowland D, Mcmahon CG, Abdo C, Chen J, Jannini E, Waldinger MD, Ahn TY. Disorders of orgasm and ejaculation in men. J Sex Med. 2010;7:1668–86.
199. Rowland D, Van Diest S, Incrocci L, Slob AK. Psychosexual factors that differentiate men with inhibited ejaculation from men with no dysfunction or another sexual dysfunction. J Sex Med. 2005a;2:383–9.
200. Rowland DL, Van Diest S, Incrocci L, Slob AK. Psychosexual factors that differentiate men with inhibited ejaculation from men with no dysfunction or with another dysfunction. J Sex Med. 2005b;2:383–9.
201. Rustamov MN, Belyaev AR, Aliev RM, Rapoport LM, Vinarov AZ. Delayed ejaculation: epidemiology, diagnostics and treatment. Urologiia. 2019:150–5.
202. Sadowski DJ, Butcher MJ, Kohler TS. A review of pathophysiology and management options for delayed ejaculation. Sex Med Rev. 2016;4:167–76.
203. Safarinejad MR, Hosseini SY. Safety and efficacy of citalopram in the treatment of premature ejaculation: a double-blind placebo-controlled, fixed dose, randomized study. Int J Impot Res. 2006;18:164–9.
204. Saitz TR, Serefoglu EC. Advances in understanding and treating premature ejaculation. Nat Rev Urol. 2015;12:629–40.
205. Saitz TR, Serefoglu EC. The epidemiology of premature ejaculation. Transl Androl Urol. 2016;5:409–15.
206. Salem EA, Wilson SK, Bissada NK, Delk JR, Hellstrom WJ, Cleves MA. Tramadol HCL has promise in on-demand use to treat premature ejaculation. J Sex Med. 2008;5:188–93.
207. Salonia A, Bettocchi C, Boeri L, Capogrosso P, Carvalho J, Cilesiz NC, Cocci A, Corona G, Dimitropoulos K, Gul M, Hatzichristodoulou G, Jones TH, Kadioglu A, Martinez Salamanca JI, Milenkovic U, Modgil V, Russo GI, Serefoglu EC, Tharakan T, Verze P, Minhas S, Sexual EAUWGOM, Reproductive H. European Association of Urology Guidelines on Sexual and Reproductive Health-2021 update: male sexual dysfunction. Eur Urol. 2021a;80:333–57.
208. Salonia A, Bettocchi C, Boeri L, Capogrosso P, Carvalho J, Cilesiz NC, Cocci A, Corona G, Dimitropoulos K, Gül M, Hatzichristodoulou G, Jones TH, Kadioglu A, Martínez Salamanca JI, Milenkovic U, Modgil V, Russo GI, Serefoglu EC, Tharakan T, Verze P, Minhas S. European Association of Urology Guidelines on Sexual and Reproductive Health-2021 update: male sexual dysfunction. Eur Urol. 2021b;80:333–57.
209. Salonia A, Maga T, Colombo R, Scattoni V, Briganti A, Cestari A, Guazzoni G, Rigatti P, Montorsi F. A prospective study comparing paroxetine alone versus paroxetine plus sildenafil in patients with premature ejaculation. J Urol. 2002;168:2486–9.
210. Salonia A, Rocchini L, Sacca A, Pellucchi F, Ferrari M, Del Carro U, Ribotto P, Gallina A, Zanni G, Deho F, Regatti P, Montorsi F. Acceptance of and discontinuation rate from paroxetine treatment in patients with lifelong premature ejaculation. J Sex Med. 2009;6:2868–77.
211. Sangkum P, Badr R, Serefoglu EC, Hellstrom WJ. Dapoxetine and the treatment of premature ejaculation. Transl Androl Urol. 2013;2:301–11.
212. Sato Y, Tanda H, Nakajima H, Nitta T, Akagashi K, Hanzawa T, Tobe M, Haga K, Uchida K, Honma I. Silodosin and its potential for treating premature ejaculation: a preliminary report. Int J Urol. 2012;19:268–72.
213. Schifano N, Capogrosso P, Boeri L, Fallara G, Cakir OO, Castiglione F, Alnajjar HM, Muneer A, Deho F, Schifano F, Montorsi F, Salonia A. Medications mostly associated with priapism

events: assessment of the 2015-2020 Food and Drug Administration (FDA) pharmacovigilance database entries. Int J Impot Res. 2022;32:S16.
214. Serefoglu EC. On-demand d-modafinil may be an effective treatment option for lifelong premature ejaculation: a case report. Andrologia. 2016;48:121–2.
215. Serefoglu EC. Post-orgasmic illness syndrome: where are we? J Sex Med. 2017;14:641–2.
216. Serefoglu EC, Cimen HI, Atmaca AF, Balbay MD. The distribution of patients who seek treatment for the complaint of ejaculating prematurely according to the four premature ejaculation syndromes. J Sex Med. 2010;7:810–5.
217. Serefoglu EC, Cimen HI, Ozdemir AT, Symonds T, Berktas M, Balbay MD. Turkish validation of the premature ejaculation diagnostic tool and its association with intravaginal ejaculatory latency time. Int J Impot Res. 2009;21:139–44.
218. Serefoglu EC, Hawley WR, Lasker GF, Grissom EM, Mandava SH, Sikka SC, Dohanich GP, Hellstrom WJ. Effect of botulinum-A toxin injection into bulbospongiosus muscle on ejaculation latency in male rats. J Sex Med. 2014a;11:1657–63.
219. Serefoglu EC, Mcmahon CG, Waldinger MD, Althof SE, Shindel A, Adaikan G, Becher EF, Dean J, Giuliano F, Hellstrom WJ, Giraldi A, Glina S, Incrocci L, Jannini E, Mccabe M, Parish S, Rowland D, Segraves RT, Sharlip I, Torres LO. An evidence-based unified definition of lifelong and acquired premature ejaculation: report of the second International Society for Sexual Medicine Ad Hoc Committee for the definition of premature ejaculation. J Sex Med. 2014b;11:1423–41.
220. Serefoglu EC, Saitz TR. New insights on premature ejaculation: a review of definition, classification, prevalence and treatment. Asian J Androl. 2012;14:822–9.
221. Serefoglu EC, Silay MS. Botulinum toxin-A injection may be beneficial in the treatment of life-long premature ejaculation. Med Hypotheses. 2010;74:83–4.
222. Serefoglu EC, Yaman O, Cayan S, Asci R, Orhan I, Usta MF, Ekmekcioglu O, Kendirci M, Semerci B, Kadioglu A. Prevalence of the complaint of ejaculating prematurely and the four premature ejaculation syndromes: results from the Turkish Society of Andrology Sexual Health Survey. J Sex Med. 2011a;8:540–8.
223. Serefoglu EC, Yaman O, Cayan S, Asci R, Orhan I, Usta MF, Ekmekcioglu O, Kendirci M, Semerci B, Kadioglu A. The comparison of premature ejaculation assessment questionnaires and their sensitivity for the four premature ejaculation syndromes: results from the Turkish society of andrology sexual health survey. J Sex Med. 2011b;8:1177–85.
224. Shanholtzer A, Stephens JR, Lauter C, Peters KM. Post orgasmic illness syndrome successfully managed with antihistamine: a case report. Urol Case Rep. 2022;45:102189.
225. Shapiro B. Premature ejaculation: a review of 1130 cases. J Urol. 1943;50:6.
226. Sharma G, Kaundal P, Pareek T, Tyagi S, Sharma AP, Devana SK, Singh SK. Comparison of efficacy of various drugs used for medical expulsive therapy for distal ureter stones: A systematic review and network meta-analysis. Int J Clin Pract. 2021;75:e14214.
227. Shebl SE, Ali S, Shokr M. Hyaluronic acid injection in the glans penis for the treatment of refractory premature ejaculation: a prospective, controlled study. Andrologia. 2021;53:e14084.
228. Shechter A, Mondaini N, Serefoglu EC, Gollan T, Deutsch F, Appel B, Gruenwald I. A novel on-demand therapy for lifelong premature ejaculation using a miniature transperineal electrical stimulator-the vPatch: an as-treated analysis. J Sex Med. 2023;20:22–9.
229. Shechter A, Serefoglu EC, Gollan T, Springer S, Meiry G, Appel B, Gruenwald I. Transcutaneous functional electrical stimulation-a novel therapy for premature ejaculation: results of a proof of concept study. Int J Impot Res. 2020;32:440–5.
230. Shi WG, Wang XJ, Liang XQ, Liu ZQ, Huang MJ, Li SQ, Ren SQ, Cao L, Meng X, Wang Z, Chen RS. Selective resection of the branches of the two dorsal penile nerves for primary premature ejaculation. Zhonghua Nan Ke Xue. 2008;14:436–8.
231. Shin D, Lee S, Yi S, Yoon SH, Cho JY, Bahng MY, Jang IJ, Yu KS. Pharmacokinetics and tolerability of DA-8031, a novel selective serotonin reuptake inhibitor for premature ejaculation in healthy male subjects. Drug Des Devel Ther. 2017;11:713–23.

232. Shindel AW, Althof SE, Carrier S, Chou R, Mcmahon CG, Mulhall JP, Paduch DA, Pastuszak AW, Rowland D, Tapscott AH, Sharlip ID. Disorders of ejaculation: an AUA/SMSNA guideline. J Urol. 2022;207:504–12.
233. Shinghal R, Barnes A, Mahar KM, Stier B, Giancaterino L, Condreay LD, Black L, Mccallum SW. Safety and efficacy of epelsiban in the treatment of men with premature ejaculation: a randomized, double-blind, placebo-controlled, fixed-dose study. J Sex Med. 2013;10:2506–17.
234. Shoshany O, Abhyankar N, Elyaguov J, Niederberger C. Efficacy of treatment with pseudoephedrine in men with retrograde ejaculation. Andrology. 2017;5:744–8.
235. Sigman M, Howards SS. Male infertility. In: Walsh PC, Retik AB, Darracott Vaughan Jr E, Wein AJ, editors. Campbell's urology. 7th ed. Philadelphia: WB Saunders Company; 1998.
236. Silbert PL, Edis RH, Stewart-Wynne EG, Gubbay SS. Benign vascular sexual headache and exertional headache: interrelationships and long term prognosis. J Neurol Neurosurg Psychiatry. 1991;54:417–21.
237. Simons JS, Carey MP. Prevalence of sexual dysfunctions: results from a decade of research. Arch Sex Behav. 2001;30:177–219.
238. Siroosbakht S, Rezakhaniha S, Rezakhaniha B. Comparative study of on-demand and daily use of sertraline in treatment of premature ejaculation: a randomized clinical trial. Asian J Urol. 2021;8:209–14.
239. Sommer F, Klotz T, Mathers MJ. Treatment of premature ejaculation: a comparative vardenafil and SSRI crossover study. J Urol. 2005;173, 202:abstract 741.
240. Spector IP, Carey M. Incidence and prevalence of the sexual dysfunctions: a critical review of the empirical literature. Arch Sex Behav. 1990a;19:389.
241. Spector IP, Carey MP. Incidence and prevalence of the sexual dysfunctions: a critical review of the empirical literature. Arch Sex Behav. 1990b;19:389–408.
242. Spector KR, Boyle M. The prevalence and perceived aetiology of male sexual problems in a non-clinical sample. Br J Med Psychol. 1986;59:351–8.
243. Stoneham MD, Everitt BJ, Hansen S, Lightman SL, Todd K. Oxytocin and sexual behaviour in the male rat and rabbit. J Endocrinol. 1985;107:97–106.
244. Strashny A. First assessment of the validity of the only diagnostic criteria for postorgasmic illness syndrome (POIS). Int J Impot Res. 2019;31:369–73.
245. Sun XZ, Deng CH, Dai YP. A clinical study of sertralin and vardenafil in the treatment of premature ejaculation complicated by erectile dysfunction. Zhonghua Nan Ke Xue. 2007;13:610–2.
246. Sun Y, Yang L, Bao Y, Liu Z, Liu L, Wei Q. Efficacy of PDE5Is and SSRIs in men with premature ejaculation: a new systematic review and five meta-analyses. World J Urol. 2017;35:1817–31.
247. Sunay D, Sunay M, Aydogmus Y, Bagbanci S, Arslan H, Karabulut A, Emir L. Acupuncture versus paroxetine for the treatment of premature ejaculation: a randomized, placebo-controlled clinical trial. Eur Urol. 2011;59:765–71.
248. Symonds T, Perelman M, Althof S, Giuliano F, Martin M, May K, Abraham L, Crossland A, Morris M. Development and validation of a premature ejaculation diagnostic tool. Eur Urol. 2007;52:565–73.
249. Takeshita J, Litzinger M. Serotonin syndrome associated with tramadol. Prim Care Companion, J Clin Psychiary. 2009;11:273.
250. Tan H, Zhou Z, Cui Y, Feng F, Zhang Y. A systematic review and meta-analysis of randomized controlled trials of "on-demand" use of tramadol vs "on-demand" use of paroxetine in the management of patients with premature ejaculation. Int J Clin Pract. 2021;75:e14825.
251. Tram M, Meyerson B, Welliver C, Inouye B. Differences in sexual adverse events for premature ejaculation medications from a public federal database. Int J Impot Res. 2023;36:515.
252. Trovão JN, Serefoglu EC. Neurobiology of male sexual dysfunctions in psychiatric disorders: the cases of depression, anxiety, mania and schizophrenia. Int J Impot Res. 2018;30:279–86.
253. Tubaro A, Polito M, Giambroni L, Famulari C, Gange E, Ostardo E. Sexual function in patients with LUTS suggestive of BPH. Eur Urol. 2001;40:19–22.

254. Tugba T, Serap U, Esra O, Ozlem C, Ufuk E, Levent EI. Features of stabbing, cough, exertional and sexual headaches in a Turkish population of headache patients. J Clin Neurosci. 2008;15:774–7.
255. Tuken M, Culha MG, Serefoglu EC. Efficacy and safety of dapoxetine/sildenafil combination tablets in the treatment of men with premature ejaculation and concomitant erectile dysfunction-DAP-SPEED study. Int J Impot Res. 2019;31:92–6.
256. Tuken M, Kiremit MC, Serefoglu EC. On-demand Modafinil improves ejaculation time and patient-reported outcomes in men with lifelong premature ejaculation. Urology. 2016;94:139–42.
257. Tupala E, Haapalinna A, Viitamaa T, Männistö PT, Saano V. Effects of repeated low dose administration and withdrawal of haloperidol on sexual behaviour of male rats. Pharmacol Toxicol. 1999;84:292–5.
258. Uckert S, Becker AJ, Ness BO, Stief CG, Scheller F, Knapp WH, Jonas U. Oxytocin plasma levels in the systemic and cavernous blood of healthy males during different penile conditions. World J Urol. 2003;20:323–6.
259. Uribe OL, Sandoval-Salinas C, Corredor HA, Martinez JM, Saffon JP. Transcutaneous electric nerve stimulation to treat patients with premature ejaculation: phase II clinical trial. Int J Impot Res. 2020;32:434–9.
260. Vallancien G, Emberton M, Harving N, Van Moorselaar RJ, Alf-One Study Group. Sexual dysfunction in 1,274 European men suffering from lower urinary tract symptoms. J Urol. 2003;169:2257–61.
261. Van Moorselaar RJ, Hartung R, Emberton M, Harving N, Matzkin H, Elhilali M, Alcaraz A, Vallancien G, ALF-ONE Study Group. Alfuzosin 10 mg once daily improves sexual function in men with lower urinary tract symptoms and concomitant sexual dysfunction. BJU Int. 2005;95:603–8.
262. Veening JG, Coolen LM. Neural mechanisms of sexual behavior in the male rat: emphasis on ejaculation-related circuits. Pharmacol Biochem Behav. 2014;121:170–83.
263. Ventus D, Jern P. Lifestyle factors and premature ejaculation: are physical exercise, alcohol consumption, and body mass index associated with premature ejaculation and comorbid erectile problems? J Sex Med. 2016;13:1482–7.
264. Walch K, Eder R, Schindler A, Feichtinger W. The effect of single-dose oxytocin application on time to ejaculation and seminal parameters in men. J Assist Reprod Genet. 2001;18:655–9.
265. Waldinger MD. The neurobiological approach to premature ejaculation. J Urol. 2002;168:2359–67.
266. Waldinger MD. Post orgasmic illness syndrome (POIS). Transl Androl Urol. 2016;5:602–6.
267. Waldinger MD, Hengeveld MW, Zwinderman AH. Ejaculation-retarding properties of paroxetine in patients with primary premature ejaculation: a double-blind, randomized, dose-response study. Br J Urol. 1997;79:592–5.
268. Waldinger MD, Olivier B. Animal models of premature and retarded ejaculation. World J Urol. 2005;23:115–8.
269. Waldinger MD, Quinn P, Dilleen M, Mundayat R, Schweitzer DH, Boolell M. A multinational population survey of intravaginal ejaculation latency time. J Sex Med. 2005a;2:492–7.
270. Waldinger MD, Schweitzer DH. Postorgasmic illness syndrome: two cases. J Sex Marital Ther. 2002;28:251–5.
271. Waldinger, M. D. & Schweitzer, D. H. 2006. Changing paradigms from a historical DSM-III and DSM-IV view toward an evidence-based definition of premature ejaculation. Part II--proposals for DSM-V and ICD-11. J Sex Med, 3, 693–705.
272. Waldinger MD, Schweitzer DH. The use of old and recent DSM definitions of premature ejaculation in observational studies: a contribution to the present debate for a new classification of PE in the DSM-V. J Sex Med. 2008;5:1079–87.
273. Waldinger MD, Schweitzer DH. Method and design of drug treatment research of subjective premature ejaculation in men differs from that of lifelong premature ejaculation in males: proposal for a new objective measure (part 1). Int J Impot Res. 2019;31:328–33.

274. Waldinger MD, Van Coevorden RS, Schweitzer DH, Georgiadis J. Penile anesthesia in Post SSRI Sexual Dysfunction (PSSD) responds to low-power laser irradiation: a case study and hypothesis about the role of transient receptor potential (TRP) ion channels. Eur J Pharmacol. 2015;753:263–8.
275. Waldinger MD, Zwinderman AH, Olivier B, Schweitzer DH. Thyroid-stimulating hormone assessments in a Dutch cohort of 620 men with lifelong premature ejaculation without erectile dysfunction. J Sex Med. 2005b;2:865–70.
276. Weintraub MP, De Mouy E, Hellstrom WJ. Newer modalities in the diagnosis and treatment of ejaculatory duct obstruction. J Urol. 1993;150:1150–4.
277. Wieder JA, Brackett NL, Lynne CM, Green JT, Aballa TC. Anesthetic block of the dorsal penile nerve inhibits vibratory-induced ejaculation in men with spinal cord injuries. Urology. 2000;55:915–7.
278. Wu T, Yue X, Duan X, Luo D, Cheng Y, Tian Y, Wang K. Efficacy and safety of tramadol for premature ejaculation: a systematic review and meta-analysis. Urology. 2012;80:618–24.
279. Xiong GG, Wu FH, Chen SH, Yao WL. Safety and efficacy of tramadol hydrochloride with behavioral modification in the treatment of premature ejaculation. Zhonghua Nan Ke Xue. 2011;17:538–41.
280. Yang DY, Ko K, Lee WK, Park HJ, Lee SW, Moon KH, Kim SW, Kim SW, Cho KS, Moon Du G, Min K, Yang SK, Son H, Park K. Urologist's practice patterns including surgical treatment in the management of premature ejaculation: a Korean Nationwide survey. World J Mens Health. 2013;31:226–31.
281. Yang J, Chu M, Qi Y, Zhang H, Yuan T, Zhou L, Cao W, Zhang C. Correlation between age and curative effects of selective dorsal neurectomy for primary premature ejaculation. Adv Clin Exp Med. 2022;31:837–45.
282. Zhang C, Quan Y, Song Y, Bai W, Li Q, Xu T, Zhang X. Efficacy and safety assessment of glandular augmentation with hyaluronic acid for premature ejaculation. Andrologia. 2022;54:e14435.
283. Zhang GX, Yu LP, Bai WJ, Wang XF. Selective resection of dorsal nerves of penis for premature ejaculation. Int J Androl. 2012;35:873–9.
284. Zhang HF, Zhang CY, Li XH, Fu ZZ, Chen ZY. Dorsal penile nerves and primary premature ejaculation. Chin Med J. 2009;122:3017–9.
285. Zhang X, Chi N, Sun M, Shan Z, Zhang Y, Cui Y. Phosphodiesterase-5 inhibitors for premature ejaculation: systematic review and meta-analysis of placebo-controlled trials. Am J Mens Health. 2020;14:1557988320916406.
286. Zhang XS, Wang YX, Huang XY, Leng J, Li Z, Han YF. Comparison between sildenafil plus sertraline and sertraline alone in the treatment of premature ejaculation. Zhonghua Nan Ke Xue. 2005;11:520–2, 525.
287. Zhou XJ, Zhang ZG, Hao L, Zhang WD, Dong BZ, Han CH. Elective microscopic resection of dorsal penile nerves for primary premature ejaculation: a clinical observation. Zhonghua Nan Ke Xue. 2013;19:1003–6.
288. Zucker I, Nackeeran S, Kulkarni N, Carto C, Madhusoodanan V, Ramasamy R. Majority of men with premature ejaculation do not receive pharmacotherapy. Int J Impot Res. 2022;35:544.

Chapter 12
Psychological Approach to Ejaculatory Disorders

Alla Satyanarayana Reddy

Ejaculatory Disorders

The culmination of sex act in a male is ejaculation and orgasm. Ejaculation (EJ) is propulsion of semen from the body to outside.

EJ is having two phases—emission and ejection. Emission is deposition of sperm and seminal fluid from testis, epididymis, seminal vesicles and prostate into prostatic urethra. Ejection (expulsion) is propulsion of this fluid from prostatic urethra outside.

Orgasm is the pleasant sensory feel that accompanies EJ.

Disturbances in EJ and orgasm are termed ejaculatory disorders (EJD) [12].

Classification of Ejaculatory D

International Consultation on Sexual Medicine (ICSM) 2015 classification of ejaculatory disorders

1. Premature ejaculation classified into lifelong, acquired.
2. Primary delayed ejaculation.
3. Acquired delayed ejaculation.
4. Retrograde ejaculation.
5. Anejaculation (antegrade ejaculation is impossible).
6. Anhedonic ejaculation (no pleasure at ejaculation).
7. Anorgasmia.
8. Hypohedonic orgasm.

A. S. Reddy (✉)
Sexual Medicine, Vinayaka Mission's University, Hyderabad, India

Vasan S S et al. (eds.), *Men's Health*,
https://doi.org/10.1007/978-3-031-76898-9_12

9. Painful ejaculation or orgasm.
10. Post-orgasmic illness syndrome.

International Classification of Diseases –11 (ICD-11) classification of EJD.
Male early ejaculation HA03.0.
Male delayed ejaculation HA03.1.
Retrograde ejaculation MF 40.3.
Other specified ejaculatory disorders HA03.Y.
Ejaculatory disorders unspecified HA03.Z.

In the ejaculatory disorders (EJD), retrograde ejaculation (RE), painful ejaculation, post-orgasmic illness syndrome (POIS) are clear-cut medical conditions. They are not addressed to in this chapter. Premature ejaculation (PE), delayed ejaculation (DE) and ejaculatory anhedonia have psychological basis or psychological consequences. These are discussed in this chapter.

Premature Ejaculation (PE)

The prevalence, aetiology, causation, definitions and classification of PE are discussed in the earlier chapter. The psychological aspects of PE are discussed here.

ICD-11 Code for.
Male Early Ejaculation HA03.0.
Male Early Ejaculation, lifelong, generalised HA03.01.
Male Early Ejaculation, lifelong, situational HA03.01.
Male Early Ejaculation, acquired, generalised HA03.02.
Male Early Ejaculation, acquired, situational HA03.03.
Male Early Ejaculation, unspecified HA03.0Z.

Historical Perspectives of PE [1]

In the earlier times sexuality and fertility were inseparable. In sexuality, impotence is the only condition considered. At the transition of nineteenth to twentieth century, the term rapid ejaculation entered the medical literature and was considered a disturbing symptom. In the first half of twentieth century, rapid ejaculation was considered a neurosis, an intrapsychic condition, the result of unresolved unconscious conflicts. Psychoanalytical psychotherapy was the treatment. In 1943, Bernhard Schapiro considered PE a psychosomatic disturbance. He identified two types of PE—Type B, a sexually hypertonic type, and Type A, a sexually hypotonic type. Type B men were treated by sedatives and Type A men were treated with nerve tonics and body rejuvenators. In the second half of twentieth century, Masters and Johnson (M&J) postulated that PE is a learned behaviour, a faulty learning in the initial sexual experiences. Behaviour therapy advocated by them was the treatment and is still in vogue. From 1990 biological factors of PE were researched. The objective assessment of ejaculation by Intravaginal Ejaculatory Latency Time (IELT) was introduced. The concept of Bernhard Schapiro was revived. Waldinger proposed Lifelong PE, Acquired PE types and two more additional subtypes—Naturally Variable PE and Premature Like PE (Subjective PE). Lifelong PE is now considered a neuroendocrine disturbance of serotonin, of a genetic predisposition, with familial transmission, and pharmacotherapy was the treatment. The ill effects of PE on the man, on his partner and on their relationship is now taken into consideration and biopsychosocial approach is practiced.

Psychological Basis of PE

Psychoanalytical View of PE

PE is a neurosis. It is an intrapsychic phenomenon. A conflict at the phallic stage of psychosexual development of the child and failure of him to resolve the conflict results in PE; this is the psychoanalytical view of PE. It is postulated that PE man harbours an unconscious sadistic feeling towards women. By ejaculating early, he is depriving the woman of sexual pleasure. Narcissism, fears of vagina causing harm to them, vicarious pleasure of losing control of urination and soiling the woman are also the views of psychoanalysts as the cause of PE. This hypothesis was never proved in clinical scenarios. Most of the men with PE are gentle loving-husbands. The psychological state of the man and his wife are the result of PE, may not be the cause of PE.

Behavioural Aspects of PE

Masters and Johnson (M&J) proposed that PE is a learned behaviour. An adolescent boy hastening masturbation not to be caught by others; an young man hurrying sex in the back seat of a car; instructions of the woman to complete sex quick at visitation to a prostitute—in similar situations at an young man's sex debut or initial sexual experiences, condition him to become a premature ejaculator. Every young man passes through this stage of sexual initiation, but why only a few of them develop PE is not answered. This is an expert opinion of M&J, but was never proved in clinical research.

Anxiety as a cause of PE is a natural explanation given by the PE man. Anxiety activating sympathetic system, reducing ejaculation threshold causing PE is the obvious explanation of the doctor. The causal link of anxiety and PE is speculative, but was not supported by evidence. Social phobia is associated with PE with an odds ratio of 2.55 when compared with general population. Alexithymia (a person has difficulty in experiencing, identifying and expressing emotions) is known to be a risk factor and maintaining factor of PE.

Consequences of PE

PE affects the person, his sex, his partner, her sex and their relationship.

On the Person

Disappointment, frustration, anger over themselves, anxiety, guilt, inadequacy, insecurity, diminished self-confidence, humiliation, fear, denial and less-frequent sexual intercourse are the sexual and psychological consequences of PE on the man. He is diffident to approach the wife for sex. He won't initiate sex for fear of her rejection; for concern not to cause her disappointment; for not to enhance his embarrassment; for his inability to face her reactions to his PE. Half of the single men are reluctant to start a new relationship or worried about maintaining the present relationship. Half of the married men with PE do less sex; lose confidence in their sexual ability; feel bad for letting their partner down. More than one-third of men have anxiety at initiation of sex.

Impact of PE on his Own Sex

Men with minimal ED hasten the ejaculation during thrusting for fear of losing erection if they delay ejaculation. Conversely, patients with PE can develop ED. General anxiety, phobia and performance anxiety in the man with PE can cause adrenaline release resulting in ED. With early ejaculation before the woman is satisfied, the man attempts to do sex second time immediately. He can't get erection in this refractory phase and brands himself as impotent. Partnered orgasmic frequency in the women is more correlated with duration of peno-vaginal intercourse, rather than (usually presumed and written) duration of foreplay. Post PE, the effort of the man to satisfy the woman by masturbation may be counterproductive, resulting in more irritation and disappointment to her or she may settle for second-best orgasm by partner's finger not by penis.

On the Partner

In PE, the man has sex problem and the partner is the sufferer of his inadequacy. The response of the partner to her husband's PE changes over time. Initially, she is hesitant to raise the problem for fear of hurting his feelings. Neither of the partners is willing to talk resulting in a collusion of silence. She may feel that he is selfish and using her as a sex vehicle. Later when she raises the problem, the husband is resultant to discuss or he denies the problem. In due course of time- she may resign to her fate; distressed; gets irritated; may demean the man; deny sex. The female sexual dysfunctions in the partners of men with PE is double to that of female partners of men without PE. PE can cause the female partner to lose sex desire; to have less subjective arousal of mind and less objective arousal of the genitals and to have vaginal dryness, sexual pain and inability to orgasm.

On the Couple

The instantaneous reaction of the couple for early ejaculation is that he feels ashamed and embarrassed; she is frustrated, angry. They turn away to weep in silence. Intimacy is lost. In due course of time, their sexual interactions become far lesser. The silence, inadequacy and disappointment in sex life lead to problems in marital life and in general life also. Majority of the couples in stable marriage set a lowered equilibrium of their sex lives.

Ejaculating before entry—Ejaculatio Ante portas—leads to unconsummated marriage, usually branded as impotent, can result in divorce. This ante portas ejaculation is one of the uncommon reasons for infertility.

Treatment-Seeking Behaviour of the Men with PE

Even though PE is widely prevalent, only 1 in 8 men consult healthcare professionals for treatment. He may have a desire to solve the problem, but not a drive to solve the problem. It is his sex problem and he can solve on his own. Embarrassment to approach the doctor; shyness to let his sexual inadequacy known to others; fear that the physician rates him poor, an inadequate man; social and economic reasons; he wants a cure for his problem, not management of the problem. It is a problem of the mind, not of the body. Don't want pill enhanced sex, but wants spontaneous good sex. On-demand drugs to be used lifelong for which he is not ready.

Common Sense Technics of Correcting PE

Before approaching a physician, almost all of the men/couple resort to common sense technics to have a relief from PE. They use nutritional supplements, native medicines and sildenafil. They try yoga, meditation and Kegels exercises. Alcohol consumption, masturbation before sex, frequent sex, extended foreplay or no foreplay are the sexual habits they develop. At sex, they practice using condoms, using delay condoms, slow thrusting, stop and start technic, deviation of the mind and special positions in sex.

Psychotherapy for PE

Even though PE is widely prevalent, in India a miniscule fraction of men with PE consult health care professional. There is no cure for PE, only management. Nine out of ten are unhappy with the treatment and expect more. Discontinuation of treatment is universal and taking medications consistently on a long term basis is a rarity. The man expects the treatment beyond an increase in IELT. Psychological interventions are designed to address the PE beyond an increase in IELT. The benefits of psychological interventions are the following: increasing the sexual confidence of the man; lowering his performance anxiety; increasing the communication with his partner and resolution of interpersonal issues in the couple.

PLIISIT Model: Each man/couple with sex problem have different levels of psychological and relational issues. Every man/couple don't need the highest level of psychological intervention. The interventions are stratified by PLISSIT model. The person/couple are **P**ermitted to talk about his problem, his perception of the problem and their expectation of the treatment. **L**imited **I**nformation is given to the client about his condition and the available treatments both medical and psychological. They are informed of the benefits of the treatment. Depending upon the aetiological diagnosis of the condition, the clients are given **S**pecific **S**uggestions- pharmacological, psychological, combined therapies. Stop-start technic, technics of foreplay and pelvic floor muscle training are the examples of this level of intervention. **I**ntensive **T**herapies like sex therapy, cognitive behavioural therapy and psychoanalytical psychotherapy are the final level of intervention.

In clinical practice of psychotherapy for EJD, everyone is given permission and limited information. Only 1 in 4 clients needs specific suggestions and only 1 in 20 needs intensive therapy.

Behavioural Technics [11]

PE is the result of abnormally rapid ejaculatory reflex; this is the concept of Semans. He advocates stop-start technic to alter the neuro-muscular mechanism of ejaculation.

Semans Stop-Start Technic

The original stop-start technic described by James S. Semans is practiced by the couple. The partners are interviewed separately to know their concepts of sex and misconceptions of PE. They are advised rest. The love play begins; followed by stimulation of the man's penis by the wife just like masturbation. When the man experiences heightened sexual sensation suggesting ejaculation is due, he informs the partner and she stops stimulating him. Once the subjective sensation of ejaculation becomes less usually in half a minute, stimulation is restarted. This cycle of stop-start is repeated till he postpones EJ. When the man is able to postpone ejaculation, the same stop-start technic is done with the help of lubricant-to give a natural feel of vaginal penetration of the man. Once the indefinite postponement of EJ is achieved at masturbation with lubricant, they are permitted to do sex. It is presumed by Semans that the ejaculatory sensation control is maintained at partnered sex also.

Minor modifications to the Semans technic were done by others. Valsalva manoeuvre to be done along with stopping the stimulation which will suppress sympathetic tone. Elevation of scrotum occurs normally prior to ejaculation. Addition of pulling the scrotum down along with stopping stimulation is another modification.

Stop-Squeeze Technic

A modification of stop-start technic called stop-squeeze technic was developed by Masters & Johnson (M&J) and they used it as a part of sex therapy. The practice of this technic is –at the height of sexual excitement, at the earliest sense impending ejaculation, stimulation is discontinued and squeeze is applied to the frenulum for a few seconds. This results in a partial loss of erection and a total loss of urge to ejaculate. Once more, the stimulation is restarted. The cycle of stop-squeeze is repeated for about three to four times until the man delays ejaculation for about 10–20 min.

M&J used the stop-squeeze technic as a part of couple sex therapy. How ever this technic can be used by an individual or the couple without penetrative sex.

Helen Singer Kaplan's Technic

Gaining voluntary control over ejaculation is the basis of this technic. Absence or deficit in voluntary control of ejaculatory reflex is the basic feature of PE. Acquisition of voluntary control of ejaculation/is similar to acquisition of voiding control of a child. Helen Singer Kaplan postulated that perception of sensation of full bladder in a child/perception of sensation of impending EJ is the key factor for acquisition of voluntary control of voiding/EJ. Failure to appreciate the sensation of impending orgasm in the man results in lack of control of EJ leading to PE.

With minimal foreplay, the man achieves erection. The wife stimulates him manually. The man focusses his attention on the erotic sensations of penile stimulation. He is instructed not to bother about his wife; not to exert voluntary, conscious control over orgasm. At premonitory orgasmic sensation, he signals his wife to stop stimulation. The orgasmic sensation disappears in a few seconds with a partial loss of erection. He signals his wife to resume stimulation. After three such cycles, the man is allowed to ejaculate. Helen Kaplan uses this technic along with sensate focus in her new sex therapy.

Cognitive Therapies of PE

The man with PE develop distorted cognitions. These maintain PE. The common cognition distortions are the following: I am a failure because I ejaculate quickly; I had a trouble to control my ejaculation yesterday, it will recur today; I know that she feels low about my competence; My wife is telling she is satisfied, because she don't want to hurt me; If I fail today my partner will leave me; I ought to, must do good sex today. These cognitive destructive distortions further aggravate the problem.

Psycho-education is the therapy to treat this distorted thinking. Limited information about the true nature of the problem and the implications of the problem relieves almost all of these misconceptions. Cognitive restructuring is rarely needed.

Psychological Management of Interpersonal Issues

PE may be the cause of interpersonal problems or interpersonal problems may be the cause of PE or it may be bidirectional. An open communication between the couple clears almost all of these misconceptions.

Resolution of the distorted cognition won't improve ejaculatory latency. Restoration of communication in the couple and resolving interpersonal issues won't improve ejaculatory latency. These aid the man and the couple to be positive to seek medical or psychological treatment of PE.

Integration of couple, cognitive and behaviour technics:

The psychological treatment for PE involves—technics to delay EJ; lessening performance anxiety, regaining sexual confidence; resolving interpersonal issues; restoring intimacy; imparting psychosexual skills.

M&J devised a structured short-term intensive therapy for all sexual dysfunctions and termed it Sex Therapy. Later Helen Singer Kaplan improvised and simplified the M&J technic and incorporated psychotherapy whenever indicated and termed it New Sex Therapy. These two technics are in practice now.

Other Non-pharmaceutical Technics for PE

Physical Exercise as a Treatment of PE [4]

EJ is a sympathetic activity. Men with EJ exhibit heightened and earlier sympathetic activation levels in both non-arousal and arousal states when compared with normal men. Men with PE have lowered parasympathetic activity and higher sympathetic/parasympathetic ratio. Resetting this imbalance can result in relief from PE.

Moderate Physical Activity

Physical activity longer than 30 min a day for at least five times a week is proved to delay ejaculation.

High-Intensity Interval Training (HIIT)

This technic involves a bout of high-intensity physical exercise followed by short recovery interval. Several such bouts are followed for 7–20 min a day for 2 weeks. Men with higher increase in heart rate during HIIT had more increase in ejaculation time.

Slow Breathing

Breathing in for 4 s through the nose and breathing out in 8 s through the mouth gives five breaths a minute. Slow breathing exercise for 7–30 min a day for 20 days increases the ejaculatory time.

Yoga

Yoga improves ejaculation time in three ways- as a moderate exercise; Vajroli Mudra, a technic similar to Kegel's exercise; and Bhastrika Pranayama a slow breathing exercise. Practicing yoga for 1 h a day for 3 months with the above exercises helps in the management of PE.

Pelvic Floor Rehabilitation

Kegels exercise

Kegels exercise is contracting the pelvic floor muscles as evidenced by closure and pulling up of anal sphincter; holding it for 3–5 s; releasing it slowly for the same time as hold; repeating ten times in a single session. Three such sessions in a day for a minimum of 3 months. The duration of holding can increase up to 10 s with training.

Pelvic Floor Muscles (PFM)

Pelvic Floor Muscles (PFM) especially Ischiocavernosus and bulbospongiosus muscles are important in the ejection (expulsion) phase of EJ and in the integrity of external urethral sphincter. PFM rehabilitation is done by physio-kinesiotherapy, trans anal probe electrostimulation and bio-feedback. In lifelong PE, a thrice weekly PFM rehabilitation regimen coupled with behaviour therapy for 12 weeks resulted in four-fold increase in IELT [6].

Transcutaneous Electrical Nerve Stimulation (TENS)

Transcutaneous Electrical Nerve Stimulation (TENS) on the perineal region causes continuous stimulation of ischicavernosus and bulbospongiosus muscles just as in plateau phase of sex, thereby preventing relaxation of these muscles resulting in delay in EJ.

A miniature perineal TENS device (patented In2 Patch) is applied to the perineum at intercourse. This gives a two-fold increase in IELT. This is an on-demand, external, noninvasive device [7]*.

Pelvic Floor Relaxation Exercise

Chronic Prostatitis (CP)/Chronic Pelvic Pain Syndrome (CPPS) is one of the aetiological factors of PE. Pelvic floor relaxation exercise is the physiotherapy for this condition. PFM relaxation exercise is a reverse Kegels exercise.

In a happy baby position (lie flat, flex the legs at hip and knee, abduct the legs and hold them) or child pose position (in the kneeling position widen the legs, bend to touch the nose to the floor) contract the pelvic floor muscles with inhalation for 2 s and push out the pelvic floor as if letting out the flatus for 10 s so that the perineal body drops down. Ten such relaxations are done three times a day for few months.

Penis Root Masturbation [2]

PE and delayed ejaculation(DE) are the extremes of EJ process. Atypical (idiosyncratic) masturbatory style is one of the reasons for DE. Training the man to do atypical masturbation can reverse the PE. Penis root masturbation is one such technic tried to manage PE.

In the privacy of their homes, sexual stimuli are given without touching glans, frenulum and distal penile shaft to get erection. Over the root of the penis involving proximal one-third of the shaft, thumb/thumbs are kept over the dorsal surface and finger over the ventral surface. Circular or to and fro movements of the thumb is made with a firm grip of the penis. Audiovisual stimulation/partner stimulating him with kiss and non-genital stimulation is done. When the man feels the urge to ejaculate, stimulation is stopped. Similar stimulation is resumed after the urge to EJ wanes. The training session is continued for 10–15 min. The training session is continued for three times a week for 3 months. The penis root masturbation can be done solo or by the partner. A three–four-fold increase in IELT is expected.

Masturbators [7]

Hypersensitivity of the glans is presumed to be the reason for quick EJ and anaesthetic creams are used to desensitize the glans at sex. Desensitization of the glans can also be done by gradually increasing the friction and vibration to the glans at masturbation. MENS training cup with five grades of tightness and strength from soft to hard is marketed. After 8 weeks of training along with behavioural technics, IELT improves two-fold.

Sex Therapy

Sex therapy is a structured, protocol-based, short-term, intensive therapeutic intervention devised by M&J. It is a couple therapy. Sex therapy consists of two parts. Sensate focus, the first part, is common to all sexual dysfunctions and the second part is designed to alleviate individual sexual dysfunctions.

Sensate Focus

Sensate focus is the focussing on the sensations generated at the touch of the partner- first non-genital organs, later genital organs, followed by sensations at sexual excitation. This facilitates nonverbal communication in the couple and relives performance anxiety. The couple reinvent their erotic zones.

The M&J Therapy for PE

The steps of therapy for PE are the following: The wife exciting the man; stop-squeeze technic of masturbation; when the man achieves some control of ejaculation, woman on the top entry and no thrusting, the man getting feel of warm moist vagina; woman on top entry and thrusting with stop-squeeze technic; lateral entry and thrusting; man on the top entry and thrusting.

Sex Therapy of Helen Kaplan for PE

The emphasis is on the identification of the sensations at impending orgasm at masturbation/ coitus. Initially, sensate focus exercises are practiced. Additionally psychotherapeutic technics are used simultaneously.

The sexual tasks done are the following: limited foreplay till erection; wife stimulates him manually; he is advised to focus on the erotic sensation and not to pay attention to his wife; when he feels impending orgasmic sensation, he instructs his wife to stop stimulation; no attempt is to be made by the man to control orgasm. After three such stop-start sessions, EJ is permitted. Later the same procedure is done with varying the speed and pressure of masturbation; later the same procedure is done with a lubricant; later woman on the top entry and doing stop-start technic; after successful woman on the top intercourse, same procedure is done in side to side penetrative sex. The therapy is concluded with man on the top sex and EJ.

Education and Coaching for PE

These are useful to address aspects of PE that are not addressed by medication. Education on the prevalence of PE, IELT in general population; correction of the misinformation received from friends, social media, internet and porn; information about the expectations of sex versus realities of sex; enlightening about their less sex frequency and restricted sex practices; correcting their maladaptive sexual practices; utility of involving the partner; information about the available medical and psychological therapies-are the psychoeducation to be imparted to the man/couple. This forms the limited information level of psychological intervention of for PE.

Formulation of Treatment Strategy of PE [11]

There is a dichotomy of treatment option for PE. Physicians are favouring pharmacotherapy and psychologists are favouring psychotherapy. The causation of PE may be exclusively biological; exclusively psychological, but the psychological consequences of PE on the man, on the woman and on the couple are also taken into consideration in formulating the treatment.

The treatment options are the following: individual treatment, couple treatment, pharmacotherapy alone, psychotherapy alone or a combination of pharmacotherapy and psychotherapy.

The International Society for Sexual Medicine (ISSM) [3] Guidelines Suggest

For lifelong PE—Lifelong PE is biologically determined and psychological factors supervene. Pharmacotherapy alone; pharmacotherapy and behaviour therapy together.

For acquired PE—There is an identifiable biological cause or a precipitating psychological/relational cause. These causative factors are treated first. Behaviour intervention; pharmacotherapy; combination of both in order of preference.

For naturally variable PE and subjective PE—Reassurance; education; psychological/behavioural treatments. Local anaesthetics and SSRIs also can be used.

For single men with PE—These men have quick EJ, are hesitant to establish a new relationship or fail to maintain the existing relationship. Pharmacotherapy and psychological counselling is the treatment.

For couple—In addition to pharmacotherapy/psychotherapy to the man, relationship problems are also addressed.

In Clinical Practice

Combined therapy offers best of both worlds. Kick-start the treatment with pharmacotherapy to have a quick result, thereby the man gaining sexual confidence. Psychotherapy helps the man and couple to maximize the gains of pharmacotherapy. It makes them proactive in seeking and continuing treatment.

Combination therapy involves sequential or simultaneous use of both pharmacotherapy and psychotherapy. The psychological interventions in combination therapy mostly address the consequences of PE. They address the avoidance of romantic relationships; avoidance of sexual interaction in the couple; restrictions in the sexual repertoire like limited foreplay; unwillingness to discuss the problem; lack of drive to get treated; having negative opinion about treatment; lack of drive to continue treatment. So the interventions are psycho-education, advices, directions and imparting technics.

Results of the Treatments for PE

No systematic studies were done on the efficacy of psychotherapy for PE. The results of psychotherapy done by experienced therapists are available, but these results are not replicated in the studies done by other therapists. Stop start therapy, M&J Sex Therapy, Helen Kaplan New Sex Therapy have given success rates of 75–80%. Maintenance of the results of these therapies on long term are not known. Amelioration of distress, acquisition of ejaculatory control which can't be quantified in studies is high in behavioural therapies and nil in pharmacotherapy.

Studies on behaviour therapy vs. drug treatment showed significant difference in IELT in favour of pharmacotherapy. When pelvic floor relaxation for PE was compared to SSRIs, the IELT was significantly more in pharmacotherapy [5].

All the studies comparing the results of pharmacological vs. combined (pharmaco and behavioural) showed consistent, but marginal improvement in IELT in favour of combined therapy. When comparing the side effects of SSRIs alone vs. combined therapy, the side effects of SSRIs alone were double to that of combined therapy. The discontinuation rate of pharmacotherapy is more. When psycho-sex education was combined with pharmacotherapy, the discontinuation of the treatment was halved.

Delayed Ejaculation

Introduction

Delayed ejaculation (DE) is marked delay in ejaculation, the extreme form of it is Anejaculation (AE). Inhibited ejaculation, retarded ejaculation, impaired ejaculation, anorgasmia are the other terms used to denote the DE. Ejaculation (EJ) and orgasm are two separate events usually occurring simultaneously, but not always. A preadolescent boy can have orgasm without ejaculation and a man can have EJ without orgasm. EJ is a physical, objective, motor phenomenon. Orgasm is a psychological, subjective, sensory, cerebral phenomenon. Anorgasmia and AE are two separate, but related conditions. The causative factors of both are similar, overlapping and hence are discussed together.

The knowledge and treatments of DE are not evidence based. They are empirical, expert opinion based. So, there is a wide variation in the prevalence, definition, causation, interventions and the results of the treatments.

Prevalence of DE

DE is prevalent, but under reported. In a sexual medicine clinic, 2% of consultations are for DE. In community based studies, around 4% have DE, but only 2% are consistently delayed ejaculators. DE is age related. Around 16% of men at 60 years of age have DE and at 80 years of age, the prevalence is doubled.

Aetiology of DE

Age, medication, psychological factors, organic diseases are the causations of DE in decreasing order of prevalence. With increasing elderly population, increasing life style diseases, corresponding increase in the usage of medications to treat these diseases, the prevalence of DE is on the rise.

Definitions of Male Delayed Ejaculation [12]

International classification of diseases-11 (ICD-11) 2022 defines DE as the "inability to achieve ejaculation or an excessive or increased latency of EJ, despite adequate sexual stimulation and the desire to ejaculate. The pattern of DE has occurred episodically or persistently over a period of at least several months, and is associated with clinically significant distress".

ICD-11 code for

Male Delayed Ejaculation is HA03.1.
Male Delayed Ejaculation Lifelong, generalised DE is HA03.10.
Male Delayed Ejaculation Life long, situational DE is HA03.11.
Male Delayed Ejaculation Acquired, generalised DE is HA03.12.
Male Delayed Ejaculation Acquired, situational DE is HA03.13 and.
Male Delayed Ejaculation Unspecified DE is HA03.1Z.

Diagnostic and Statistical Manual of Mental diseases-5 (DSM-5) defines DE as a marked delay in ejaculation or marked infrequency or absence of ejaculation. The disorder must be present in 75% or more of partnered sexual encounters and persistent over at least the last 6 months. To qualify as a dysfunction, the man must not desire delay of ejaculation and he must experience personal distress. The code for DE is 302.74. The DE can be Lifelong or Acquired; Generalised or Situational.

Fourth International Consultation on Sexual Medicine (ICSM) 2015 definition:

Primary DE-A lifelong experience of inability to ejaculate in all or almost all (75–100%) occasions of coital activity which causes distress.

Acquired DE-A distressing lengthening of ejaculatory latency that occurs in most (>50%) coital experiences after a period of normal ejaculatory function and/or a clinically meaningful change that results in distress.

The time quantification of delay in ejaculation is not defined in any of these definitions. Studies on IELT showed a range of 0–45 min. The median IELT is 5.4 min. Two standard deviations from this median is 21–23 min. An arbitrary time frame of 25–30 min is set to recognise the condition.

Causation of Delayed Ejaculation

Physiological

Age: Age is a risk factor for DE. The prevalence of DE in elder men is 8–16 times higher than in young men. Progressive slowing of all bodily functions with age; less physical stamina to do sex for long periods of time; increase in medical diseases that cause DE; use of medications to treat these medical diseases; progressive neuronal loss resulting in less sensory and motor neural function- delays ejaculation in elder men.

Organic Causes of DE

Autonomic, somatic motor, sensory nerves are involved in EJ. A damage to these nerves cause DE.

Diabetic autonomic neuropathy is the commonest medical cause of DE. Multiple sclerosis, spinal cord injury also results in DE. Damage to the pelvic nerves as in pelvic irradiation, radical prostatectomy and para aortic lymph node dissection also causes DE.

Cognition and emotions are essential for orgasm. So any psychiatric disease can cause DE.

Hypogonadism, hypothyroidism and hyperprolactinemia result in DE. Reversal of these endocrine states restores EJ.

Prostatic pain, orchalgia and genital tuberculosis are uncommon causes of DE.

Congenital anomalies of Mullerian ducts can block EJ.

Drug-induced delay or absence of ejaculation is the commonest organic cause of DE. Serotonin delays EJ and dopamine promotes EJ. So, any psychiatric medication which increases serotonin and decreases dopamine results in DE. SSRI, MAO inhibitors, anti-psychotics, anti-epileptics, Chlordiazepoxide, Opiates, Tramadol delays EJ. Alcohol, Marijuana also prolong ejaculatory latency. 5-alpha reductase inhibitors like Finasteride, Dutasteride impair testosterone metabolism to cause DE. Alfa blockers affect autonomic system resulting in DE. Similarly Anti-hypertensives like Guanethidine, Reserpine, Prazosin, Methyl dopa and Labetolol interfere with EJ process and delays EJ [8, 9].

Because of their widespread nature, diabetes mellitus, psychiatric disease, psychiatric drugs, and prostatic diseases along with their treatments are the commonest reasons for DE. But all of these cause ED also. So, when there is erection problem, ejaculatory problems are side lined and not complained of.

Psychological Causes of DE

Psychogenic ejaculatory and orgasmic disorders are more common than organic ejaculatory disorders.

Models of EJ and EJD

The ejaculation and ejaculatory disorders are explained by two major clinically important models.

(a) Each man is having a naturally determined ejaculatory thresh hold. With excitation, when the man reaches this thresh hold EJ ensues. This ejaculatory thresh hold is ultrashort in lifelong PE and unduly long in DE/AE. Other acquired variables or situations act over this predetermined ejaculatory latencies causing some changes in these thresh holds.
(b) Sexual tipping model of Perelman: In sex there are excitatory and inhibitory factors each with biological and psychological components. Ejaculation ensues when the scale tilts to excitation. Excitatory factors outweighing inhibitory factors hastens EJ. Inhibitory factors outweighing excitatory factors leads to delay in ejaculation.
(c) Subjective arousal and objective arousal: At sex a man can have objective arousal (physical arousal) manifested as erection; can have subjective arousal (mental arousal) commonly described as horny. Both are necessary for EJ and orgasm. In coitus, a man with objective arousal without subjective arousal can't have mental excitation necessary for EJ. He fails to ejacul0ate and fails to achieve orgasm. This is classically manifested at sex with sildenafil. Sildenafil-induced vaso congestive erections if not accompanied by mental excitation results in delay in EJ.

Sexual Orientation Problem as a Reason for DE

Some men are asexual. For them sex is a nonentity. They don't have any sex interest. Homosexual men have sexual interest in men. These asexual, homosexual men after marriage with a girl are obligated to do sex without their wish. At sex, even if they have erection and do penetrative peno-vaginal thrusting mechanically, they don't have mental arousal causing delay in or no EJ. Some men are Autosexual, meaning their sexual interest is directed to themselves. They prefer masturbation to partnered sex. They can EJ at masturbation. After marriage, they rarely initiate and rarely participate in sex. In vaginal sex, they fail to achieve stimulus necessary for EJ and have AE. Normally men fantasise a girl at masturbation. But these men have to fantasise their solo masturbation at sex with a woman to get erection and EJ.

Paraphilia of a man is a definite reason for DE. He can't express his paraphilia, he can't get over these paraphilia, she resents these paraphilia.

Psychoanalytical and Psycho-Dynamic Factors of DE

Some men with DE/AE have—unconscious, unexpressed anger; are unwilling to receive pleasure; don't have interest to have children; have fear of loss of semen; have fear of female genitalia; have hatred towards women; don't want to give pleasure of motherhood to women. Some men feel that semen is an excreta, dirty; don't want to spoil or soil the woman with semen. All of these intra psychic phenomenon leads to DE.

Poor body image, anxiety, depression are associated with DE.

Cultural Factors in the Causation of DE

Semen is precious. It has to be conserved. Conserved semen can be converted to body, mind and spiritual energy. Loss of semen is the root cause of many bodily and mental illnesses—These are cultural values of some communities. Young men who are indoctrinated with these, are candidates for DE. Sex is a holy act; sex is for procreation only; practicing sex for recreational purposes is a sin; celibacy is to be cherished—some religions preach this. Men brought up with this religious orthodoxy are prone to develop DE.

Interpersonal Aspects of DE

Forced marriages; couples from different sociocultural values; couples with different sexual preferences and poor communication of their sexual preferences to their partners; couples without romance; couples with communication/relational conflicts— men in these situations are predisposed to DE and the same factors maintain DE.

Patient-partner anger is a major contributor to DE. Anger of the man towards his wife and their marriage is the major anti-aphrodisiac for a man. He rarely initiates sex. When obligated to do sex on her initiation or for fertility, he may achieve erection, does a mechanical thrusting and fails to ejaculate.

Behavioural Aspects of DE

In men who consult doctor for DE, men who are able to ejaculate with masturbation, but not in vaginal sex is the commonest presentation. 75% of DE men fall into this category. Even in the men who ejaculate with masturbation but not at vaginal sex, some can ejaculate with their own hand only, not with wife's hand.

Ejaculation is a learned behaviour is the proposition of Masters & Johnson (M&J). For young men doing sex more frequently and for longer time is considered a measure of their sex prowess. Adolescents who in the initial stages of their life learn to prolong their masturbation time by stop start or other common sense technics are more prone to have DE in married life. Frequent masturbation more than three times a week and multiple masturbations in quick succession in the same day are associated with DE.

Masturbation Technics and DE

To and fro movement of the hand encircling the penis is the commonest way of masturbation. This is similar to coital thrusting. Men who practice masturbation by this technic can easily transition from masturbation to vaginal sex. Youngsters who practice masturbation to ejaculation in uncommon ways—rubbing against the bed, thumping over pillows, tossing the penis up and down, pill rolling movement of fingers over foreskin, stroking a particular spot on the glans or frenulum- may not be able to transition to peno-vaginal thrusting, leading to loss of erection or AE.

Fantasy

Ejaculation is the result of friction and fantasy. Men at masturbation can fantasise anything—normal fantasy, abnormal fantasies, forbidden/fantasies. The content of the fantasy can be a person, object, position, movement or a situation. These fantasies can't be realised in partnered sex. Without their wild, weird fantasies, they are not aroused mentally and can't ejaculate. At masturbation, the grip firm or soft, speed slow or fast, the technic of masturbation and the fantasy at masturbation can vary greatly among individuals. Idiosyncratic masturbation is the term coined to describe this varied masturbation.

Pornography and DE

Men who does masturbation while viewing porn, who never do masturbation without porn are prone to have ED and DE. Men who are conditioned to masturbate and ejaculate with varied, vulgar, violent, hardcore sex acts done by a voluptuous woman can't be stimulated by a simple softcore wife. This results in DE. An young man on a week end, viewing porn for hours, stroking the penis intermittently, postponing ejaculation is vulnerable to develop DE.

Situational Reasons of DE

The man may be able to ejaculate with one partner, may not with another partner; may be able to ejaculate with the same partner in one situation, but not in another situation. Failure to give semen sample at infertility assessment, failure to ejaculate during ovulation days is the classical example of situational DE.

Reactions of the Couple to the Man's DE

With prolonged sex, the man is exhausted, fails to ejaculate and discontinues sex, eventhough he is having strong erection. Guilt, loss of self-worth, feeling that he is less of a man, depression are the consequences of DE. Some men may fake orgasms to avoid discomfort. Men with DE in the initial stages of marriage use condom, fake orgasm, end coitus and resort to solitary masturbation later. The DE comes to light at fertility. In due course of time, the DE man loses erection during thrusting. This ED is secondary to DE.

The woman for a while enjoys prolonged sex, compliments him for his sex prowess. Later she feels physical discomfort and soreness in vagina. She gets irritated, and sex becomes an ordeal for her. The woman may think that she is less attractive, not able to excite him. She may think that he is attracted to some other woman; using his semen somewhere else. Accusations of infidelity are common.

Diagnosis and Evaluation of DE

DE is a complaint, condition and a self-made diagnosis. Men who discontinue sex after few minutes of thrusting because of boredom; men who are easily exhausted at vaginal thrusting discontinue sex. Men who lose erection during thrusting(ED) also brand themselves as anejaculators. Woman with a quick orgasmic response brand their husbands as DE, even if they are ejaculating in the normal time.

A man who is not able to ejaculate after continuous thrusting with good erection, for a minimum of 20 min measured by a stop watch is to be confirmed as DE.

DE/AE has to be differentiated from Retrograde Ejaculation (RE)/ Aspermia. In DE/AE, there is no EJ, no orgasm, no loss of erection. In RE, there is orgasm, followed by loss of erection, no visible ejaculation, and sperm in post-coital urine specimen. In Hypospermia/Aspermia, there is orgasm, followed by loss of erection and no or a drop of semen.

Enquiry should be made about situational DE. EJ or no EJ at different scenarios-solitary masturbation, masturbation in front of wife, masturbation by wife; coital sex; at blow job, at anal sex, at vaginal sex; with every partner or with some partners; consistently with every sex act or occasionally—gives a clue to the psychopathology of DE. Enquiry to his masturbatory style, fantasies, porno usage; low libido, sexual orientation; frequency of sex vs masturbation—is to be done. The information is to be corroborated by the wife. His attitude towards marriage, wife, having children; his mental involvement during sex is to be elicited from wife [10].

Interview, examination and investigations targeted to the organic causes of DE/AE is to be done.

In clinical practice two groups of men present with DE/AE. Young man not able to ejaculate in newly married life; husband referred by infertility centre for his inability to ejaculate; elder man complaining of ejaculatory disorder after some years of normal ejaculatory function.

Management of DE/AE

DE/AE with organic pathology: discussed in another chapter.

The Psychotherapeutic Technics

The technics adopted in the treatment of the DE man/ couple are—(1) Psychosexual education. (2) Reduction of ejaculatory performance anxiety. (3) Increasing genitally focussed stimulation. (4) Retraining masturbatory technics. (5) Realignment of sexual fantasies.

Age-Related DE

Psychosexual education and reassurance is the treatment. As men age, there is lengthening of ejaculatory latency, lengthening of refractory period; less frequent, less intense orgasms; less volume, less forceful ejaculations. Imparting this knowledge and making him to accept the realities of sex life with ageing is the solution. Making him to enjoy the travel, than the destination relieves his performance anxiety at EJ and can restore EJ.

Sexual Orientation

For men with DE because of homosexual orientation: Imparting knowledge about the reason for his sex DE, about his marital life; allowing him to choose dyssyncratic marriage/divorce-is to be done. However when forced to ejaculate at fertility management, usage of homosexual fantasy at coitus with wife may result in EJ.

Pornography-Induced DE

At least one-third of men who masturbate for at least 1 h a day while viewing porn have DE/AE at partnered sex. Stopping masturbation temporarily or delinking masturbation and porn viewing can restore ejaculations.

Fantasy as a Cause and Treatment of DE

Every man uses fantasy at masturbation. The fantasy may be over a girl, over an object, about a sexual activity, at a sexual situation. Identifying the fantasy that resulted in ejaculation at masturbation and using the same fantasy at coital sex can result in coital ejaculation. When the man is able to ejaculate at sex with fantasy, he regains sexual confidence. Weaning him away slowly from fantasy dependant EJ at sex is possible later.

Men with DE with Idiosyncratic Masturbatory Technics

Retraining the man about masturbatory style and technic is the treatment. For example, a man who can ejaculate by rubbing the penis against bed, but not by hand stroking of the penis—making him ejaculate by rubbing over the back of the wife, later by rubbing over her thigh, later by rubbing over vulva, later by rubbing over her introitus and finally by vaginal intercourse are the progressive steps of retraining.

Men with Lifelong AE/Anorgasmia

In these men there is no ejaculatory response in any situation throughout life. They might have had nocturnal ejaculations. The treatment is in two steps- EJ at masturbation; EJ at coital sex.

The psychotherapeutic steps are the following: The man identifies his sexual preferences and identifies his arousal preferences; communicating these preferences to the wife; the wife masturbates him with his preferred arousal method; the man uses his fantasies of sex when the wife is masturbating him. This results in ejaculation at masturbation.

Men with Coital Anorgasmia

Men who are able to ejaculate at masturbation but not in penetrative sex and men who are lifelong anejaculators, who achieved EJ by masturbation with the above technic are included in this treatment regimen. This technic devised by M&J and modified by Helen S. Kaplan involves—sensate focus as the preliminary step. This results in identification of their erogenous zones; identification of their arousal methods; removal of performance anxiety; building communication and bonding between the couple.

The second step is sexual tasks.

M& J Technic for DE

The couple learn the sensate focus exercises. The wife stimulates the man, specifically asking verbal or physical direction in stimulation technics that are appealing to the male. Because of lengthy masturbatory time, moisturising lotions are used. Achieving EJ with wife's hand is the first step of success. The next step is —the husband is stimulated manually by the wife. As the male approaches the stage of ejaculatory inevitability, rapid, woman on the top entry is done. Then vigorous thrusting is done by the woman forcing EJ. In due course of time, the length of manual stimulation is made lesser and vaginal thrusting is made more. Finally ejaculation solely by woman thrusting from above is achieved. The final step is man on the top entry, thrusting to ejaculation.

Helen Singer Kaplan Technic

Sensate focus exercises is the first step. Then the couple engage in foreplay and mutual manual and oral stimulation; next-foreplay, manual stimulation, orgasm for the woman, but male ejaculation is forbidden; next- the same stimulation and male ejaculation; next- penile stimulation is done by the woman close to the vaginal entrance with her secretions as lubricant; next- at the point of ejaculatory inevitability, vaginal entry and ejaculation; gradually, the man enters the wife with lower level of manual stimulation and does longer intra vaginal thrusting to have ejaculation.

If there is a problem of insufficient stimulation at peno-vaginal thrusting, bridge manoeuvre is done. In this technic, the distal half of the penis enters vagina and thrusting is done. The proximal part of the penis is outside the vagina and the woman does manual stimulation of the proximal half of the penis with her fingers. Simultaneous peno-vaginal thrusting of the distal half of the penis and manual stimulation of the proximal half of the penis results in EJ.

Results of the Treatment

M&J with his psychotherapeutic technic of sensate focus and masturbation, coital technic could achieve success in 82% of cases. Others reported success rates of 70–80%. Around 20% of men are able to have intravaginal ejaculations consistently in 6 weeks. Others are able to achieve EJ intermittently not consistently. For some men, even after achieving intravaginal ejaculation, masturbatory orgasm may be their preferred choice over coital orgasms.

Anhedonia

Ejaculatory Anhedonia / Pleasure dissociative orgasmic dysfunction.

Ejaculatory anhedonia is EJ without pleasure/orgasm.

This disorder is rare. Systemic studies on this condition are not done. Expert opinion about the causation of this problem are low desire in man; decreased dopamine; hypothyroidism, hypogonadism, hyperprolactinemia; psychiatric diseases, psychotropic medications. Addiction to opioids, alcohol and heroin also may be the reasons. Over-dosage of pyridoxine is a reason for anhedonia and discontinuation of B6 supplementation can relieve the problem. Past psychological trauma, sex abuse and cultural prohibitions of pleasure at sex are the psychological reasons for anhedonia. Yohimbine and dopamine agonists like amanatidine, cabergoline, aripiprazole and L-Dopa are the medical treatments.

References

1. Waldinger MD. Evolution of the understanding of premature ejaculation: historical perspectives. Europ Urol Suppl. 2007;6:762–76.
2. Ma G-C, et al. Regular penis-root masturbation, a novel behavioural therapy in the treatment of primary premature ejaculation. Asian J Androl. 2019;21:631–4.
3. McMahon CG, et al. Standard operating procedures in the disorders of orgasm and ejaculation. J Sex Med. 2013;10:204–29.
4. Santtila CNP. Effects of physical exercise interventions on ejaculation control. Sex Med Rev. 2024;12:106–13.
5. Cooper K, et al. Behavioral therapies for management of premature ejaculation: a systematic review. Sex Med. 2015;3:174–88.
6. Rodrı'guez JE, Marzo JC, Piqueras JA. Efficacy of Sphincter Control Training (SCT) in the treatment of premature ejaculation, a new cognitive behavioral approach: a parallel-group randomized, controlled trial. PLoS One. 2019;14(2):e0212274.
7. Shechter A, Gruenwald I. New technologies developed for treatment of premature ejaculation. IJIR: Your Sex Med J;1–6.
8. McMahon CG, Jannini E, Waldinger M, Rowland D. Standard operating procedures in the disorders of orgasm and ejaculation. J Sex Med. 2013;10:204–29.
9. Shin DH, Spitz A. The evaluation and treatment of delayed ejaculation. Sex Med Rev. 2014;2:121–33.
10. Sadowski DJ, et al. A review of pathophysiology and management options for delayed ejaculation. Sex Med Rev. 2016;4:167e176.
11. Althof SE. Psychosexual therapy for premature ejaculation. Transl Androl Urol. 2016;5(4):475–81.
12. Otani T. Clinical review of ejaculatory dysfunction. Reprod Med Biol. 2019;18:331–43.

Further Reading

13. Kathryn S. K. Hall et al. (2022) Principles and practice of sex therapy, 6th edition. The Gulford Press. ISBN 97863543397, pp 134–1796.
14. Jannini EA, editor. Premature ejaculation. Cham: Springer, ISBN 9788847026469.
15. IsHak WW, editor. The textbook of clinical sexual medicine. Cham: Springer. ISBN 9783319525389
16. Masters WH, Johnson VE. Human sexual inadequacy. North Las Vegas, ISBN 9784871877015: Ishi Press International.
17. Kaplan HS. The new sex therapy. New York: Times Books.: ISBN 0812905024.

Part III
Sexually Transmitted Diseases

Chapter 13
Summary of Sexually Transmitted Diseases

K. Hanumanthayya and Fahim L. H. Rajiwate

Introduction

Sexually transmitted diseases (**STD**) are common all over the world, and the history of STD is as old as history of human race. European doctors in 1918 introduced the term **Venereal Diseases** (**VD**), and were discussing and treating only five diseases. They are (1) Syphilis, (2) Chancroid, (3) Granuloma Venereum, (4) Lymphogranuloma Venereum, and (5) Gonorrhea. Doctors all over the world understood that these five diseases are communicable diseases, which get transmitted during the act of sex. They convinced the **WHO** that during the act of sex, in addition to the five VDs mentioned, other infections present in genital mucous membrane of one partner will get transmitted to other sex partner. Hence all infections transmitted during the act of sex are to be included under the term VD. WHO re-designated the term VD to *Sexually Transmitted Diseases (STD)* in 1974, included all the infections transmitted during the act of sex. Early 1980s, all over the world the new disease HIV/AIDS started spreading and people were scared of this new STD. People started equating any skin lesion on genitalia with HIV/AIDS. WHO realized the fear of people and in 1997, re-designated the term STD to *Reproductive Tract Infections (RTI)*. To control the spread of HIV/AIDS, WHO realized that portal of entry of HIV, and portal of exit of HIV, is mainly the active STDs. To control the HIV/AIDS transmission immediate treatment of STDs is essential, once inflammation of STDs is resolved, inflammatory cells (macrophages) disappear from the lesion, HIV will neither enter the body nor come out to infect the sex partner.

K. Hanumanthayya
Department of Dermatology, Venereology and Leprosy, Sri Devaraj Urs Medical College, Kolar, Karnataka, India

F. L. H. Rajiwate (✉)
Ankur Healthcare / Raja Rajeswari Medical College and Hospital, Bangalore, Karnataka, India

Vasan S S et al. (eds.), *Men's Health*,
https://doi.org/10.1007/978-3-031-76898-9_13

Macrophages of inflammatory zone take up the HIV from surface to the interior of the body (*portal of entry*), and also bring out HIV from interior of the body to the surface (*portal of exit*). Accurate clinical diagnosis of STDs is around 60 to 70%. Patients may present with multiple STDs and secondary infections, and the treatment of the one of the STD can be missed, and laboratory investigations for all STDs not always available. Hence to solve this problem, WHO introduced *Syndromic Case Management of STDs (SCM)*. Syndromic Case Management of STDs is simple; every health professional can manage all STDs effectively.

VD denotes the venereal origin (Venery means Goddess of love, act of sex).

STD denotes the mechanism of infection.

RTI denotes the anatomical region of the body involved.

Prevalence of STDs

"**1 million curable STDs are reported every day.**" Sex is a basic instinct of all living organisms. Around the world, many men and women engage in sexual activity, often with multiple partners. However, awareness about proper genital hygiene remains limited, leading to an increased risk of sexually transmitted diseases (STDs). Hence STDs are prevalent all over the world. Sexually transmitted diseases (STDs) encompass a range of infections caused by bacteria, viruses, fungi, protozoa, or ectoparasites, transmitted through sexual contact (Table 13.1). Today specific antibiotics are available; most of the bacterial STDs are under control. Clinicians will be

Table 13.1 Classification of STDs [1–3]

Bacterial infections	Syphilis—*Treponema pallidum*
	Chancroid—*Haemophilus ducreyi*
	Granuloma venereum (donovanosis)—*Klebsiella granulomatis*—(*Calymmatobacterium granulomatis*)
	Lympho granuloma Venereum—*Chlamydia trachomatis* (L1, L2, L3)
	Gonococcal urethritis—*Neisseria gonorrhea*
	Non-gonococcal urethritis—*Mycoplasma hominis*
	Non-gonococcal urethritis—*Ureaplasma urealyticum*
Viral infections	Herpes genitalis—Herpes simplex virus 1 or 2
	Warts (condyloma accuminata)—Human papilloma virus
	Molluscum contagiosum—Pox group virus
	AIDS—Human immunodeficiency virus (HIV)
	Hepatitis—Hepatitis B virus
Protozoal infections	Vaginitis –*trichomonas vaginalis*
	Amoebiasis—*Entamoeba histolytica*
	Giardiasis—*Giardia lamblia*
Fungal infections	Vaginitis & balano posthitis –*Candida albicans*
Ectoparasites	Pediculosis (pubic lice)—*Phthirus pubis*
	Genital scabies—*Sarcoptes scabies*

treating viral and fungal STDs today, and the incidence is increasing. STDs may go untreated because of social stigma. Active STD lesions will have more inflammatory cells; hence they are portal of entry and portal of exit for HIV. To curb the spread of Human Immunodeficiency Virus (HIV), it is crucial to address and treat sexually transmitted diseases (STDs) with urgency and prioritization. Today the ideal treatment for STDs is "**Syndromic Case Management of STD**" (Table 13.2).

1. Syphilis Syphilis is oldest venereal diseases in medical records. Syphilis is a bacterial infection caused by the spirochete TP. The clinical features are multiple and different from one patient to another patient and from today's clinical presentation to tomorrow's presentation, hence it has been called the "**great imitator and mimicker**" among all medical diseases. Initially TP was virulent and killed millions of people all over the world. Today TP is less virulent, the disease is manageable, and the organism is sensitive to all antibiotics. Although the prevalence has come down, new cases are being reported. Syphilis infects all the organs of the body, it shows alternate periods of activity for some time, and clinical latency for many days and months, and it is transmissible to offspring.

Syphilis can be discussed under two headings: (1) **acquired syphilis** and (2) **congenital syphilis**. Acquired syphilis is further subdivided into (a) **early infectious phase** (first 2 years of infection) and (b) **late non-infectious phase** (after the end of 2 years). Early acquired syphilis begins with entry of TP, body reacts with TP, after the incubation period of 9–90 days, a painless, indurated, clean and well circumscribed single ulcer develops, with regional lymphadenitis. This tissue reaction to TP is called **primary stage**. Patient may take treatment, or he may neglect, then the lesion resolves locally, but TP will be multiplying and reach every organ of the body.

About 6–8 weeks after the appearance of ulcer, there is an immune response to TP, which is the **secondary stage**. During secondary stage, every organ of the body is infected and inflamed, and clinical signs mimic every disease described in medical literature. Hence syphilis is called **the greatest imitator** in medicine. The clinical signs last for 3–9 months. After few days of clinical latency, again clinical signs will reappear and this stage is called **recurrent phase**. Till the end of second year,

Table 13.2 Case approach to STDs management

Three approaches to diagnosing and treating STDs [1–3]	
Different approaches	Explanation
1. Etiologic approach	1. Laboratory investigation to find out the cause of the disease 2. Treat accordingly
2. Clinical approach	1. Good history and examination of patient, considering symptoms and signs of the patient, arriving at diagnosis 2. Treat accordingly
3. Syndromic approach	1. Consider the group of symptoms and group of signs common to few diseases make a syndrome 2. Treat all the diseases, which can cause the syndrome. Use multiple drugs to treat all diseases

clinically patient will be inactive, but TP are active in the body, this stage is called **early latent stage**. At the end of second year, patient will be not infective to other person, but TP have settled in one of the body structure, it may be skin, bones, muscles, any viscera including brain. Clinically patient will not show any activity. This stage is called **late latent syphilis**. After a clinical latency period of 5–10 years (or up to 20 years), the body may suddenly develop destructive inflammation in an organ. This condition is known as the tertiary stage of syphilis, characterized by gummas. Heart and brain are affected in the tertiary stage and quaternary stage and are called **cardiovascular syphilis** and **neurovascular syphilis**.

Congenital Syphilis The TP enters the fetal body through the umbilical cord directly, hence fetus will not develop primary stage; from day 1 the fetus will have symptoms and signs of secondary syphilis. Lesions of congenital syphilis can be grouped into: (a) **Early Congenital Syphilis**—first 2 years of life, the skin and mucous membrane lesions are infective. The clinical features resemble those of the secondary stage of acquired syphilis. (b) **Late Congenital Syphilis**—at the end of 2 years, the clinical features are not infective. The Gumma is identical with those of tertiary stage of acquired syphilis. (c) The **stigmata**—all the lesions are scars and deformities of primary and secondary syphilitic lesions. They are no longer active lesions. Many of them are distinctive and can be easily recognized.

The organism TP is a very thin, hair-like coiled motile bacteria, size: length 6–20 microns and breadth 0.1–0.18 microns. TP has slow and steady royal movements and can be easily spotted among non-pathogen Treponema (they will have jerky and fast movement). It has regular coils which help in identifying from other non-pathogenic and pathogenic Treponema. Minimum number of organisms required for successful infection is 57 organisms. Biological multiplication time is 30 h. The content of outer membrane of TP is rich in phospholipid (**20% of dry weight**).

Transmission of syphilis is mainly by sexual contact. Sometimes it may spread via contaminated blood, through the placenta, and accidentally to health professional.

Diagnostic Workup for a Suspected Case of Syphilis

1. Good history and examination of genitals and entire body,
2. Microscopic examination for the evidence of TP—Dark field microscope and direct fluorescent microscope (DFA-TP) are used to demonstrate TP.
3. Serological tests for syphilis (STS) arethe following: (a) Non-Treponemal tests (antigen—cardiolipin, cholesterol, and lecithin, and antibody—reagin IgM & IgG). Complement fixation tests—Wassermann reaction and Kolmer test. Flocculation tests—Venereal Disease Research Laboratory test (VDRL), Rapid Plasma Reagin test (RPR), Automated Reagin Test (ART). (b) Specific STS (Antigen—entire organism or components and antibodies—specific antibodies).

These include the TP Immobilization Test (TPI), FTA-ABS Test, TPHA, MHA-TP, and HATTS.

4. ELISA.

Treatment will be as per chart (syndromic case management of syphilis).

2. Chancroid Chancroid is also called soft chancre (**soft sore**), is caused by streptobacillus called Haemophilus ducreyi. The organism is transmitted during heterosexual act, mainly men suffer (men to woman ratio is 25:3). Incubation period is 2–5 days. The ulcers are superficial, shallow, and painful and well demarcated multiple ulcers on genitalia. The organisms enter the lymph nodes and cause unilocular abscess. Sometimes phimosis and Para phimosis may develop. Today with the availability of good antibiotics, the prevalence has come down. Multiplex PCR (M-PCR), is very sensitive method (laboratories stopped culturing organisms routinely), the procedure amplifies DNA of H ducreyi, TP, HSV-1 & HSV-2, hence easy to diagnose all three conditions from given sample. The histopathology of ulcer consists of three zones overlying each other and shows characteristic changes. The three zones are (1) the superficial necrotic zone, (2) the middle vascular zone, and (3) the deeper cellular zone. In the past an Intradermal test was done, called "**Ito-Reenstierna test.**"

3. Granuloma Inguinale It is also called Granuloma Venereum and Donovanosis. The term granuloma means tumor of granulation tissue. Clinically the ulcer is well demarcated and consists of beefy red granulation tissue, bleeds on touch. This bacterial STD caused by Klebsiella granulomatis (Calymmatobacterium granulomatis), is less infective to sexual partner. Charles Donovan discovered this organism in India in 1905. Dr. Rajam and Rangayya wrote a monograph on this disease, published by WHO. Morphological variants are (1) Classical fleshy exuberant type, (2) Hypertrophic type, (3) The sclerotic or cicatricial type, and (4) The destructive, necrotic, phagedenic type. The incubation period is 8–80 days. The organisms do not enter the lymphatic channels; hence lymph nodes do not get involved. Sometimes subcutaneous nodules develop, appear like lymph nodes, and are called "**pseudo bubo.**" Ulcer may get superadded anaerobic infection (fusospirillary organisms), resulting in destruction and necrosis of the tissue called, "**phagedenic ulcer.**" Diagnosis is done by (1) clinical history and examination, (2) tissue smear from the ulcer to see the bacteria, (3) Biopsy, (4) Serological tests—Complement fixing test and skin tests, (5) culture of the organism, and (6) A special test called "Colorimetric Detection System" for klebsiella granulomatis has been developed. Rarely malignant changes develop in chronic long standing cases.

4. Lymphogranuloma Venereum It is also called Lymphogranuloma inguinale, and Durand Nicolas Favre disease. LGV is a STD targets the lymphatic system. Causative agents are L1, L2, and L3 serovars. Initial lesion at the site of inoculation is small negligible ulcer. Soon organisms spread to regional lymph nodes and inflammatory process begins; star-shaped abscess are formed in the lymph nodes. Soon the adjoining lymph nodes get infected, individual lymph nodes get enlarged, and star-shaped abscess develops in every lymph node. Hence it will be "**multilocu-**

lar abscess." In 2000, an epidemic of lymphogranuloma venereum (LGV) emerged among HIV-positive individuals using crack cocaine in the Bahamas. It later spread to Europe, the United Kingdom, and Australia, particularly affecting homosexual men (MSM) and presenting as symptomatic proctitis. As Chlamydia cannot synthesize their own ATP (lacks enzymes), they are dependent on host cells for their ATP and nutrition, and hence they are called "**Energy parasites.**" Chlamydia can be grouped into 15 serological variants (based on monoclonal antibody assay). (1) Serovars A, B, Ba, C cause trachoma. (2) Serovars D, E, F, G, H, I, J, K cause genital tract infection. (3) Serovars L1, L2, L3 cause LGV. LGV mainly affects the lymphatic system. The LGV causes inflammation and thrombosis of lymph vessels, and inflammation of surrounding tissue. Infected lymph nodes rapidly enlarge, infiltrated by inflammatory cells including neutrophils. Neutrophils cause discrete abscesses; the inflammation spreads to capsule, adjoining lymph nodes and skin. The abscesses of the lymph nodes break open on skin as multilocular sinuses.

The inflammatory process gradually regresses over weeks, leading to healing characterized by extensive fibrosis. This fibrosis disrupts the normal structure of lymph vessels and lymph nodes. There is stagnation of the protein rich fluid in the subcutaneous tissue; clinically it is seen as non-pitting edema, later enlargement of the part, called "**elephantiasis.**" The fibrotic process also constricts the blood vessels, resulting in necrotic ulceration of the enlarged tissue called "**esthimone.**"

Incubation Period 7–70 days

Complications are (1) Inguinal syndrome, (2) Genital syndrome, (3) Anorectal syndrome, (4) Esthiomene, (5) Urethro-genito-perineal syndrome, and (6) Penoscrotal elephantiasis. The manifestation in men can be in the form of (1) Ram horn penis, (2) Saxophone penis, both being the result of chronic, massive edema of the penis. Stricture of the urethra, prostatitis, seminal vesiculitis and epididymo-orchitis may occur. In women, chronic edema leads to enlargement of the vulva (**elephantiasis**) often referred to as "**Esthiomene.**" Fistulae involving the rectum and vagina, Fistulae involving the Urethra and vagina, Cervix and vagina or vulva may occur in women. Carcinoma of the rectum is known to develop in 2–5% cases of rectal stricture due to LGV.

The Intradermal Test for LGV Is Frei Test

5. Urethritis Urethritis is the inflammation of urethra, presenting as burning sensation while passing urine and purulent discharge from urethra. The causative agent is *N. gonorrhea*. Nowadays *C. trachomatis* and other pathogens like *Ureaplasma urealyticum*, *Mycoplasma genitalium*, and *Trichomonas vaginalis* cause urethritis.

Rarely some other organisms may infect. Non-infective causes include catheterization, preexisting urethral stricture, and dehydration.

The Incubation Period: From 2 to 5 days

Anterior two-third of urethra is called anterior urethra, gonococci infects and results in inflammation. Initially patient will notice slight mucoid discharge from urethra, and in a day or two mucoid discharges will change to purulent discharge. The patient will feel discomfort and burning sensation while passing urine, the discharge becomes thick and foul smelling, and contamination of glans penis and prepuce will result in balanoposthitis. Infection spreads to the posterior urethra and bladder, and Tyson's glands.

Gonococcal infection in female presents as mild to moderate burning sensation while passing urine. Patient feel increased desire to void urine, and she feel urgency to void urine. Gonococci infect single layered epithelium, as the vagina is lined by multilayered stratified epithelium it escapes. The cervical canal and fallopian tubes are lined by single layer epithelium, both are infected and inflamed. On speculum inspection, discharge from cervix is seen, and severe pain will be felt in lower abdomen due to fallopian tube inflammation. In men having sex with men (**MSM**), rectal infection is common. People practicing oral sex suffer from pharyngeal infection.

Complications in men include extension of infection from anterior urethra to posterior urethra, infection of Cowper's glands and Tyson's glands, epididymis, acute or chronic prostatitis, seminal vesicles and periurethral abscess. **Complications in women** include Salpingitis and Bartholin's gland abscess. **Complication in infants** is Ophthalmia Neonatorum. Metastatic complications are (1) Disseminated gonococcal infection, (2) Gonococcal arthritis, (3) Meningitis, and (4) Endocarditis.

Laboratory diagnosis: (1) Microscopy for gonococci, (2) The culture on (a) modified Thayer Martin medium (MTM), (b) Chacko Nayar Medium, (c) Martin Lewis medium, (d) New York City medium (NYC). (3) Serological tests are (a) the complement fixation test, (b) latex agglutination immunofluorescence and anti-surface pili assays; (c) Nowadays, Nucleic Acid Amplification Tests (NAATs) are commonly used for the initial screening of gonorrhea and chlamydia.

6. Herpes genitalis Genital herpes simplex virus infections are common STDs; the incidence is increasing. It is caused by the DNA virus called Herpesvirus hominus type 2. In few patients, type 1 is isolated. The incubation period is 5–14 days. HSV infects the epidermal cells; edema of the cytoplasm produces "**ballooning degeneration,**" giant cells formed from keratinocytes, intranuclear inclusion bodies called "**Cowdry bodies Type A.**" Intercellular edema and degeneration of epidermal cells produces vesicles in the epidermis (genitals). The first episode of herpes in nonimmune (seronegative) person is called "**True primary.**" The first episode of herpes in an immune person (seropositive, infected by another virus type) is called "**Nonprimary.**" HSV after infecting epithelial cells spreads to the peripheral nervous system, travels along the axon and reaches posterior root ganglion and remain as latent virus. Periodically HSV latent stage gets reactivated travels down along the sensory nerves and multiplies in skin and produces "**Recurrent genital herpes.**" Latent virus gets reactivated spontaneously, or due to immunosuppression, fever, other infections. In primary genital herpes, systemic symptoms like fever, headache, and myalgia are common and are severe. Secondary infections may manifest as cellulitis and pyoderma. Sometimes complications like aseptic meningitis and transverse myelitis are reported. **Recurrent genital herpes** is mild and the patient will have prodromal symptoms. **Genital herpes in pregnancy** may spread to neonate during delivery. **Neonatal herpes** is a serious and frequently fatal disease.

Laboratory tests for the diagnosis of HSV are (1) Tzanck smear, (2) Viral culture, (3) Serology, and (4) PCR. Rarely biopsy is done. Tzanck smear is bedside test, viral culture is confirmatory test. Commonly serological tests are done. The tests are (1) ELISA, (2) CFT, and (3) Western Blot tests. ELISA and CFT detect circulating antibodies to HSV-1 and HSV-2 (IgG and IgM). Western Blot test distinguishes between HSV 1 & 2. In few laboratories HSV PCR test is also done.

7. Human Papilloma Virus HPV causes infection of anal and genital skin and mucosa. They are also called "**Condyloma Acuminata.**" The incidence is slowly increasing. HPV is double-stranded DNA virus, and is epidermotrophic. Almedia et al., showed cutaneous warts can infect genital mucosa, but genital warts cannot infect glabrous skin. HPV enter the genital mucosa, after the incubation period of 1–8 months, raised verrucous papules and nodules or pedunculated lesions develop, sometime few lesions coalesce to form **cauliflower like growths**.

In men, the warts appear on glans, coronal sulcus, frenulum, penile shaft, scrotum, and anal orifice.

In women, warts are seen in the posterior part of the introitus, labia, perineum, and perianal area. HPV genotyping identifies specific viral types, which are likely to progress to genital cancer.

More than 100 different genotypes of HPV are detected. Of these, 45 genotypes infect genital epithelium. Serovar 16 and 18 can cause cervical cancer, serovar 6 and 11 cause **condylomata acuminata** and **Giant condyloma of Buschke and Lowenstein tumor** (locally malignant tumor). Oncologists are of the opinion that **serovar 6, 11, 16, 18, 31, 33, 45, 52, and 58 strains can initiate cervical cancer**. The HPV vaccine is widely administered worldwide to prevent cervical cancer is practiced. There are three types of HPV vaccines. They are (1) **Gardasil 9** (9 vHPV effective against 6, 11, 16, 18, 31, 33, 45, 52, and 58 strains), (2) Quadrivalent vaccine (**Gardasil 4** (Gardasil 4, 4vHPV effective against serovar 6, 11, 16 & 18), (3) Bivalent vaccine (2vHPVare **Cervarix** and **Cecolin** are effective against strains 16, and 18). Serum Institute Pune has introduced **quadrivalent vaccine** called "Cervavac" effective against strains 6, 11, 16, and 18.

Treatment is either with (1) Podophyllin, (2) Cryotherapy with liquid nitrogen, or (3) Surgical excision.

8. Molluscum contagiosum MC is a benign skin infection, infective agent is a pox group of virus called MC virus. **Incubation period is 2 weeks to 6 months**. It is characterized by pearly colored smooth papules and nodules with central depression called **umblication**. They vary from 2 to 5 mm. they are broadly grouped into three groups. They are (1) **common MC**, found on the face, trunk and limbs of children, (2) **sexually transmitted lesions** found over genitalia, lower abdomen, and inner thighs, and (3) **giant MC found in AIDS patients** and is recalcitrant for treatment. The treatment options are the following: (1) Physical removal (cryotherapy, curettage, and LASER therapy), (2) Cimetidine, (3) Podophyllin resin application, potassium hydroxide, 3% salicylic acid, tretinoin, and cantharidine, and (4) ART for AIDS patients.

9. Postnatal and perinatal mortality Untreated chlamydial infections will have ill effects on both mother and baby. Pregnant woman may have preterm labor, early rupture of membranes, and stunted growth of baby. The new born, while descending through birth canal, is exposed to eye and lung infections. Ten to fifteen percent of chlamydial infections and gonorrhea will develop lower abdominal pain (PID). Inflammation in lower abdomen will cause irreparable damage of the fallopian tube and uterus. This can lead to infertility and ectopic pregnancy. Gonorrhoeae will cause ophthalmia neonatorum in new born, and child will have blindness. Syphilis will cause congenital syphilis during pregnancy or at the time of labor. HIV may spread vertically during pregnancy, or horizontally during lactation. The best ways to reduce chances to get STDs during pregnancy are (1) Avoid sex during pregnancy (avoid oral, anal and vaginal sex), (2) Mutual monogamy, (3) use condoms, (4) vaccination against Hepatitis B, HPV, (5) Regular antenatal checkup and necessary treatment.

10. Genital candidiasis Vulvo Vaginal Candidiasis is common during sexually active age, pregnancy, when on hormones, diabetes, immunocompromising conditions like HIV, and immunosuppressive therapy like steroids. The symptoms are pruritus in vulva, vaginal pain, dyspareunia, burning sensation while passing urine, and abnormal vaginal discharge.

Candida infection of male genital tract is called candida balanitis (balanitis means glans penis infection), candida posthitis (posthitis means prepuce infection) and balanoposthitis (inflammation of both glans penis and prepuce). Patient will feel pain and burning sensation over glans penis, and inner surface of prepuce. Abnormal discharge from preputial sac, sometimes prepuce may be inflamed, erythematous, and edematous, difficult to retract the prepuce, called **phimosis**. Sometimes, it is difficult to bring back the retracted prepuce called **paraphimosis**.

Diagnosis of candidiasis is (1) demonstration of candida in KOH preparation, and (2) culture of candida on Sabouraud's dextrose agar and blood agar. Candida infection is an opportunistic infection. Hence, while treating candida, underlying cause is also to be treated (diabetes or immunosuppressive therapy).

11. Ectoparasites Ectoparasites affecting the genitalia are (1) **pubic lice** and (2) **genital scabies**. Pubic lice infestation occurs during sex act. It is caused by *Pediculosis pubis*, also called Phthirus pubis (**crab lice**). Crab lice are smaller than body lice or head lice. They are 1.3–2 mm long, with three pairs of legs. Crab lice feed on human blood two to four times a day. They bury their body in infundibulum of the hair follicle. Female louse copulate with male louse, and after 1 week start laying 2–3 eggs (nits) per day for 2 weeks. The eggs hatch in 6–7 days, into nymph and then into adult louse. Adult louse live for 1 month. They also infest axillary hairs and eye lashes. Symptoms are itching in pubic region, demonstration of nits attached to the hair shaft, and adult lice. Discolored skin called "**maculae ceruleae**" are brownish red macules of 1 × 1 to 1 × 2 cm subcutaneous blood, secondary to lice bite. Lice do not survive outside the human body, and they die in 24–48 h. Treatment is 1% permethrin lotion application, and to be repeated after 1 week to kill nits. Tab Ivermectin 12 mg is the ideal drug, which has to be repeated after 1 week to kill nits.

Pre-packed STI/RTI kits syndromic case management of sexually transmitted diseases [1–3]

Kits	STD syndrome	Color	Contents of the kits
Kits 1	The diseases considered under this syndrome are: 1. urethral discharge (UD), 2. cervical discharge (CD), 3. Ano rectal discharge (ARD), 4. pain scrotal swelling (PSS), 5. presumptive treatment (PT)	Gray	1 tablet of 1 g azithromycin and 1 tablet of 400 mg Cefixime
Kits 2	The disease considered under this syndrome is: 1. Vaginal discharge (VD)	Green	1 tablet of 2 g Secnidazole and 1 tablet of 150 mg fluconazole
Kits 3	The disease considered under this syndrome is: 1. Genital ulcer disease (GUD) (non-herpetic ulcer)	White	1 vial of 2.4 mega units of Benzathine penicillin, + 1 ampule of 10 ml sterile water + 1 needle of 21 gauge + 1 disposable syringe of 10 ml. + 1 tablet of 1 g azithromycin
Kits 4	The disease considered under this syndrome is: 1. Genital ulcer disease (GUD) (non-herpetic ulcer). Allergic to penicillin	Blue	1 tablet of 1 g azithromycin and 30 capsules of doxycycline 100 mg

(continued)

Pre-packed STI/RTI kits syndromic case management of sexually transmitted diseases [1–3]			
Kits	STD syndrome	Color	Contents of the kits
Kits 5	The disease considered under this syndrome is: Herpes genitalis	Red	21 tablets of 400 mg acyclovir
Kits 6	The disease considered under this syndrome is: Pain in the lower abdomen (pelvic inflammatory disease PID)	Yellow	1 tablet of 400 mg Cefixime and 28 tablets of 400 mg metronidazole and 28 capsules of doxycycline 100 mg
Kit 7	The disease considered under this syndrome is: Swelling in the inguinal region (inguinal bubo)	Black	42 capsules of doxycycline 100 mg and 1 tablet of 1 gm azithromycin

Similarly, scabies also causes itching around genitalia, scratch marks, papules, vesicles, pustules, and sometimes burrows are also seen. Treatment given for pediculosis is effective.

Presumptive treatment (PT): treatment of clinically suspected cases without or prior to results from confirmatory tests.

Syndromic case management of STIs (Table 13.3) will be suitably modified based on STI surveillance and other related information. WHO eventually included all the syndromes (Table 13.4) suggested by the venereologists and has put forth the updated list [1–3].

Conclusion Sex is a basic instinct of all living animals. Everyone will indulge in sexual activity during reproductive age group. Sexual hygiene, monogamy, monoandry, and condom use will prevent STDs. If a person suffers from any of the STDs, they should come forward for the treatment. They should be properly counselled, investigated fully, and treated adequately along with all their sex partners. Bacterial STDs are on decline, viral and fungal STDs are on rise. Syndromic Case Management of STDs is a very effective method to stop the spread of AIDS disease.

Table 13.3 Syndromic approach to management of STDs

Syndromic Case Management (SCM) of Sexually Transmitted Diseases [1–3]
SCM is based on consensus opinion of venereologists and physicians all over the world.
The treatment recommended in SCM is very simple, a doctor working in Primary Health Center and a doctor working in Tertiary Center can give treatment to STD patient during the first visit itself, grouping the patient in one of the syndrome and offering the treatment recommended for that syndrome.
The aim is to treat all organisms causing that syndrome with multiple drugs. In SCM few extra drugs are used, use of extra drugs is justified, keeping in mind HIV infection. As STDs are main cause for HIV transmission, SCM will treat STDs during the first visit itself.

Duties of doctor treating STDs, as per SCM are:
1. Winning the confidence of the patient, good counselling (take the help of counsellor), convince him to take treatment, bring all sex partners for examination and treatment, importance of monogamy and monoandry, use of condoms, and regular follow-up.
2. Detailed history of sexual behavior.
3. Physical examination of the patient and sex organs.
4. Grouping into one of the syndrome and offering appropriate treatment.
5. Advise him to get HIV and VDRL tests and other necessary tests.

Syndrome	**Causative organisms**
1. Urethral discharge syndrome.	*N. Gonorrhea*, *C. Trachomatis* D to K, *T. Vaginalis*
2. Vaginal discharge syndrome.	*N. Gonorrhea*, *C. Trachomatis* D to K, *C. Albicans*, *G. Vaginalis*, herpes simplex, *trichomonas vaginalis*, mycoplasma
3. Genital ulcer disease syndrome.	*T. Pallidum*, *H. Ducreyi*, *C. Trachomatis* D to K, *K. Granulomatis*, HSV
4. Inguinal bubo.	*C. Trachomatis* (L1, L2, L3), *H. Ducreyi*
5. Pain in lower abdomen (PID).	*N. Gonorrhea*, *C. Trachomatis* D to K, *C. Albicans*, *G. Vaginalis*, anaerobic bacteria, mycoplasma,
6. Scrotal swelling.	*N. Gonorrhea*, *C. Trachomatis* D to K,
7. Oral and anal STI.	*N. Gonorrhea*, *C. Trachomatis* D to K, *C. Albicans*, *G. Vaginalis*, herpes simplex, *trichomonas vaginalis*, mycoplasma, *T. Pallidum*,

Table 13.4 Syndromes included in WHO STDs list

No.	Syndromes
1	Male urethritis
2	Lower abdominal syndrome in women: Vaginitis/cervicitis/urethritis
3	Genital ulceration
4	Proctitis/colitis
5	Salpingitis
6	Epididymitis/orchitis
7	Abnormal growths (Condyloma accuminata), Molluscum contagiosum,
8	Infertility and ectopic pregnancy
9	Postnatal and perinatal mortality
10	Hepatitis and hepatic carcinoma
11	Genital carcinoma
12	Acquired immunodeficiency syndrome (AIDS)

Acknowledgement We would like to express our gratitude to all the teachers, especially Dr. N Krishnamurthy (venereologist), Dr. P S Shankar (physician), and Dr. S J Nagaloothimath (pathologist), who nurtured our knowledge that made us write this chapter. WHO guidelines also helped to prepare this chapter.

References

1. WHO Guidelines. Guidelines for the management of symptomatic sexually transmitted infections, June 2021.
2. K P. Sexually transmitted diseases. In: Park's textbook of preventive and social medicine. 26th ed. Pune: Banarsidas Bhanot Publishers; 2021. p. 314–84.
3. Kishore J. Sexually transmitted diseases control program. In: National Health Programs of India. New Delhi: Century Publications; 2022. p. 298–310.

Chapter 14
Sexually Transmitted Infections

Murugan Sankaranantham

STIs are a group of infections, not a single disease, caused by various types of different organisms like bacteria, virus, protozoa, fungus, and parasites. When the name was VD, it comprised of only a handful of diseases, whereas today more than 30 diseases are included under this category. The list is growing day by day after the inclusion of Ebola virus, zika virus infection and the monkey pox.

We all know that organisms can be transmitted through various means like airborne, food-borne, through water, through direct contact, and vector-borne. But certain diseases are transmitted preferably through sexual contact. Sexually transmissible organisms are either highly fragile or can live only in body fluids alone. Certain organisms prefer to live in warm, moist atmosphere with a facultative anaerobic condition, which prevails in human genitals. They cannot withstand heat, dryness and atmospheric oxygen concentration. Certain others prefer to live only in the presence of human body fluids like blood, semen, vaginal fluid, and internal body fluids like peritoneal fluid and CSF. Human saliva, tears, urine, and sweat are not able to transmit the infection as the viral load is very minimal. On repeated exposure, human breast milk can transmit the infection. Skin–to-skin contact during coitus also promotes the transmission of certain ectoparasitic infections. Otherwise, transmission through casual contacts and through fomites is extremely rare. The sexual act promotes minor abrasions which facilitate the transmission of organisms or through any type of exchange of body fluids. Almost all the STIs including HIV

M. Sankaranantham (✉)
Department of Dermatology and Venereology, Sree Mookambika Institute of Medical Sciences, Kulaskaram, Kanyaakumari District, India

STI/HIV Medicine and Sexual Medicine, Shifa Hospitals, Tirunelveli, Tamilnadu, India

Indian Association for the Study of Sexually Transmitted Diseases and AIDS (IASSTD and AIDS), Chennai, India

Tirunelveli, Tamil Nadu, India

Vasan S S et al. (eds.), *Men's Health*,
https://doi.org/10.1007/978-3-031-76898-9_14

are transmitted through sexual contact in 75–85% or more. Other modes of transmission of these infections are through transfusion of blood and blood products, through sharing sharp objects like needle (including tattoos), dildos, and shaving razors, and through vertical transmission from infected mothers to children. Accidental infection through needle exposure and fluid exposure are very rare. These infections are not transmitted through mosquito bites or other blood sucking insects. Mosquito saliva contains an enzyme called as lysozyme which is inimical to HIV and hepatitis virus. The insects suck the blood but do not inject the blood. Moreover, STI organisms do not multiply in the body of these insects as those of malaria or filaria, and these organisms are not present in mosquito saliva, which will be injected into the host vessel while biting (acts as an anticoagulant in the proboscis of these insects).

Sexual route does not imply peno-vaginal contact alone. Sexual orientations are different from person to person. All types of penetrative activities have the risk of the transmission of these organisms, though there are variations of intensity.

GOA: Genito-genital contact -heterosexual activity

Oro-genital contact—cunnilingus, felatio.
Ano-genital contact—sodomy.
Ano-oral contact—rimming and annilingus.

Among these, anogenital contact carries more risk for the transmission of HIV/STI than peno-vaginal contact, as vagina is designed for sex (elasticity, distensibility and lubrication) which are lacking with anal canal. Anal canal and rectum are more vulnerable for injury during coitus, and exchange of body fluids happen easily each and every time. Oral sex carries low risk for HIV/STI, Other types of sexual activity like breast sucking and kissing have negligible risk for transmission, and masturbation and hugging have almost no risk [1].

Presence of genital ulcers and inflammation facilitate the transmission of virus like HIV and HBV. So prevention and early intervention of STIs will reduce the transmission rates of HIV and HBV.

STIs Are Classified as:

1. Bacterial STIs—Syphilis caused by *Treponema pallidum*, Gonorrhea caused by *Neisseria gonorrhea*, Chancroid caused by *Hemophilus ducryei*, Granuloma Inguinale caused by *Calymmatobacterium granulomatis* or *Klebsiella granulomatis*, Lymphogranuloma Venereum and Nongonococcal urethritis caused by *Chlamydia trachomatis*, Bacterial Vaginosis caused by *Gardenerella vaginalis* and other Nongonococcal urethritis causing organisms like *Mycoplasma hominis, Mycoplasma genitalium* and *Ureaplasma urealyticum*.
2. Viral STIs—Genital Herpes caused by Herpes Simplex Type 2 and rarely HSV1, Genital warts caused by Human Papilloma virus (HPV), AIDS caused by Human immunodeficiency virus (HIV 1 and 2), Molluscum Contagiosum caused by Pox group of viruses, Hepatitis caused by Hepatitis B, C and rarely A virus (HBV, HCV, HAV), Zika virus, Ebola virus, and Money Pox virus diseases.
3. Protozoal STIs—*Trichomonas vaginalis*, *Entamoeba hystolytica*, *Giardia lambia*.

4. Parasitic diseases—Ectoparasites—Genital Scabies caused by *Sarcoptes scabiei* or *Acarus scabiei*, Louse infestation caused by *Pediculosis pubis* or *Pthirus pubis. Endoparasites - Ascaris lumbricoid (round worm) and Enterbius Vermicularis (pin worm)*
5. Fungal infections—*Candida albicans* and Non-*Candida albicans* infections causing vulvo-vaginitis and balanoposthitis.

STIs are mostly manifested with three common symptoms—**BUD**—**B**ubo (Inguinal swelling), **U**lcers (In and Around Genital and anus) and **D**ischarges -urethral, vaginal, and anal.

STI Genital Ulcers can be caused by Syphilis, Chancroid, Granuloma Inguinale, LGV, Herpes Simplex and Genital scabies.

STI Genital Discharges can be caused by Gonorrhea, Nongonococcal organisms,—Can cause urethral discharges and vaginal discharges whereas bacterial vaginosis can cause vaginal infection.

STI Bubo—can be caused by Chancroid and Lymphogranuloma Venereum.

STI growth—Genital warts caused by HPV.

Syphilis, Gonorrhea and HIV are considered as Major STIs and others are Minor STIs as the complications of major STIs are not only confined to the site of inoculation, but also elsewhere in the body.

Syphilis—Syphilis is classified as acquired syphilis and congenital syphilis (vertical transmission).

Acquired syphilis is classified into early and late syphilis—Syphilis within 2 years duration is called as early syphilis and syphilis beyond 2 years is called as late syphilis. As per CDC guidelines, syphilis within a year is called as early syphilis and more than a year is called as late syphilis. Early syphilis includes primary, secondary, and early latent syphilis, and late syphilis includes late latent syphilis and tertiary syphilis.

Congenital syphilis is classified into early, late congenital syphilis and stigmata.

Primary syphilis is characterized with presenting genital ulcers otherwise called as chancre. The incubation period is 10–100 days. The first manifestation in syphilis is the Primary chancre characterized with a solitary genital or anal ulcer (according to the type of sexual act), usually painless, ham (Brownish red or raw meat colored), with clean floor and well-defined edges, not tender, not bleed on manipulation, indurated base. The inguinal glands will be enlarged bilaterally, discrete, not tender, and shotty in appearance (Figs. 14.1, 14.2 and 14.3). This ulcer even without treatment or with inadequate treatment, may heal within a month or more, but the individual may likely proceed to secondary syphilis after 6–8 weeks or likely to go for late manifestations (benign tertiary or Gumma and/or cardiovascular, central nervous system syphilis or ocular syphilis) after 3–10 years or more or tend to remain without any manifestation (Latent syphilis). Early syphilis is diagnosed by demonstrating *Treponema pallidum* by dark field microscope or by serology as well the late syphilis. Nonspecific tests (VDRL and RPR) are useful for the assessment of prognosis, whereas the specific test is useful in confirming the diagnosis. The specific tests (TPHA, FTA- ABS) once reactive remain reactive forever even after the complete treatment.

The treatment for early syphilis is single Injection of Benzathine Penicillin 2.4 megaunits. If the individual is sensitive to Penicillin, Capsule Doxycyclin

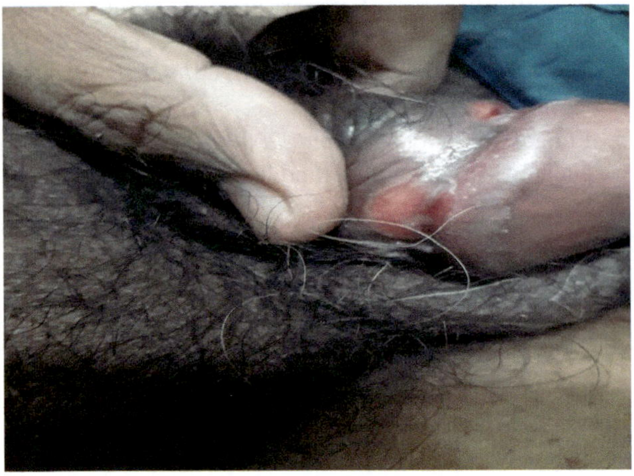

Fig. 14.1 Chancre

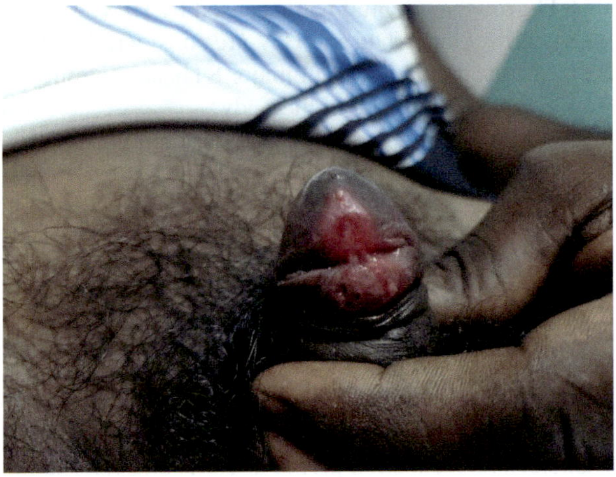

Fig. 14.2 Kissing chancre

100 mg twice daily for 14 days or Injection Ceftrixone 1 g IM daily for 2 weeks. For late syphilis, Injection Benzathine Penicillin 2. 4 megaunits weekly once for 3 weeks or Doxycyclin or Ceftrixone (in case of allergy to peniciilin) for 3 weeks.

The sexual partner should be examined, investigated for syphilis and other STIs and treated accordingly. The patient also has to be investigated for other STIs and has to be managed accordingly.

Chancroid—Another ulcer producing condition. Incubation period is 3–7 days. Multiple, tender ulcers with slightly irregular edges or undermined edges with yellow color floor with necrotic debris and red halo, bleeds on manipulation and not indurated. Sometimes these ulcers unite together to form a big confluent ulcer (Fig. 14.4). Always associated with tender inguinal adenitis (usually unilateral, may go for bilateral). Single node may become abscess formation. The abscess will rupture and will leave a large ulcer (Giant chancroid). The treatment is Tablet

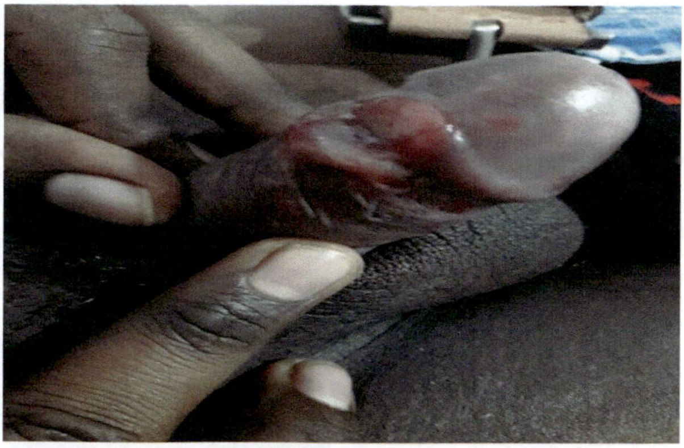

Fig. 14.3 Typical primary chancre

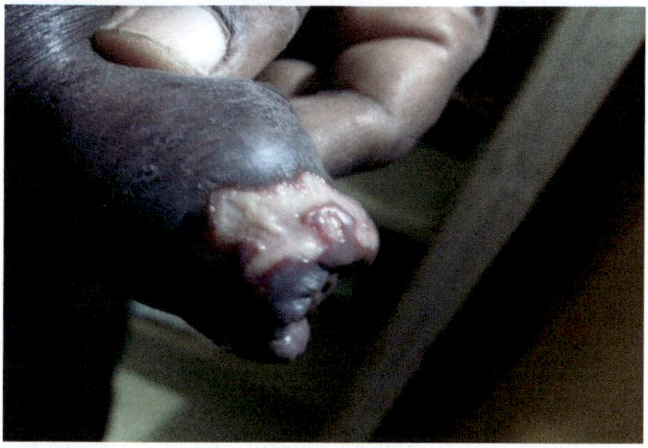

Fig. 14.4 Chancroid

Azithromycin 1 g orally as a single dose or tablet Ciprofloxacin 500 mg twice daily for 3 days. The organisms can be demonstrated with Gram's stain by demonstrating gram negative bacilli arranged in school of fish appearance.

Granuloma Inguinale—Incubation period varies from 2 weeks to 2 months, single or multiple painless ulcers bright pink or reddish color, slightly raised from the surface with fleshy exuberant granulation tissue (Fig. 14.5). Usually, lymph nodes will not be involved except in mixed infection or with secondary infection. The treatment of choice is capsule Doxycyclin 100 mg twice daily or tablet Azithromycin 1 g weekly once for 3 weeks or till complete healing occurs. Diagnosis confirmed by demonstrating the organisms in tissue smears inside mononuclear cells (GreenBlatt- Pund cells) by Leishman's or Giemsa Stain as safety pin appearance or telephone handle appearance due to absorption of the bipolar stain.

Lymphogranuloma Venereum—The primary ulcer in LGV is tiny and evanescent appear after a week, usually go unnoticed. The patient used to present with painful inguinal swelling 3 weeks after the exposure. The inguinal nodes will be very tender, matted, may rupture with sinus formation. Multilocular swelling, so after the rupture of the swelling, it will not lose its size unlike that of Chancroidal

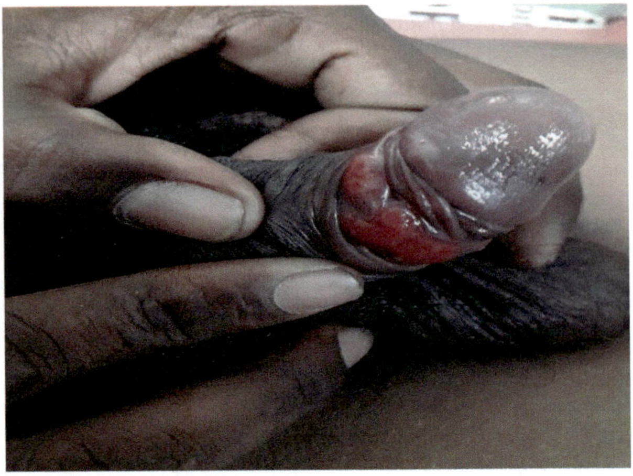

Fig. 14.5 Granuloma Inguinale

bubo. The glands above the inguinal ligament and below inguinal ligaments are involved. They exert a pulling effect and form a "Groove sign or Green Blatt sign"; as mentioned already it is caused by *Chlamydia trachomatis* serovars L1, L2, L3. Can be diagnosed by PCR test for *Chlamydia trachomatis*. LGV can be treated with capsule Doxycyclin 100 mg twice daily for 3 weeks or Tablet Azithromycin 1 gm once weekly for 3 weeks.

Genital Herpes—Mainly caused by Herpes Simplex virus 2 and rarely HSV 1 also can cause manifestations especially following oral sex. Incubation period is around 7 days. The patient may feel prodromal symptoms like spells of fever, itchy, or insect crawling sensation at the site of entry of the organisms followed by tiny grouped vesicles which will rupture and gives rise to multiple grouped tiny superficial ulcers which may be painful or not (Figs. 14.6, 14.7 and 14.8) . It is a self-limiting disease. Primary episode may last for 10–14 days whereas recurrent attacks (recurrence is a rule in majority) will last for not more than a week or so. In the presence of HIV infection, HSV lesions behaves differently, with tiny grouped lesions coalesced together to form a large lesion which can mimic Granuloma Inguinale or even malignant ulcers and have poor tendency for spontaneous healing. Treatment with acyclovir (400 mg thrice daily for 5–7 days) or with Famcyclovir (250 mg twice daily) or with Valacyclovir 1 g twice daily for a week will reduce the severity.

Low-dose antivirals can be administered as suppressive doses for a year or more if the recurrences are more than six episodes in a year.

Genital Scabies—When you find genital ulcers with intense itching (Impetigenous) (Fig. 14.9), it could be due scabies, and the contact history and other sites of involvement will confirm the diagnosis. It can be treated with antihistamines and applications of scabicidal drugs from neck to foot weekly once for 2–3 weeks. Simultaneous treatment for all contacts is a must to have a good result. Antibiotics are indicated for the management of secondary infection.

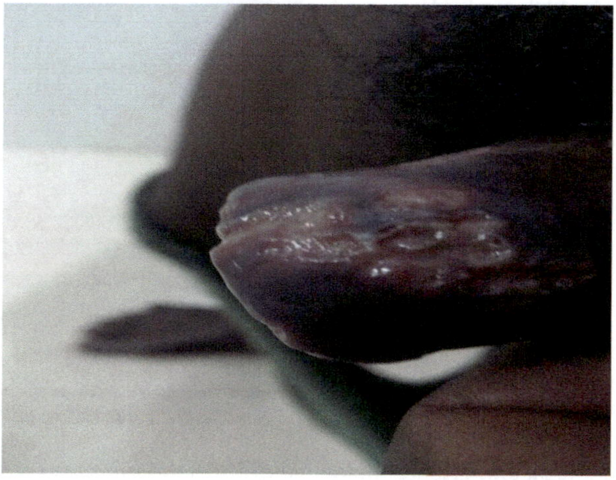

Fig. 14.6 Genital Herpes (groped ulcers}

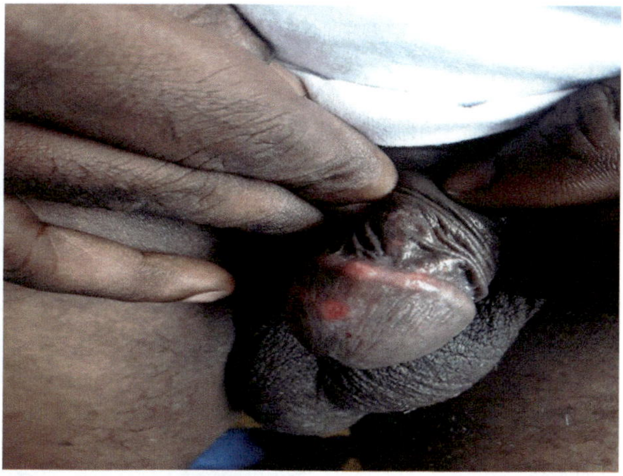

Fig. 14.7 Genital herpes (grouped ulcers)

Gonorrhea—It is a sexually transmitted disease with a short incubation period of 3–7 days. Patient will have burning sensation during micturition with a profuse, greenish white discharge (Figs. 14.10 and 14.11). The urinary meatus will be inflamed and the patient may have pain during erection. Gram's stain on the smear from the urethral discharge will reveal intracellular Gram-negative Diplococci called as *Neisseria conorrhea*. It can be preferably be treated with a statum dose of tablet Cefixime 400 mg or with a single Injection of Ceftrixone 500 mg. Partner and contact treatment is very important for complete cure and not to leave untreated any contact.

Nongonococcal urethritis—Incubation period for NGU is 21 days. Caused by different organisms like *Chlamydia trachomatis* (serovars D to k) and *Mycoplasma hominis*.

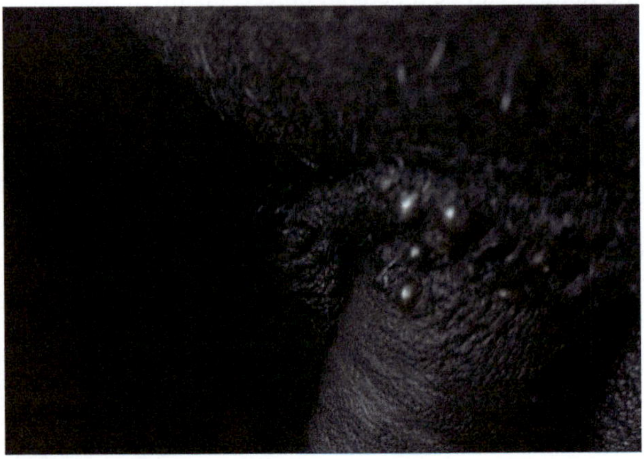

Fig. 14.8 Genital Herpes (grouped vesicles)

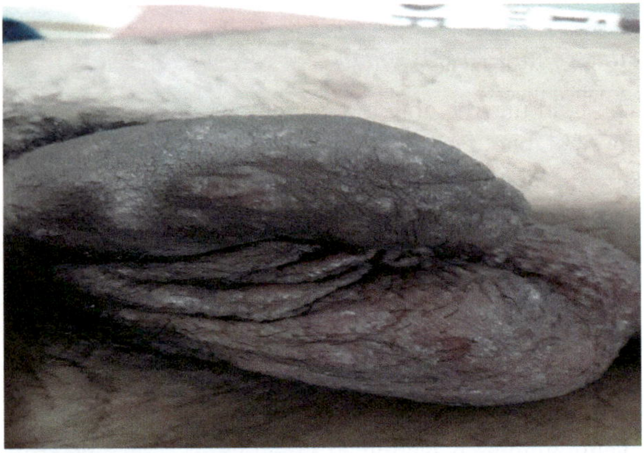

Fig. 14.9 Genital scabies

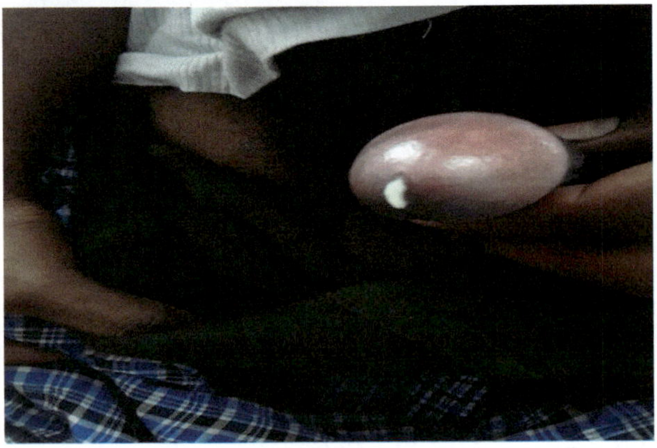

Fig. 14.10 Urethral discharge

Ureaplasma urealyticum—Patient may have mild burning sensation during micturition and a mucoid or mucopurulent discharge. This will respond to Capsule Doxycyclin 100 mf twice daily for 2 weeks. Tablet Azithromycine 2 g single dose also will be effective.

Trichomonas vaginalis infection rarely causes symptoms in men. When the spouse or contact is having the infection, the individual has to be treated with Tablet Metranidazole 2 g statum dose. Tablet Metranidazole can also be used in the dose of 400 mg thrice for 7 days,

Candida albicans—It is one of the commonest yeast fungal infections manifested a balanoposthitis in men and vulvovaginitis in women. Balanoposthitis marked over the prepuce with reddening, soddening, and fissuring of the margin of the preputial skin (Fig. 14.12). Prolonged oral broad-spectrum antibiotics, diabetes mellitus, pregancy, oral contraceptive tablets, other debilitating diseases, and cytotoxic drugs can precipitate candida balanoposthitis. Controlling the predisposing factors to the maximum extent and antifungal antibiotics like tablet fluconazole 150 mg statum dose is recommended along with topical antifungal antibiotic creams like Clotrimazole or Miconazole. Sexual abstinence for 3 weeks is advisable.

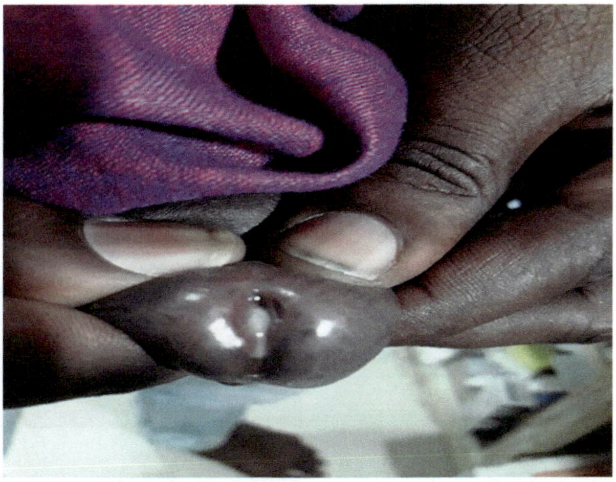

Fig. 14.11 Gonococcal urethritis

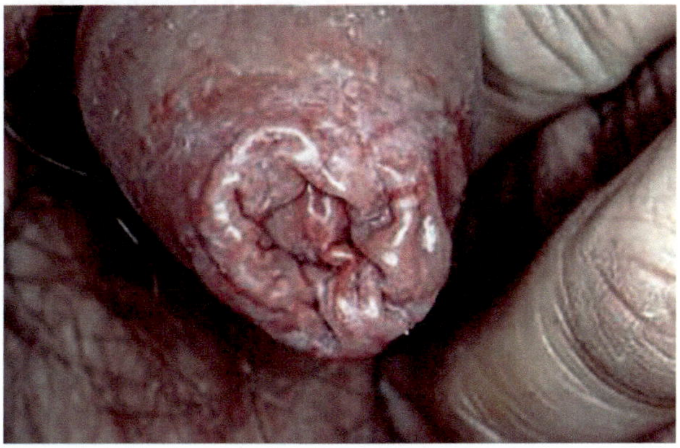

Fig. 14.12 Monilial balanoposthitis

Bacterial vaginitis will not cause severe symptoms but the fishy odor following intercourse will be a nuisance. Capsule Ampicillin 500 mg thrice daily or Tablet Metranidazole in the dose of 400 mg thrice daily for a week will clear the problem.

Genital warts—Incubation period varies from 2 months to 6 months**.** This may be tiny and multiple raised lesions or a cauliflower like lesions either pinkish or greyish in appearance (Figs. 14.13 and 14.14). Warts can also occur over the perianal area following anal sex (Fig. 14.15). It can be ablated either by chemical cauterization or with cryo-surgery. Especially for intraluminal lesions cryo is the best. For chemical cauterization, 25% podophyllin resin in alcohol or tincture benzoin can be used. This should be a physician initiating treatment as the excess use will result in severe irritant balanoposthitis. Protecting the normal area with some bland ointments, Podophyllin applied over the lesion and instructed the patient to wash the application with plain water within 3–4 h. Weekly twice application will remove the lesions within few weeks according to the number of lesions and size of the lesions.

Partner treatment, safe sex advice, contact tracing, and sex education are very important in the management of STIs to avoid a new infection, to avoid further complications, and to avoid the HIV transmission. Regular follow-up clinically and serologically (wherever it is needed) and the **treatment adherence** as advised by the physicaian also should be stressed in the management of these diseases. All these measures will ensure a total cure from these STIs.

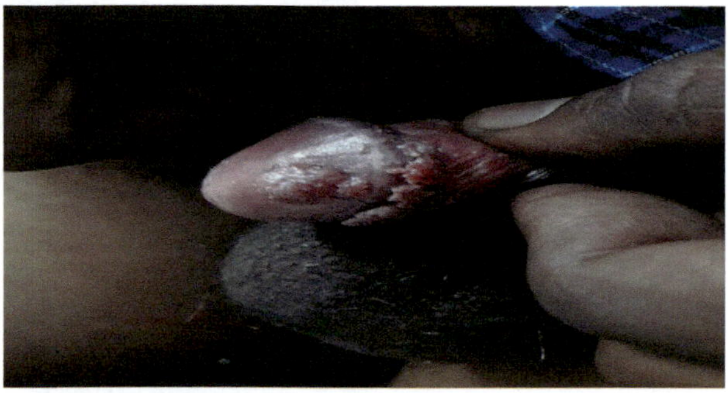

Fig. 14.13 Genital warts

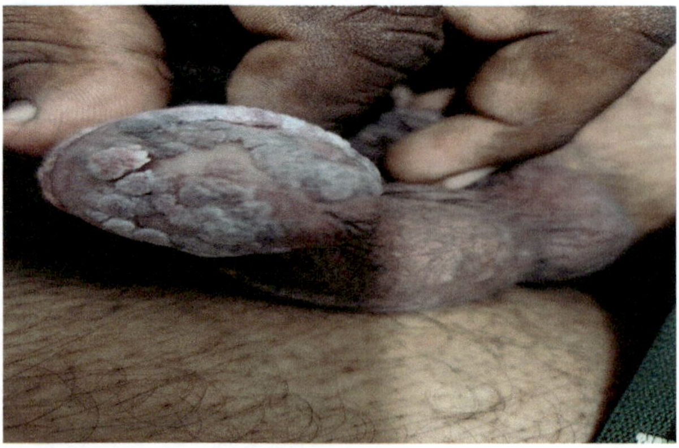

Fig. 14.14 Genital warts

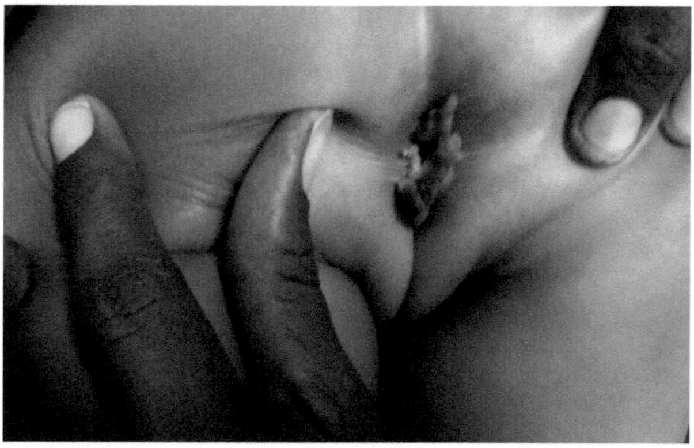

Fig. 14.15 Anal wart

Reference

1. https://www.cdc.gov/hiv/risk/estimates/riskbehaviors.html

Chapter 15
Sexual Health and Genital Care

Murugan Sankaranantham

Importance of Sexual and Reproductive Health

Sexuality is a natural and healthy part of living. Next to food and sleep, **sex** is the prime need for all living creatures.

For human beings, the function of propagation and procreation is associated with pleasure and recreation. At the same time sex organs are always not exhibited like other organs of our body. Naturally hidden things elicit more attractions, curiosity and an interest to explore. Due to restrictions in society, it is neither well discussed nor taught in curriculum and that leads to lot of myths and misconceptions. Sex is a subject often neglected and not discussed both in schools and society. Parents and teachers as well hesitate to talk about genital and sex problems to their wards. Medical curricula also neglect very much these aspects. There is no separate specialty in the medical field and so the knowledge about this subject lacks very much even among medical professionals and at the same time problems in this regard among the public are increasing day by day due to the progress of technologies and changes in life style, social permissiveness and culture. This is high time to consider a separate specialty in the field of Sexual health and reproductive medicine. The myths and misconceptions prevailing in society lead to sexual dysfunction, **non consummation** of marriage, marital disharmony and ends ultimately with broken

M. Sankaranantham (✉)
Department of Dermatology and Venereology, Sree Mookambika Institute of Medical Sciences, Kulaskaram, Kanyaakumari District, India

STI/HIV Medicine and Sexual Medicine, Shifa Hospitals, Tirunelveli, Tamilnadu, India

Indian Association for the Study of Sexually Transmitted Diseases and AIDS (IASSTD and AIDS), Chennai, India

Tirunelveli, Tamil Nadu, India

Vasan S S et al. (eds.), *Men's Health*,
https://doi.org/10.1007/978-3-031-76898-9_15

marriages, divorce and suicide. Any abnormality seen over the genitals evokes lot of anxiety and fear.

Men and women are **complimentary sexes**, and not opposite sexes. Like a cup and saucer, they form a single unit. The function of this unit is reproduction. **Man gives 'love' to get 'sex' whereas woman gives 'sex' to get 'love'. When a marriage is considered as 'HOLY' and motherhood is also considered 'HOLY', then how can be the genitals considered as dirty and sexual act as obscene?**

As per **WHO, sexual Health** provides physical, mental and social well-being in relation to sexuality.

The Concept of Sexual Health Includes

1. Capacity to enjoy and control sexual and reproductive behavior in accordance with social and personal ethics.
2. Freedom from fear, shame, guilt, false beliefs and other psychological factors, inhibiting sexual responses and impairing sexual relationships.
3. Freedom from organic disorders, diseases and deficiencies that interfere with sexual and reproductive functions.

Reproductive Health

Reproductive health is defined as a state of complete physical, mental and social well-being and not merely the absence of disease, infirmity in all matters related to the reproductive system and its functions and processes.

It includes:

1. A satisfying and safe sex life free from the fear of diseases and free from coercion and violence.
2. The capacity to reproduce and the freedom to decide if, when and how often to do so; that is access to both infertility service on one hand and contraceptive services on the other.
3. Access to safe, effective, affordable and acceptable methods of family planning of their choice.
4. Access to safe and affordable abortion facilities.
5. Safe child bearing.
6. Access to services for prevention and care of reproductive health problems; both gynecological and obstetrical in a culturally sensitive manner.
7. Special attention to adolescents' reproductive health.

In all these aspects both partners must be in a position to make decisions on their own (Empowerment) and the partner should be in a position to respect the decision of the other.

I want to quote Dr. T. S.S Rao's (the famous psychiatrist from Karnataka) words at this juncture: **"An ideal wife is the one who is not expecting an ideal husband". This could be vice versa also!**

Benefits of Sex

SEX is good for you in many ways and the health benefits extend beyond the Bedroom.

It relieves stress, lowers blood pressure, boosts immunity, provides exercise, burns calories, improves cardiovascular health, boosts self-esteem, strengthens your well-being, improves Intimacy, helps to bind family-bonds, reduces pain, reduces the risk of prostatic carcinoma, strengthens the pelvic floor and helps you to relax and sleep better.

Reasons for Sex Problems

During sex, mind and body have to coordinate together. The individual's mind has to be focused on the partner's body and on sexual pleasure alone and it should not get diverted. If the individual is not able to focus his mind on these, then he or she will not be able to complete the '**sexual response cycle**' and this will end up in sex problems. **Failure to complete the first coitus (could be situational)** will also lead to sex problems. This situational problem might be due to misconceptions, poor esteem, disliking of partner, pressure on performance, social pressure, bad odour, halitosis, guilty complex, anxiety, fear of being caught, fear of STIs/HIV, pregnancy, lack of time and hurry, uncongenial place, lack of adequate privacy and faulty position etc. Some other causes are upbringing, religious taboos, misinterpretations by parents, friends, elders etc., depression, low self-esteem, lack of personal relations or conflicts, childhood traumatic experience or child sex abuse, stress at home or work and inconsistent meeting hours between couples due to work schedule, disliking (spouse, sex, odour), liking towards altered behaviour, lack of stimuli or monotony (elderly and middle aged), **5 'S'**—Smoking, Scotch, Sugar, Stress, Sedentary Life and poor orientation due to lack of friends or due to low IQ.

Points to Ponder

Erection is not at one's will as other voluntary actions.

Semen is not a precious thing. The semen is like that of any other secretions of the body like saliva or tears.

Frequency of sex may be likely to vary with person to person, depends on their age and duration of the acquaintance with that particular partner or duration of marriage. Don't compare with others.

Intercourse and masturbation do not cause weakness: During intercourse or masturbation, the tension in muscles raises. Heart beat increases. Tachypnoea occurs. Because all of these, the individual will become fatigue which will be relieved by rest and a meal and he will regain his energy back. This is just tiredness and interpreted as weakness mistakenly. Nobody can perform more than what is possible as one cannot eat more than sufficient. The body know its limits and can regulate the same. So sexual activity will not lead to weakness.

Homosexuality is not unnatural. Nowadays it is neither considered as unnatural, nor as deviation, but as a normal variation.

Comments from friends at schools and colleges, comments from sex partner/s can affect the sexual function of an individual. It may sometimes be worsen by relatives, family members attitudes, lawyers blame when it becomes a legal issue and sometimes by the treating doctors even.

Non-consummation of marriage is increasing nowadays. Longer the duration of this unconsummated state among the couples creates problems with deep impact and becomes difficult to resolve. In these cases the individual, who was blamed, would lose hope and the partner will lose the trust with him. If they seek help within few months, we can solve their problems easily. I had seen a couple with 19 years of non-consummation after their marriage.

Patients will expect advice from their physicians with regards to resuming sex during pregnancy, after delivery, hysterectomy and following surgeries, circumcision, myocardial infarction, heart surgeries, arthritis etc., as sex is an important function for all human beings. Those physicians and surgeons must address these issues when they discharge these individuals and the partners appropriately.

As there is social pressure or need to have a baby, there is an urge to prevent unwanted pregnancy also. A woman's ability to choose, whether and when to become pregnant, has a direct impact on her health and well-being. Family planning allows spacing of pregnancies and can delay pregnancies in young women as there are increased risks of health problems and risk of death from early childbearing. It prevents unintended pregnancies, including those of older women who face increased risks related to pregnancies and congenital anomalies. **Family planning also reduces the need for unsafe abortion.** Family planning is the key to slowing unsustainable population growth and the resulting negative impacts on the economy, environment, and national and regional development efforts.

There are many ways to avoid pregnancies. **Abstinence from sex is the surest way to avoid pregnancies**. But this will not be possible and not necessary at all times. There are a number of different methods and it is important to choose one that best meets your needs and circumstances.

Considerations when choosing contraception should include accurate information about the effectiveness in pregnancy prevention, health issues which may limit some choices, ease to use, side effects including changes in usual periods, benefits other than contraception, cost and availability, reversibility and protection against sexually transmissible infections (STIs).

So sexual health and reproductive health are equally important like that of any other system of the body for a happy and peaceful life for everyone in this world. Sex education in schools and colleges and if installed as a separate specialty in our medical colleges will have a definite role in improving this issue and it should be stressed as a priority issue.

Genital Care

Sex organs are not exhibited like our other organs. Naturally hidden things elicit more attraction and curiosity to explore. At the same time, due to the restrictions in the society, it is neither well discussed nor taught either in schools or colleges which result in lots of myths and misconceptions. Sex has a lot of benefits like relieves the stress, lowering the blood pressure, boost immunity, provides exercise, burns calories, improves cardiovascular health, boosts self-esteem and wellbeing, improves intimacy between people, reduces the risk of prostatic carcinoma and helps you to relax and sleep well. At the same time, sex is subjected to risk when it is not streamlined in the correct channel. When we are not planning it properly it may result in unwanted pregnancies, repeated abortions, and when having multi-partner sex, or sex with unknown partner, the individual is vulnerable for infections transmitted through the sexual route which are called as Sexually Transmitted Infections (STIs) {(Venereal Diseases (VD) in olden days after the God of Love VENUS in Greek mythology and Sexually transmitted Diseases (STD)}. To have a pleasant and healthy sexual life, one should know their genitals to an extent, care their genitals and keep their genital hygiene to the maximum.

Male external genitals are penis and scrotum. Penis has a shaft and glans penis (separated by Coronal sulcus). Glans penis is covered by a fold of skin called as Prepuce or foreskin. This foreskin is retractable normally. In few people foreskin could not be retractable since birth and this condition is called as **phimosis**. This inability to retract the foreskin may be congenital or acquired (secondary to infection or inflammation or growth).

Smegma is an off-white cheesy collection (modified sebaceous secretion) secreted by a pair of glands (**Tyson's glands**), situated on either side of the frenum on both sides. In humans, these glands are vestigial in nature and has no function. These collections are more abundant in adolescents and in young adults. It will spontaneously cease to secrete upon ageing. It has carcinogenic property, so has to be cleaned properly, preferably daily. The incidence of carcinoma of the Cervix and the penis is almost 'nil' in Jews community and negligible in Muslim community as they have circumcision (removal of the foreskin) ritually on religious basis (Immediately after birth in Jews and during childhood in case of Muslim community). At the same time, prepuce is rich with sensory nerve endings and very sensitive and have an important role in the sexual act and a source of sexual pleasure for the individual and his partner. So routine circumcision is not to be encouraged. But we have to stress the importance of cleaning of the sub-preputial space and coronal sulcus daily to all the male population and children have to be trained to retract and clean their penis daily from childhood onwards as one brushes his teeth. Many people do not know that prepuce is retractable. If at all, they clean only the tip of glans. We are coming across cases with infection or growth in elderly people, who never bother or never attempt to retract their foreskin. The foreskin has to be retracted completely, exposing the coronal sulcus and to be cleaned daily with ordinary plain water. The presence of smegma for years is a risk for carcinoma and the uncleaned prepuce is vulnerable for infection. Presence of any ulcers, growth or swelling will result in inflammatory phimosis. Congenital phimosis and preputial adhesions are definite indications for circumcision whereas in inflammatory phimosis, the underlying causes should be attended properly and after the completion of treatment, circumcision can be planned if necessary. This sub-preputial space can get infected and inflamed with anaerobic organisms like Fuso-spirochaetes (*Borrelia vincenti*, Refringens or balanitidis along with fusiform bacilli). Betalactam antibiotics along with the tablet Metronidazole for adequate duration along with regular and frequent cleaning. It will be difficult to clean the phimotic prepuce. In such a situation, we have to instruct the individuals to follow this procedure: Stretch the foreskin beyond the glans penis and pass the urine after closing the preputial orifice, then let it out. This procedure has to repeated not less than thrice during every act of micturition. This act will help to clean the space and the antibiotics will act better and the patient will benefit quickly. Women also have smegma collection (Not marked) around the labial folds and over the clitoral hood.

Hypospadias (Urethra opens at the ventral aspect of the penis and **Epispadias** (urethra opens on the dorsal aspect of the glans penis) are congenital anomalies. The incidence of Hypospadias (is around 3%in a urology clinic and 25% in a STI clinic) is more common than Epispadias. In hypospadias individuals, the urethra will be shorter than in normal individuals and it will be devoid of the terminal 12 mm portion of the squamous epithelial lining of the urethra which offers protection against bacterial infection in normal individuals. So, the hypospadias individuals are more vulnerable for infections and reported more in a STI clinic. The degree of hypospadias varies with individuals. Glandular hypospadias is more common and the penile, peno-scrotal and perineal hypospadias are rare, but associated with infertility as they are not able to deposit the sperms into the vagina during intercourse. Because of the shorter urethra, it exerts a force during erection and produces a ventral curvature during erection, which is called **Chordee**.

During erection of penis on stimulation, there will be a scanty mucoid secretion appearing at tip of penis (through urethral orifice) which is called as pre-ejaculatory fluid or precum or prosemen. It is secreted by **Litre's glands** (mucus secreting glands situated over the roof and side walls of urethra) and Cowper's glands. It helps in eliminating the acidic deposits over urethral floor after the prolonged years of passing urine which is inimical to viable spermatozoa and ensures the safe delivery of semen inside the vagina of the partner. It also provides lubrication for the preputial movements over the glans and also removes the debris on the floor of urethra. Some individuals after noticing this secretion for the first time, imagine as urethral discharge of STD origin and becomes venerophobic, or semen leaked out earlier which will result in sexual dysfunction. Actually, it a boon to mankind and not to be worried. We have to educate our future generations in this regard also.

For a happy sexual health, one should take care their genitals as if we are brushing our teeth daily to maintain our oral health. Many men don't know that the prepuce can be retracted and they never visualized their coronal sulcus at all till their dusk of life in spite of having children and regular sex due to lack of proper sex education either at school or college level. But this will not be healthy always. The unattended genital hygiene would result in infection, Smegma-lith and even carcinoma of their own and of their partners. So genital hygiene in men (Fig. 15.1) is very important.

Male Genital Hygiene

- Teach everyone since childhood onwards (school days) that the foreskin of penis is retractable.
- The retraction has to be demonstrated to everyone that they can visualize the coronal sulcus.
- Smegma and female genital secretions (after an intercourse) tend to collect on the coronal sulcus and extend over glans penis.
- The space underneath the foreskin can act as a platform for infections.
- Coronal sulcus has never been seen by many men even in their late 60s, but say they used to clean.
- The space underneath the foreskin has to be cleaned daily during bathing as we brush daily our teeth.
- Prefer plain water for cleaning rather than using soap and water.
- If anyone has problem in retracting the foreskin they have to report to their doctors.

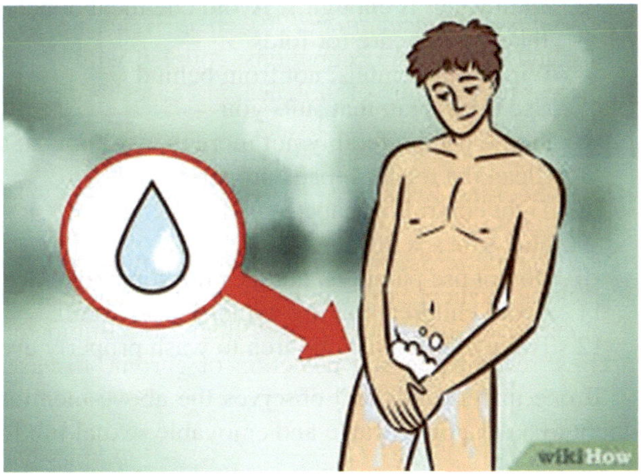

Fig. 15.1 Importance of genital hygiene

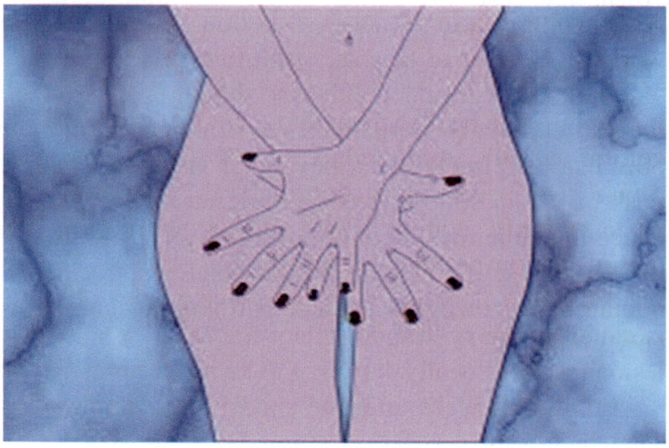

Fig. 15.2 Importance of female genital hygiene

- Phimosis is a condition in which they cannot be able to retract their foreskin—Could be congenital or acquired secondary to infection and Inflammation.
- Congenital phimosis has to be corrected by circumcision. Otherwise the individual is susceptible for infections and possibly malignancy in later years.
- Unhygienic penis is harmful not only to the individual but also to his sex partner.
- Pissing and washing after coitus will do well for everyone.

To maintain a happy and healthy sexual life, the female partners of men also have to care for their genitals and hygiene (Fig. 15.2).

Female Genital Hygiene

- **Take care of yourself….**
- **Avoid unnecessary trouble…..**

1. Wash your genitals, every time you use toilets
2. Plain water is enough… Avoid chemical douche
3. Take special care for folds
4. Wipe your genitals, not from behind
5. Use the napkin that suits you.
6. Single pad preferably not more than 4 hours at a stretch
7. Clean the reusable pads properly
8. Tight control of diabetes mellitus…
9. Play safe sex always
10. Do not use pampers, huggies for hours together
11. Avoid children playing without inner wears
12. Train your female children to wash properly every time.

If one understands and observes the above-mentioned points, there will be no doubt to have a pleasurable and enjoyable sexual life for ever.

Chapter 16
Diagnostic Armamentarium in Sexually Transmitted Diseases

Akshay Samagani

Introduction

Sexually transmitted diseases (STDs) are one of the significant health issues among sexually active men. The diagnosis of STDs such as genital ulcer diseases is usually clinical, yet investigations play an important role in the confirmation, atypical presentations, adequate treatment and follow-up.

Genital Ulcer Diseases

Common genital ulcer diseases include syphilis, chancroid, herpes genitalis, lymphogranuloma venereum and donovanosis. All these have varied clinical presentations. Following are commonly used bedside tests. Sterile swabs are used to collect specimen such as discharge or exudates from the floor of the ulcer. They are easy-to-do and inexpensive tests aiding in quick diagnosis.

- Gram stain: crystal violet, iodine, alcohol and safranin are used to identify bacteria.
- Tzanck smear: 10% Giemsa stain is used to identify viral etiology like herpes genitalis.
- Darkground microscopy: unstained/transparent organisms are illuminated with transverse beam of light creating a dark background.

A. Samagani (✉)
Department of Dermatology, Venereology and Leprosy, RajaRajeswari Medical College and Hospital, Dr. M.G.R. Educational and Research Institute, Bangalore, India

Vasan S S et al. (eds.), *Men's Health*,
https://doi.org/10.1007/978-3-031-76898-9_16

Syphilis

Organism: *Treponema pallidum* (sp.)
Clinical Presentation:
Primary syphilis: single indurated, painless ulcers with lymph node (LN) involvement (painless).
Secondary syphilis: psoriasiform skin lesions and oral ulcers.
Tertiary syphilis: cardiac and neural system involved.
Specimen: Exudates from ulcers or lymph node aspirate.
Microscopy/Immunofluorescence:
Darkground microscopy: Spiral motile *Treponema pallidum* with corkscrew and angular movements.
Serology: Seropositivity after 4–6 weeks.

- Non-treponemal test: **VDRL** (significant if >1:16), RPR, TRUST.
- Specific blood test: **TPHA/TPPA** (confirmatory), TPI, IgM antibody tests.
- Most sensitive and earliest to be positive (3 weeks): IgM FTA Abs.
- Others: ELISA.

Molecular Techniques: Polymerase Chain Reaction (PCR), RT-PCR.
Skin Biopsy: In atypical cases such as HIV.

Herpes Genitalis/Simplex

Organism: *Herpes simplex virus* (HSV 2 > HSV 1).
Clinical Presentation: Grouped vesicles with multiple painful ulcers/erosions.
Tender Inguinal lymph node involvement.
Specimen: Disruption of vesicles—swabs from ulcer floor (Dacron swabs).
Microscopy/Immunofluorescence:
Tzanck smear: Multinucleated giant cells, ballooning degeneration.
Culture: Human diploid fibroblast cell/HeLa or McCoy cell culture. Green Monkey Kidney Cell medium
Serology: ELISA, Western blot.
Molecular Techniques: PCR.
Skin Biopsy: In atypical cases such as HIV.

Chancroid

Organism: *Hemophilus ducreyi.*
Clinical Presentation: Solitary/few painful ulcers with ragged edges and discharge. Inguinal lymph node enlargement with tenderness is seen.

Specimen: Swabs from ulcer floor, LN aspirate.
Microscopy/Immunofluorescence:
Gram stain: Gram negative coccobacilli: School of fish/rail road/tram track appearance.
Culture:
Gonococcal agar base +2% bovine hemoglobin +5% fetal calf serum.
Mueller-Hilton agar base with 5% chocolate horse blood.
Dermal tests: Ito-Reenstierna Test is an intradermal test where a cutaneous reaction as an inflammatory papule of 0.5–1 cm size, within 48 hrs following an intradermal injection of vaccine consisting of killed *H. ducreyi* is considered positive.
Serology: Enzyme Immuno-Assay, immunoblot test, Complement fixation test.
Molecular techniques: Multiplex PCR.

Lympho-Granuloma Venereum (LGV)

Organism: *Chlamydia trachomatis* (L1, L2, L3).
Clinical presentation: Solitary painless papule/vesicle/pustule/ulcer with painful/painless LN enlargement (Groove Sign) with or without proctitis.
Specimen: Swabs from ulcer floor, LN aspirate.
Microscopy/Immunofluorescence:
Micro-IF, IF, Giemsa and iodine staining methods- inclusion bodies in WBC.
Culture:
Cell line: HeLa-229, McCoy, Yolk sac, Human diploid fibroblast cells
Serology: Complement fixation test (titer $\geq$1:64).
Molecular Techniques: PCR.

Donovanosis/Granuloma Inguinale

Organism: *Klebsiella granulomatis*.
Clinical Presentation: Solitary or multiple painless ulcers without LN involvement (pseudo bubo).
Specimen: Swabs from ulcer floor—crush the specimen between two clinical slides (Rajam Rangaiah method).
Microscopy/Immunofluorescence:
Giemsa stain: Intracellular Donovan bodies in mononuclear cells—safety pin appearance.
Culture: Heat-inactivated fetal calf and peripheral blood mononuclear cells.
Molecular Techniques: PCR.
Skin Biopsy: Crush the biopsy specimen and stain with Giemsa stain (Greenblatt and Barfield method). Histopathology shows plasma cell infiltrate.

Urethral Discharge

Organisms: *Neisseria gonorrhea, Escherichia coli, Chlamydia trichomatis*, etc.
Clinical Presentation: Mucopurulent/purulent/greenish discharge usually associated with dysuria.
Specimen: Urethral meatal swab to be obtained.

- Discharge deposited on external genitalia.
- >2–3 h post voiding or OVERNIGHT SAMPLE.
- 'Milk' the penis on ventral part, from base to tip 3–5 times.

Microscopy/Immunofluorescence:
Gram stain:

- Urethral discharge: ≥2 polymorphonuclear (PMN) cells per oil immersion field.
- First void urine sediments: ≥10 PMN per high-power field.

Culture:

- Modified Thayer Martin medium: *Neisseria gonorrhea.*
- Cell culture: McCoy, HeLa cell lines:

Sample collection: Columnar cells of urethra devoid of mucopurulent discharge for the detection of Chlamydia trichomatis.
Serology:

- Complement fixation test.
- Direct fluorescent antibody test.
- Enzyme immunoassay (EIA) in non-gonococcal urethritis.

Nucleic Acid Hybridization Techniques (preferred for the diagnosis due to high sensitivity)—PAGE 2 assay by Genprobe (FDA approved).
Molecular Techniques: PCR, Transcription-mediated amplification, Ligase chain reaction.

Anogenital Warts

Organism: *Human papilloma virus* (HPV).
Most common (90%): HPV 6 and 11.
High risk: HPV 16 and 18.
Clinical Presentation: Epitheliotropic/verruciform growth over external genitalia caused by human papilloma virus.
Diagnosis is clinical with urethroscopy/anoscopy/dermascopy.
Histopathology:

Koilocytes—mature keratinocytes with large hyperchromatic nuclei and perinuclear halo present in outer epidermal layers.

HIV

Organism: *Human Immunodeficiency Virus* (HIV).
Clinical manifestations: Varied clinical presentations depending on the staging.
Salient Features of HIV Infection:

- Infection begins at day 0.
- HIV- RNA plasma appears first—10 days after infection, peaks about 30 days after infection, decreases until about 40 days and plateaus.
- Acute phase of infection is defined as time between appearance of HIV-RNA before HIV is detectable by immunoassays, lasts between 5 and 40 days after RNA appears.
- HIV p24 antigen can be detected by fourth-generation assays 15 days after infection and peaks at 30 days after infection and undetectable by 45 days.
- IgM HIV becomes detectable by third-generation immunoassays about 22 days after infection and have an initial peak after 35 days of infection. Later decreases until 38 days when IgG becomes detectable by second generation immunoassays.
- IgG antibodies increase until 38 days when IgG becomes detectable by second generation immunoassays.
- IgG antibodies increase until 45–50 days after infection, then can be detected by first generation immunoassays.

HIV Tests

Laboratory tests employed for the diagnosis of HIV infection may be classified into the following groups:

Antibody-Based Tests

Screening Tests

ELISA (ENZYME LINKED IMMUNOSORBENT ASSAY)—most widely used with high sensitivity.

- First generation- whole viral lysate.
- Second generation—recombinant antigen.
- Third generation—synthetic peptide.

- Fourth generation- antigen + antibody (simultaneous detection of HIV Antigen and antibody)—HIV duo.

Note: Antibody can be detected in a majority of individuals within 6–12 weeks after infection using the earlier generation of assays. But it can be detected within 3–4 weeks when using newer third-generation ELISA due to their ability to detect p24 antigen. The fourth-generation ELISA will be of value in detecting early infection. The window period can be shortened to 2 weeks using p24-antigen assay. The principles of ELISA are classified as indirect, competitive, sandwich and capture assay.

RAPID Tests

- Dot blot assays/tridot.
- Particle agglutinantion.
- HIV spot and comb tests.
- Fluorimetric microparticle technologies.

Supplemental or Confirmatory Tests

Western blot
It is more specific assay. In this, antibodies against numerous proteins are detected.

- Env (gp160, gp120, and gp41).
- gag (p55, p24, and p17),
- pol (p66, p51, p31).

Immunofluorescent assay (IFA).
Line immunoassay.
Radio-immuno-precipitation assay.

Other Tests

P24 antigen test.
Culture (peripheral blood mononuclear cells).
Polymerase chain reaction (PCR)- HIV RNA or proviral DNA.

Alternative to Classical Tests

Oral fluid (saliva) HIV tests- ORAQUICK ADVANCE RAPID HIV TEST.
Urine tests—Ig G antibodies.

Table 16.1 The conditions causing false positive and false negative results

False positive results	False negative results
Autoimmune disorders	Window period (up to 3 months)
Haematological malignancies(plasmocytoma)	Immunosuppressive therapy
Alcoholic hepatitis	Replacement transfusion
Connective tissue disorders	B-cell dysfunction
Acute rheumatic fever	Malignant disorder
Multiple pregnancies	Late-stage disease (immune collapse)
Multiple transfusions	Technical error
Post-vaccination including HIV vaccine	
Chronic renal failure	
Positive rapid plasma regain test	
Technical errors, etc.	

Drug Susceptibility Tests

Drug susceptibility test to be considered if there is no significant reduction in viral load and improvement of CD4 count at the end of 6 months of anti-retroviral therapy.

The conditions causing false positive and false negative results are as follows. (Table 16.1).

•

Newer Techniques for Differentiation of Acute and Chronic Infections

(i) *Serological Testing Algorithm for Recent HIV Seroconversion (STARHS)*: By deliberately combining highly sensitive with less sensitive antibody i.e. a sensitive commercial assay and a customized, less-sensitive (*LS or "detuned"*) version of this assay, it is possible to identify the specimen from a recently infected individual.

(ii) *Capture enzyme immunoassay*: Principle is based on relative proportion of anti- HIV IgG antibodies on the total IgG antibodies present in a specific volume of serum.

(iii) *Drug Resistance Tests*: Resistance is the ability of a virus to multiply rapidly in patients taking medications. It consists of genotypic and phenotypic testing.

(iv) *Coreceptor Tropism Analysis*: It determines the type of cellular coreceptor (either CCR5 or CXCR4) that an HIV-infected individual's dominant viral population uses to gain access to host cells.

(v) *Human Leukocyte Antigen Testing*: It should be performed before initiating abacavir-based therapy, as there is genetic predisposition to development of abacavir hypersensitivity.

Bibliography

1. Caruso G, Giammanco A, Virruso R, Fasciana T. Current and future trends in the laboratory diagnosis of sexually transmitted infections. Int J Environ Res Public Health. 2021;18(3):1038.
2. Prabhakar P, Narayanan P, Deshpande GR, Das A, Neilsen G, Mehendale S, Risbud A. Genital ulcer disease in India: etiologies and performance of current syndrome guidelines. Sex Transm Dis. 2012;39(11):906–10.
3. Roett MA, Mayor MT, Uduhiri KA. Diagnosis and Management of Genital Ulcers. Indian J Clin Pract. 2013;24(6):507–15.
4. Fearon M. The laboratory diagnosis of HIV infections. Can J Infect Dis Med Microbiol. 2005;16(1):26–30.
5. Murphy G, Parry JV. Assays for the detection of recent infections with human immunodeficiency virus type 1. Euro Surveill. 2008;13(36):18966.

Chapter 17
Case Scenario in Sexually Transmitted Diseases

K. Hanumanthayya, Fahim L. H. Rajiwate, and Hanumanthayya Keloji

Every patient entering OPD will have his/her own story to narrate. With information at a click away, patients verify their symptoms on the internet. They also expect us to believe them and treat as per their assumption. We as clinicians have learnt over years to listen to them attentively, but also to take correct decision in terms of investigation to arrive at a diagnosis and treat accordingly and appropriately (sometimes it is difficult to convince such patients with internet knowledge). This chapter includes some noteworthy cases to discuss.

Case 1

A 40-year-old female, senior and high placed bank manager of a nationalized bank comes to OPD with history of having pigmentation of both hands and feet for a month. It is not troubling her, but all her assistants and bank customers were asking her, what has happened to her hands. Hence she had come for consultation. She consulted a physician who made a preliminary diagnosis of tuberculosis of adrenal glands, and pigmentation of both her hands and feet are secondary to adrenal gland insufficiency (Figs. 17.1, 17.2 and 17.3) and was investigated accordingly. The investigations were negative. On further detailed history, she is a sexually active woman with unprotected sexual activity with multiple partners. On investigation [HIV (PCR), HBsAg, HCV, VDRL, VDRL, TPHA], her TPHA test was found to be

K. Hanumanthayya · H. Keloji
Dermatology Department, Sri Devaraj Urs Medical College, Kolar, Karnataka, India

F. L. H. Rajiwate (✉)
Ankur Healthcare / Raja Rajeswari Medical College and Hospital, Bangalore, Karnataka, India

Vasan S S et al. (eds.), *Men's Health*, https://doi.org/10.1007/978-3-031-76898-9_17

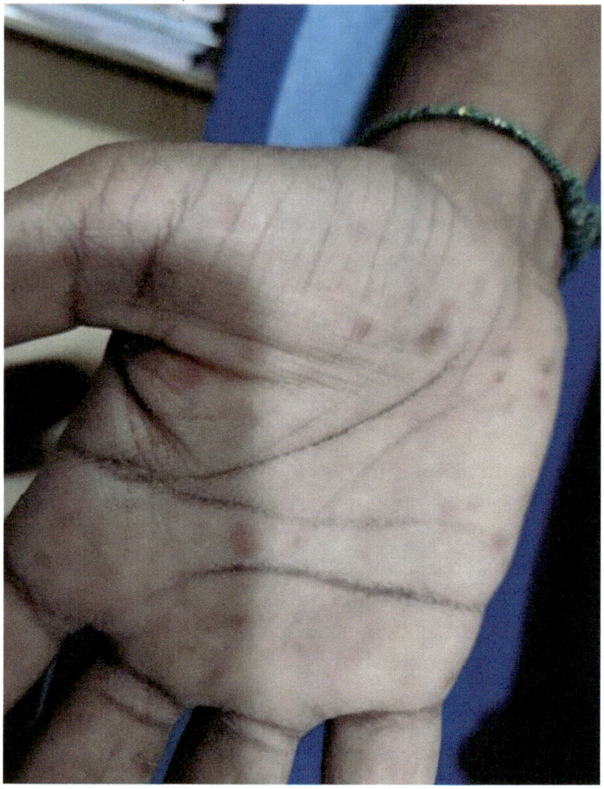

Fig. 17.1 Macular pigmentation of hands. (Photo courtesy Dr. Murgan S)

positive, and other parameters were negative. Inj. BBenzathine Penicillin 24 lakhs [12 lac in each buttock] was given deep intramuscularly, after test dose. Three doses at weekly intervals. The lesions regressed fully.

Case 2

In one of our clinical meetings, a case was discussed. The patient was our own medical colleague. He came to medical OPD, with the pain in the chest of 1 month duration. The clinician asked for X ray of the chest. A lytic lesion was seen in the sternum and few ribs, and his provisional diagnosis was multiple myeloma. I asked him two questions: (1) Has the sexual history been taken, and (2) Was VDRL test done? All my colleagues were angry as it was questioning the integrity of colleague. Finally, it was agreed upon and VDRL test was performed. VDRL test came positive. Inj. Benzathine Penicillin 24 lakhs [12 lac on each buttock] was given deep intramuscularly, after a test dose. Three doses were given at weekly intervals, lesions regressed fully. Lytic lesions are common in flat bones, and sclerotic lesions are common in long and stout bones in secondary syphilis.

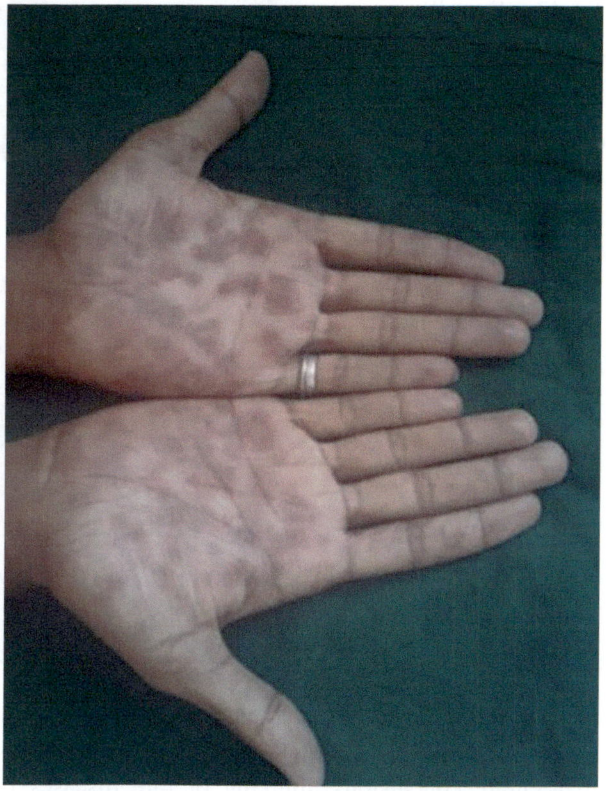

Fig. 17.2 Macular pigmentation of hands. (Photo courtesy Dr. Hanumanthayya)

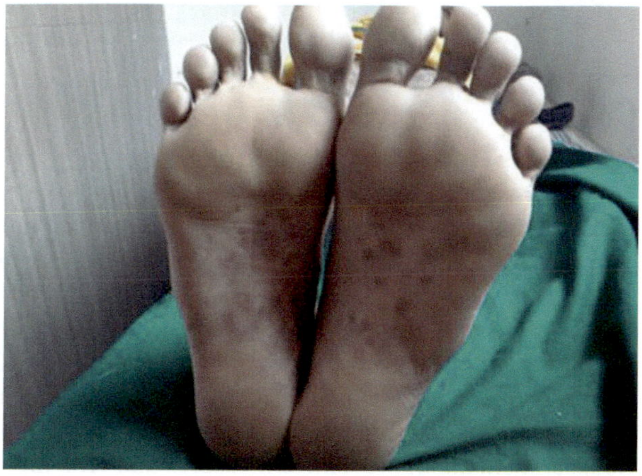

Fig. 17.3 Macular pigmentation of feet. (Photo courtesy Dr Hanumanthayya)

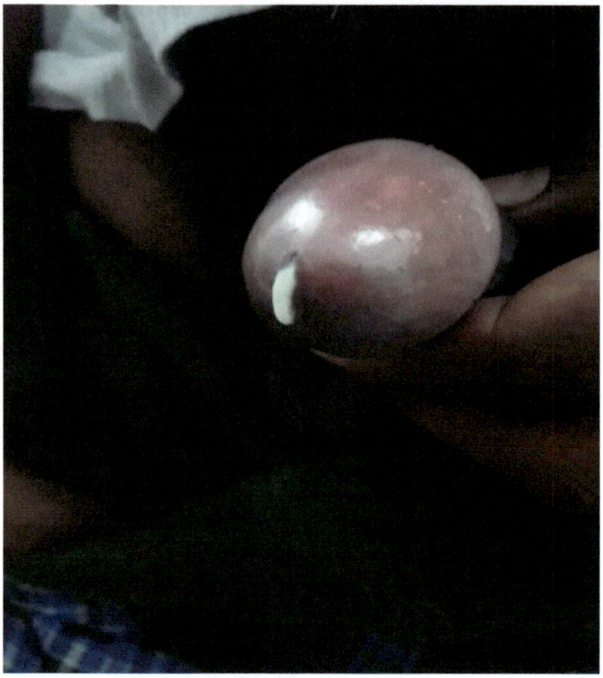

Fig. 17.4 Frank Pus Oozing Per Urethra

Lesson learnt: We are most likely to be correct when considering common diseases first. While considering rare presentations of common diseases may still lead to accurate conclusions, thinking of rare diseases rarely results in the correct diagnosis.

Case 3

A 21-year-old college student came to OPD with the complaints of passing buttermilk like discharge from his genitals. On examination of his genitals, frank pus was coming from urethra (Fig. 17.4). Pus examined under microscopy showed plenty of neutrophils and intracytoplasmic gram-negative diplococci were present. A diagnosis of gonorrhea was made. Patient received Inj. Ceftriaxone 250 mg intramuscular, Cap Doxycycline 100 mg bid for 7–10 days with sexual counselling.

Lesson learned: STD patients will be giving peculiar history, do not scold them, listen patiently, and analyze clinical symptoms, signs carefully, and treat them. Counsel them about preventive measures and HIV infection.

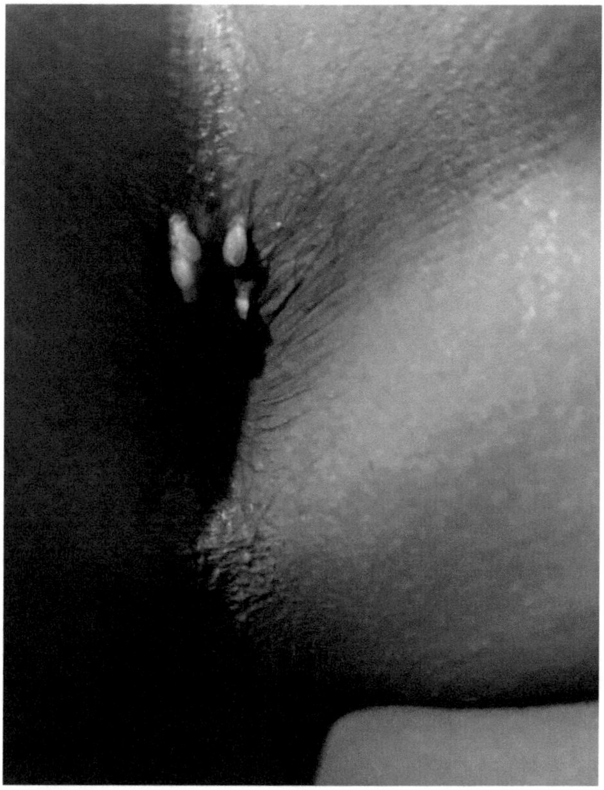

Fig. 17.5 Perianal viral warts

Case 4

A group of software employees were referring the internet, analyzing their symptoms and making their own diagnosis. They were suggesting in the clinic to believe their diagnosis and treat them accordingly. Many a times, it will become difficult to convince such persons and the conversation ends up in argument. A member of this group came to OPD with the complaint of pain during defecation, and he feels a mass in the anal and perianal lesion. On examination, anal fissure, and viral warts in perianal region were noted (Fig. 17.5). On detailed sexual history. He revealed the following: (1) All the members are homosexuals (one member is bisexual) with multiple partners of unprotected intercourse. (2) All of them took one tablet of 500 mg Azithromycin or 100 mg Doxycycline (to prevent STDs), one tablet of 10 mg Diazepam (to calm the brain), and one tablet of 500 mg Paracetamol (not to have body pain). After the medication they indulge in anal sex. In counseling, it was explained that Azithromycin and Doxycycline are effective only against bacterial infections and do not protect against viral or fungal STDs. Anal fissure was treated with SITZ bath in the anus and for viral wart topical application of Podophylline once in 3 days for 3–4 sessions or till lesions settle, whichever is later.

Part IV
Men's Health Clinic

Chapter 18
What Is Men's Health and Why Is It Gaining Popularity?

Vasan S S

Introduction

Men's health is a specialized field of medical practice and research focused on health issues uniquely affecting men. This includes both physical and mental health concerns, spanning from specific diseases and conditions to broader lifestyle and behavioral factors. The increasing focus on men's health is driven by recognition of gender-specific health disparities and the need for tailored healthcare approaches to improve outcomes for men. This section provides a detailed overview for medical professionals, highlighting the key aspects and recent developments in this growing field.

Definition and Scope

Men's health encompasses the study, diagnosis, prevention, and treatment of conditions that are either unique to men or more prevalent among them. This includes but is not limited to:

- *Cardiovascular Diseases*: Conditions such as coronary artery disease, heart attacks, and strokes are leading causes of mortality among men [1].
- *Reproductive and Sexual Health*: Issues such as erectile dysfunction, prostate health, and infertility.
- *Mental Health*: Higher rates of suicide, substance abuse, and reluctance to seek mental health care [2].

Vasan S S (✉)
Ankur Healthcare, Bangalore, Karnataka, India
e-mail: vasan@ankurhealthcare.com

Vasan S S et al. (eds.), *Men's Health*,
https://doi.org/10.1007/978-3-031-76898-9_18

- *Cancers*: Higher incidence of prostate, lung, and liver cancers in men [3].

Key Statistics

1. *Life Expectancy Gap*: On average, men have a shorter life expectancy than women. In the United States, for example, men live approximately 5 years less than women [4].
2. *Chronic Diseases*: Men are more likely to suffer from chronic conditions such as hypertension, diabetes, and cardiovascular diseases at younger ages compared to women [5].
3. *Mental Health*: Men account for 75% of all suicides in the United States, reflecting significant mental health challenges [6].

Factors Driving the Popularity of Men's Health

Increasing Awareness and Advocacy

- *Health Campaigns*: Public health campaigns and men's health organizations have raised awareness about the importance of preventive care and early diagnosis. Movements like Movember have been instrumental in promoting awareness of prostate cancer, testicular cancer, and mental health issues among men [7].

Gender-Specific Research

- *Biomedical Research*: There has been a surge in gender-specific research, leading to a better understanding of how diseases affect men and women differently. This has highlighted the need for tailored treatments and preventive strategies [8].

Social and Cultural Shifts

- *Changing Norms*: Societal shifts towards recognizing and addressing men's health issues have encouraged men to seek medical help. Breaking down stigmas associated with masculinity and health care has been crucial in this process [9].

Health Disparities

- *Addressing Inequalities*: Health professionals and policymakers are increasingly focused on addressing health disparities that negatively impact men's health, including socioeconomic factors, access to healthcare, and educational outreach [10].

Economic Impact

- *Workplace Health*: The economic burden of poor men's health on productivity and healthcare systems has prompted businesses and governments to invest in men's health initiatives [11].

Recent Developments and Initiatives

Personalized Medicine

- *Genomic Research*: Advances in genomics and personalized medicine are providing new insights into male-specific health issues and enabling more precise treatments [12].

Digital Health

- *Telemedicine and Apps*: The rise of digital health platforms has made healthcare more accessible to men, who may be less likely to visit traditional healthcare facilities. These platforms offer convenient ways to manage health, including mental health support [13].

Preventive Health Programs

- *Screening and Vaccination*: Increased focus on preventive health measures, including regular screenings for common male cancers and vaccinations, has been shown to improve outcomes [2].

Mental Health Initiatives

- *Community Programs*: Initiatives aimed at reducing the stigma around mental health and providing support through community-based programs are gaining traction [14].

Policy and Advocacy

- *Government Initiatives*: Governments are implementing policies to address men's health issues more effectively, including funding research and health programs specifically targeted at men [15].

Conclusion

Men's health is an essential and expanding area of medical practice that addresses the unique health challenges faced by men. The growing popularity of men's health is driven by increased awareness, targeted research, cultural shifts, and recognition of the economic impact of men's health issues. Medical professionals play a critical role in advancing this field through continued research, patient education, and the implementation of gender-specific health interventions. By focusing on the distinct needs of men, healthcare providers can significantly improve health outcomes and quality of life for this population.

References

1. American Heart Association. Heart disease and stroke statistics—2020 update: a report from the American Heart Association. Circulation.
2. Centers for Disease Control and Prevention (CDC). National Vital Statistics Reports, Vol. 69, No. 12; 2020.
3. National Cancer Institute. Cancer Stat Facts: Prostate Cancer; 2021.
4. Centers for Disease Control and Prevention (CDC); 2021.
5. World Health Organization (WHO). Global TB Rep 2020; 2020.
6. American Foundation for Suicide Prevention. Suicide statistics; 2020.
7. Movember Foundation. About Movember; 2020.
8. Harvard Health Publishing. Men's health: what you need to know; 2018.
9. Mahalik JR, Burns SM, Syzdek M. Masculinity and perceived normative health behaviors as predictors of men's health behaviors. Soc Sci Med. 2007;64:2201.
10. Healthy People 2020. Men's health; 2019.
11. World Economic Forum. The economic burden of poor health; 2018.
12. Collins FS, Varmus H. A new initiative on precision medicine. N Engl J Med. 2015;372:793.

13. Bashshur RL, et al. The empirical foundations of telemedicine interventions for chronic disease management. Telemed J E Health. 2016;20(9):769–800.
14. National Institute of Mental Health. Men and mental health; 2020.
15. Department of Health and Human Services. Men's health equity and policy; 2019.

Chapter 19
Mens Health: Unique Health Challenges in Southeast Asia and the far East

Vasan S S

Introduction

The Southeast Asia and Far East regions face distinct health challenges shaped by a combination of genetic, environmental, socioeconomic, and cultural factors. This chapter provides a detailed overview of these unique health challenges, aiming to inform medical professionals about the epidemiological trends, disease burdens, and healthcare needs in these regions.

Epidemiological Overview

Southeast Asia and the Far East are home to over two billion people, with diverse populations and varying health profiles. Rapid urbanization, economic growth, and lifestyle changes have significantly influenced the health landscape. Understanding these trends is crucial for developing effective public health strategies.

Vasan S S (✉)
Ankur Healthcare, Bangalore, Karnataka, India
e-mail: vasan@ankurhealthcare.com

Vasan S S et al. (eds.), *Men's Health*,
https://doi.org/10.1007/978-3-031-76898-9_19

Communicable Diseases

Tuberculosis (TB)

- *Prevalence*: The WHO reports that Southeast Asia accounts for 44% of global TB cases, with significant burdens in countries like India, Indonesia, and the Philippines [1].
- *Challenges*: High population density, HIV coinfection, and drug-resistant TB strains complicate control efforts.

Dengue Fever

- *Incidence*: The region experiences recurrent dengue outbreaks, with over one million cases reported annually [2].
- *Vector Control*: Challenges in managing mosquito populations and climate change exacerbate the spread.

Malaria

- *Burden*: While malaria incidence has declined, it remains a significant problem in rural and border areas, particularly in Myanmar, Laos, and Cambodia [3].
- *Drug Resistance*: Resistance to artemisinin-based therapies poses a significant threat.

Hepatitis B and C

- *Prevalence*: High rates of chronic hepatitis B and C infections are seen in the region, leading to liver cirrhosis and cancer [4].
- *Prevention and Treatment*: Efforts focus on vaccination, blood safety, and antiviral therapies.

Noncommunicable Diseases (NCDs)

Cardiovascular Diseases

- *Risk Factors*: High prevalence of hypertension, diabetes, and smoking contribute to cardiovascular diseases. In China and India, NCDs account for 80% of deaths [5].
- *Prevention*: Strategies include promoting healthy diets, physical activity, and controlling tobacco use.

Diabetes

- *Epidemic*: Southeast Asia is experiencing a diabetes epidemic, with the International Diabetes Federation estimating 88 million diabetics in the region [6].
- *Management*: Improved screening, public awareness, and access to insulin and other treatments are critical.

Cancer

- *Common Types*: Liver, lung, and stomach cancers are particularly prevalent, influenced by factors like hepatitis infections, smoking, and dietary habits [7].
- *Screening and Treatment*: Early detection and access to cancer treatments remain key challenges.

Environmental and Occupational Health

Air Pollution

- *Impact*: Cities like Beijing, Delhi, and Jakarta face severe air pollution, linked to respiratory diseases and cardiovascular mortality [8].
- *Interventions*: Policies aimed at reducing emissions from vehicles and industry are crucial.

Occupational Hazards

- *Industries*: High-risk industries, including mining, construction, and manufacturing, contribute to occupational injuries and diseases.
- *Regulations*: Strengthening workplace safety regulations and enforcement is essential.

Nutritional Challenges

Undernutrition

- *Children*: Malnutrition remains a critical issue, with stunting affecting 30% of children under five in some areas [9].
- *Programs*: Nutritional interventions and food security programs are necessary to combat undernutrition.

Overnutrition

- *Obesity*: Concurrently, rising obesity rates due to sedentary lifestyles and high-calorie diets are contributing to NCDs [5].
- *Public Health Campaigns*: Initiatives to promote balanced diets and physical activity are required.

Mental Health

Stigma and Access

- *Barriers*: Cultural stigma and limited access to mental health services hinder effective treatment.
- *Interventions*: Community-based mental health programs and destigmatization efforts are vital.

Suicide Rates

- **Statistics:** Countries like South Korea and Japan report high suicide rates, influenced by socioeconomic pressures and mental health issues [10].
- **Prevention:** Enhanced mental health support and crisis intervention strategies are needed.

Infectious Disease Control and Immunization

Vaccine-Preventable Diseases

- *Programs*: Immunization programs have significantly reduced diseases like polio and measles, but coverage gaps remain.
- *Strategies*: Expanding vaccine access and addressing vaccine hesitancy are critical.

Emerging Infectious Diseases

- *Surveillance*: Strengthening disease surveillance and response systems is crucial in managing outbreaks like SARS, MERS, and COVID-19 (WHO, 2020).
- *Preparedness*: Regional cooperation and public health infrastructure improvements are necessary for better preparedness.

Conclusion

The Southeast Asia and Far East regions face unique and complex health challenges that require tailored public health strategies. Medical professionals must consider the socioeconomic, environmental, and cultural contexts when addressing these issues. By enhancing disease surveillance, promoting preventive health measures, and improving healthcare access and quality, significant strides can be made in improving the health outcomes of these populations.

References

1. World Health Organization (WHO). Global Tuberculosis Report 2020; 2020.
2. World Health Organization (WHO). Dengue and severe dengue; 2019.
3. World Health Organization (WHO). World Malaria Report 2018; 2018.
4. World Health Organization (WHO). Hepatitis B and C; 2020.
5. International Diabetes Federation (IDF). IDF Diabetes Atlas; 2019.
6. GLOBOCAN. Cancer Today; 2020.
7. Health Effects Institute (HEI). State of Global Air 2019; 2019.
8. UNICEF. The State of the World's Children 2019; 2019.
9. World Health Organization (WHO). Noncommunicable diseases; 2020.
10. World Health Organization (WHO). Suicide in the world: Global Health Estimates; 2019.

Chapter 20
Why Is Male Life Span Lower Than Women's? Insights for Southeast Asia

Vasan S S

Introduction

Across the globe, men tend to have shorter life expectancies than women. This disparity is particularly pronounced in Southeast Asia, where cultural, socioeconomic, and biological factors interplay to affect male health outcomes. This chapter explores the reasons behind the shorter male life span in Southeast Asia, supported by relevant data, and provides guidelines for medical professionals to address these issues.

Life Expectancy Disparities in Southeast Asia

In Southeast Asia, the life expectancy for men is consistently lower than that for women. According to the World Bank data [1], the average life expectancy at birth for men in Indonesia is 69 years, compared to 73 years for women. Similar trends are observed in other countries within the region, such as Thailand and Vietnam.

Vasan S S (✉)
Ankur Healthcare, Bangalore, Karnataka, India
e-mail: vasan@ankurhealthcare.com

Vasan S S et al. (eds.), *Men's Health*,
https://doi.org/10.1007/978-3-031-76898-9_20

Key Factors Contributing to Lower Male Life Expectancy

Biological Differences

- *Genetic and Hormonal Factors*: Men are more prone to certain genetic disorders and have higher levels of testosterone, which has been linked to riskier behaviors and higher mortality rates [2].
- *Immune System Differences*: Women generally have stronger immune responses, contributing to lower infection rates and better recovery outcomes from diseases [3].

Behavioral Factors

- *Risk-Taking Behaviors*: Men are more likely to engage in risky behaviors such as smoking, excessive alcohol consumption, and unsafe driving, leading to higher rates of accidents and lifestyle-related diseases [4].
- *Violence and Occupational Hazards*: Higher involvement in physically demanding and hazardous occupations, coupled with a higher likelihood of being victims or perpetrators of violence, increases mortality risks for men.

Health-Seeking Behavior

- *Reluctance to Seek Medical Help*: Cultural norms often discourage men from seeking medical care, leading to delayed diagnosis and treatment of diseases [5].
- *Preventive Care*: Men are less likely to participate in preventive health screenings, resulting in late detection of chronic diseases such as hypertension and diabetes.

Noncommunicable Diseases (NCDs)

- *Cardiovascular Diseases*: Men have a higher prevalence of heart disease and stroke compared to women. In Southeast Asia, cardiovascular diseases are a leading cause of death among men [3].
- *Cancer*: Higher rates of tobacco use contribute to lung, liver, and oral cancers, which are more prevalent in men. The Global Cancer Observatory [6, 7] reports higher incidence rates of liver and lung cancers in men in Southeast Asia.

Communicable Diseases

- *Infectious Diseases*: Men are more susceptible to certain infectious diseases due to occupational exposures and lifestyle factors. For example, tuberculosis incidence is higher among men in countries like Indonesia and the Philippines [8].

Socioeconomic Factors

- *Access to Healthcare*: Economic barriers and lower health literacy among men can limit access to quality healthcare services.
- *Education and Employment*: Lower educational attainment and employment in high-risk industries contribute to poorer health outcomes.

Reproductive Health

- *Infertility*: Male infertility can be a significant issue, influenced by environmental factors, lifestyle, and occupational hazards.

Limited Access to Andrology Services: Access to specialized reproductive health services might be limited, impacting men's ability to seek help for fertility issues.

Specific Malignancy Risks

Men in Southeast Asia face a higher risk of certain malignancies compared to women:

- *Lung Cancer*: Due to higher smoking rates, men are significantly more likely to develop lung cancer. According to the International Agency for Research on Cancer (IARC), lung cancer incidence in men is twice that of women in many Southeast Asian countries.
- *Liver Cancer*: Men are at a higher risk of liver cancer, partly due to higher rates of hepatitis B and C infections and alcohol consumption. The IARC reports that liver cancer incidence in men in Southeast Asia is one of the highest globally.
- *Oral Cancer*: High rates of tobacco and betel nut chewing among men in the region lead to a greater incidence of oral cancers.

Hospitalization Risks

Men are more likely to be hospitalized for certain conditions:

- *Injuries and Accidents*: Higher involvement in manual labor and risk-taking behaviors result in more frequent hospitalizations due to injuries and accidents [4].
- *Cardiovascular Events*: Men are more prone to acute cardiovascular events such as heart attacks and strokes, leading to higher hospitalization rates for these conditions.

Access to Healthcare

Men face unique barriers to accessing healthcare:

- *Economic Barriers*: Financial constraints can limit access to necessary healthcare services. Men in lower socioeconomic strata may prioritize family needs over personal health expenditures.
- *Health Literacy*: Lower health literacy among men can result in a lack of awareness about available healthcare services and the importance of regular check-ups.
- *Cultural Norms*: Cultural expectations and norms often discourage men from seeking medical help, viewing it as a sign of weakness.

Men's Health—Healthcare Access and Utilization

Men's Health

- *Limited Access to Healthcare*: In rural areas, access to healthcare facilities can be limited, resulting in delayed diagnoses and treatment.
- *Reluctance to Seek Medical Help*: Cultural norms and gender roles may discourage men from seeking medical advice, leading to a lack of preventive care.

Women's Health

- *Healthcare Services*: Women utilize healthcare services more frequently, partly due to reproductive health needs.
- *Preventive Screenings*: Women are more likely to seek preventive care and participate in health screenings such as mammograms and Pap smears.

Lifestyle Factors

Diet and Nutrition

- *Traditional Diets*: Traditional diets in some regions may be high in unhealthy fats and sugars, contributing to an increased risk of chronic diseases like heart disease and diabetes.

Substance Use

- *Smoking and Alcohol*: High rates of smoking and alcohol consumption are prevalent in some areas, leading to respiratory diseases and other health risks.

Chronic Diseases

Cardiovascular Diseases

- *Heart Disease*: Heart disease is a significant concern, exacerbated by lifestyle factors like smoking and poor diet.

Conclusion

Men's health in Southeast Asia and the Far East faces unique challenges due to cultural, environmental, occupational, and lifestyle factors. Addressing these challenges requires a multifaceted approach, including culturally sensitive health education, improved access to healthcare, workplace safety improvements, and targeted interventions to address chronic diseases and mental health issues. Additionally, reducing stigma

Guidelines for Medical Professionals

Promote Preventive Health Measures:

- *Screenings and Vaccinations*: Encourage regular health checkups and screenings for hypertension, diabetes, and cancers. Promote vaccination against hepatitis B and HPV.
- *Health Education*: Provide targeted health education focusing on the importance of preventive care and healthy lifestyle choices.

Address Behavioral Risks:

- *Smoking Cessation Programs*: Implement programs to reduce tobacco use among men, including counseling and nicotine replacement therapies.

- *Alcohol and Substance Abuse*: Develop interventions to reduce alcohol consumption and substance abuse, incorporating both medical and psychological support.

Enhance Access to Healthcare:

- *Affordable Services*: Advocate for policies that make healthcare services more affordable and accessible to men, particularly in rural areas.
- *Workplace Health Programs*: Collaborate with employers to implement workplace wellness programs that include regular health screenings and health promotion activities.

Improve Mental Health Services:

- *Mental Health Awareness*: Increase awareness about mental health issues and reduce the stigma associated with seeking mental health care.
- *Support Services*: Provide accessible mental health services, including counseling and psychiatric care, tailored to the needs of men.

Foster Health-Seeking Behavior:

- *Community Engagement*: Engage community leaders to promote positive health-seeking behaviors among men.
- *Cultural Sensitivity*: Develop culturally sensitive health interventions that address the specific needs and preferences of men in Southeast Asia.

Conclusion

The lower life expectancy of men in Southeast Asia is a multifaceted issue influenced by biological, behavioral, and socioeconomic factors. By understanding these underlying causes and implementing targeted health interventions, medical professionals can help improve the health outcomes and life expectancy of men in the region. Enhancing preventive care, addressing behavioral risks, and improving access to healthcare are essential steps in bridging the life expectancy gap between men and women.

References

1. World Bank. Life expectancy at birth, total (years) – Indonesia; 2020.
2. Gandhi M, Aweeka F, Greenblatt RM, Blaschke TF. Sex differences in pharmacokinetics and pharmacodynamics. Annu Rev Pharmacol Toxicol. 2017;44:499–523.
3. Klein SL, Flanagan KL. Sex differences in immune responses. Nat Rev Immunol. 2016;16(10):626–38.
4. World Health Organization (WHO). Noncommunicable diseases country profiles 2018; 2018.
5. Galdas PM, Cheater F, Marshall P. Men and health help-seeking behaviour: literature review. J Adv Nurs. 2015;49(6):616–23.
6. The Global Cancer Observatory. Cancer Today; 2018.
7. International Agency for Research on Cancer (IARC). Global Cancer Observatory; 2018.
8. World Health Organization (WHO). Global Tuberculosis Report 2020; 2020.

Chapter 21
Prioritizing Men's Health: Key Elements for Longevity and Wellness

Vasan S S

As medical professionals, our mission extends beyond treating illnesses; it encompasses promoting overall well-being and longevity. In this pursuit, understanding and addressing the unique health needs of men is paramount. Despite advances in medicine, men still have a shorter life expectancy compared to women. However, proactive management of key health elements can significantly impact longevity and quality of life. This chapter aims to delve deeper into these key elements, providing comprehensive strategies backed by evidence and references.

Cardiovascular Health

Cardiovascular disease (CVD) remains the leading cause of death among men globally, claiming approximately 1 in 4 male lives. Men are more prone to CVD due to factors like hypertension, high cholesterol, smoking, obesity, and sedentary lifestyle.

Management Strategies

- Encourage regular aerobic exercise, aiming for at least 150 min per week, to improve cardiovascular fitness and reduce the risk of CVD.
- Promote a heart-healthy diet rich in fruits, vegetables, whole grains, lean proteins, and unsaturated fats, while minimizing intake of saturated and trans fats, sodium, and added sugars.

Vasan S S (✉)
Ankur Healthcare, Bangalore, Karnataka, India
e-mail: vasan@ankurhealthcare.com

Vasan S S et al. (eds.), *Men's Health*,
https://doi.org/10.1007/978-3-031-76898-9_21

- Monitor and manage blood pressure and cholesterol levels through lifestyle modifications such as dietary changes, weight management, smoking cessation, and, if necessary, pharmacological interventions.

Prostate Health

Prostate conditions, including benign prostatic hyperplasia (BPH) and prostate cancer, are prevalent among men, especially with advancing age. Prostate cancer is the second most common cancer in men globally, with significant morbidity and mortality if not detected early.

Management Strategies

- Encourage regular prostate cancer screenings, typically recommended for men aged 50 and older, using prostate-specific antigen (PSA) testing and digital rectal examination.
- Provide thorough education to patients regarding the benefits, limitations, and potential risks associated with prostate cancer screening to facilitate informed decision-making.
- Highlight the importance of lifestyle factors, including maintaining a healthy weight, engaging in regular physical activity, and consuming a diet rich in fruits, vegetables, and antioxidants, which may reduce the risk of prostate cancer progression

Stroke Risk Assessment

Stroke is a significant cause of morbidity and mortality in men, with risk factors including hypertension, diabetes, smoking, obesity, and physical inactivity. Early identification of stroke risk factors and implementation of preventive measures are essential for reducing the burden of stroke in male populations.

Assessment Strategies

- Utilize validated risk assessment tools such as the Framingham Stroke Risk Score or the American Heart Association/American Stroke Association's Life's Simple 7 to estimate individual stroke risk based on age, sex, blood pressure, cholesterol levels, diabetes status, smoking status, diet, and physical activity.

- Conduct noninvasive screenings such as blood pressure measurements, lipid profiles, and blood glucose testing during routine healthcare visits to identify modifiable risk factors for stroke.
- Educate patients about the signs and symptoms of stroke, emphasizing the importance of seeking immediate medical attention if they experience sudden onset of facial drooping, arm weakness, or speech difficulty, which are hallmark signs of stroke.

Fracture Risk Assessment

Osteoporosis and fragility fractures are significant concerns in aging male populations, contributing to morbidity, mortality, and impaired quality of life. Identifying individuals at high risk of fracture allows for early intervention and preventive measures to reduce fracture risk.

Assessment Strategies

- Use validated tools such as the Fracture Risk Assessment Tool (FRAX) to estimate individual 10-year fracture risk based on age, sex, body mass index, previous fracture history, parental history of hip fracture, smoking status, alcohol consumption, glucocorticoid use, and secondary osteoporosis conditions.
- Perform noninvasive bone mineral density (BMD) testing using dual-energy X-ray absorptiometry (DXA) scans to assess bone density and identify individuals with osteoporosis or osteopenia who are at increased risk of fracture.
- Administer self-administered questionnaires such as the Osteoporosis Self-Assessment Tool for Men (OSTAM) to screen for fracture risk based on age, weight, height, and history of previous fractures.

Mental Health

Men are less likely than women to seek help for mental health issues, leading to underdiagnosis and inadequate treatment of conditions such as depression, anxiety, and suicide risk.

Management Strategies

- Integrate mental health screenings into routine healthcare visits, particularly for high-risk populations such as veterans and middle-aged men.
- Foster an environment of open communication to reduce stigma surrounding mental health issues and encourage men to seek help when needed.
- Offer evidence-based treatments, including psychotherapy, medication, and lifestyle interventions, tailored to address the specific mental health needs of male patients.

Sexual Health

Sexual dysfunction, including erectile dysfunction (ED) and low testosterone levels, can significantly impact men's quality of life and interpersonal relationships.

Management Strategies

- Conduct comprehensive evaluations for men experiencing sexual health concerns, including a detailed medical history, physical examination, and appropriate laboratory testing.
- Offer evidence-based treatments for ED and low testosterone, including lifestyle modifications, medications such as phosphodiesterase type 5 (PDE5) inhibitors and testosterone replacement therapy, and psychosexual therapies.
- Address underlying medical conditions such as diabetes, hypertension, and cardiovascular disease that may contribute to sexual dysfunction through targeted management and lifestyle interventions.

Conclusion

By aggressively managing key elements of men's health, including cardiovascular health, prostate health, mental health, testicular health, and sexual health, medical professionals can play a pivotal role in improving longevity and overall well-being in male patients. Through evidence-based interventions, proactive screening, and patient education, we can empower men to prioritize their health and lead fulfilling lives.

Further Reading

1. World Health Organization. Global Health Observatory (GHO) data: top 10 causes of death; 2017. Retrieved from https://www.who.int/gho/mortality_burden_disease/causes_death/top_10/en/
2. American Cancer Society. Key statistics for prostate cancer; 2021. Retrieved from https://www.cancer.org/cancer/prostate-cancer/about/key-statistics.html
3. Centers for Disease Control and Prevention. Suicide Mortality in the United States, 1999–2019; 2020. Retrieved from https://www.cdc.gov/nchs/products/databriefs/db398.htm
4. American Cancer Society. Key statistics for testicular cancer; 2021. Retrieved from https://www.cancer.org/cancer/testicular-cancer/about/key-statistics.html
5. Mayo Clinic. Erectile dysfunction; 2020. Retrieved from https://www.mayoclinic.org/diseases-conditions/erectile-dysfunction/diagnosis-treatment/drc-20355782
6. American Heart Association/American Stroke Association. Stroke risk factors; 2020. Retrieved from https://www.stroke.org/en/about-stroke/stroke-risk-factors
7. Framingham Heart Study. Framingham stroke risk score; 2021. Retrieved from https://framinghamheartstudy.org/fhs-risk-functions/stroke-risk/
8. National Osteoporosis Foundation. Fracture Risk Calculator (FRAX®); 2021. Retrieved from https://www.nof.org/prevention/fracture-risk-calculator/
9. Kanis JA, et al. Development and use of FRAX® in osteoporosis. Osteoporos Int. 2008;19(4):385–97.
10. Osteoporosis Canada. Osteoporosis Self-Assessment Tool for Men (OSTAM); 2021. Retrieved from https://osteoporosis.ca/osteoporosis-self-assessment-tool-for-men-ostam/

Chapter 22
Men's Health: Preventive Diagnostics

Vasan S S

Blood Tests and Non-invasive Tests

In preventive health diagnostics for men, blood tests are essential in assessing the risk for heart attacks, fractures, strokes, malignancies (cancers), and sexual health issues. These blood tests, combined with other noninvasive assessments, help healthcare professionals identify risk factors early and provide targeted interventions. Below are the most relevant blood tests for each risk category, along with their utility in guiding health decisions.

Blood Test for Cardiovascular Health Risk

To evaluate cardiovascular health and the risk of heart attacks, these blood investigation are crucial:

- *Lipid Profile*: Measures cholesterol levels, including LDL (bad cholesterol), HDL (good cholesterol), total cholesterol, and triglycerides.
- *High-Sensitivity C-Reactive Protein (hs-CRP)*: Indicates inflammation, which is a risk factor for cardiovascular disease.
- *Fasting Glucose and Hemoglobin A1c (HbA1c)*: Assesses blood sugar levels to detect diabetes or prediabetes, which increases heart attack risk.
- *Homocysteine Levels*: Elevated homocysteine is associated with a higher risk of heart disease.

Vasan S S (✉)
Ankur Healthcare, Bangalore, Karnataka, India
e-mail: vasan@ankurhealthcare.com

Vasan S S et al. (eds.), *Men's Health*,
https://doi.org/10.1007/978-3-031-76898-9_22

- *Natriuretic Peptides (e.g., BNP or NT-proBNP)*: Indicators of heart stress, used to assess heart failure risk.

Fracture / Bone Health Risk Blood Tests

These blood tests are used to assess bone health and fracture risk:

- *Serum Calcium and Vitamin D*: Critical for bone health; low levels can indicate a higher fracture risk.
- *Parathyroid Hormone (PTH)*: Helps regulate calcium; elevated levels may suggest bone metabolism issues.
- *Alkaline Phosphatase*: An enzyme related to bone turnover; abnormal levels can indicate bone diseases.
- *Bone-Specific Alkaline Phosphatase (BSAP)*: A more specific test for assessing bone formation activity.

Stroke Risk Blood Tests

Blood tests that help evaluate stroke risk and related factors include:

- *Lipid Profile*: High cholesterol and triglycerides are risk factors for stroke.
- *Fasting Glucose and HbA1c*: High blood sugar increases the risk of stroke.
- *Blood Pressure Measurement*: Although not a blood test, high blood pressure is a significant risk factor for stroke.
- *Complete Blood Count (CBC)*: Can detect conditions like anemia or polycythemia, which can influence stroke risk.

Malignancy (Cancer) Risk Blood Tests

These blood tests are used for cancer screening and risk assessment:

- *Prostate-Specific Antigen (PSA)*: Elevated PSA can indicate prostate cancer risk.
- *Carcinoembryonic Antigen (CEA)*: A marker used to detect certain types of cancer, including colorectal cancer.
- *Alpha-Fetoprotein (AFP)*: Often used to screen for liver cancer.
- *CA-125*: Used to detect ovarian cancer, but can also be indicative of other cancers.
- *CA 19-9*: A marker for pancreatic cancer.

Sexual Health Risk Blood Tests

To assess sexual health risks, particularly related to hormonal balance and cardiovascular health, these blood tests are relevant:

- *Testosterone Level*: Low testosterone can affect sexual function and libido.
- *Luteinizing Hormone (LH) and Follicle-Stimulating Hormone (FSH)*: Can indicate issues with hormonal regulation.
- *Estradiol*: An estrogen hormone; high levels in men can suggest hormonal imbalances.
- *Prolactin*: Elevated prolactin can reduce libido and cause erectile dysfunction.
- *Thyroid-Stimulating Hormone (TSH)*: Thyroid issues can affect sexual function.

Conclusion

Blood tests play a crucial role in preventive diagnostics for men's health. By combining these tests with other noninvasive assessments, healthcare professionals can identify and address risks early, reducing the likelihood of severe outcomes like heart attacks, fractures, strokes, cancer, or sexual dysfunction. If you have concerns about any of these risks, speak with your healthcare provider to discuss the most appropriate tests and preventive measures.

Men's Health Preventive Diagnostics: Blood Tests and Noninvasive Assessments

In preventive health diagnostics for men, blood tests are indispensable tools for assessing the risk of heart attacks, fractures, strokes, malignancies (cancers), and sexual health issues. Combined with noninvasive assessments, these tests help healthcare professionals identify risk factors early and provide targeted interventions. Below are the most relevant blood tests for each risk category, along with their utility in guiding health decisions.

Heart Attack Risk Blood Tests

To evaluate cardiovascular health and the risk of heart attacks, consider the following blood tests:

- *Lipid Profile*: Measures cholesterol levels, including LDL (bad cholesterol), HDL (good cholesterol), total cholesterol, and triglycerides.

- *High-Sensitivity C-Reactive Protein (hs-CRP)*: Indicates inflammation, a significant risk factor for cardiovascular disease.
- *Fasting Glucose and Hemoglobin A1c (HbA1c)*: Assesses blood sugar levels to detect diabetes or prediabetes, which increases heart attack risk.
- *Homocysteine Levels*: Elevated homocysteine is associated with a higher risk of heart disease.
- *Natriuretic Peptides (e.g., BNP or NT-proBNP)*: Indicators of heart stress, used to assess heart failure risk.

Fracture Risk Blood Tests

To assess bone health and fracture risk, consider the following blood tests:

- *Serum Calcium and Vitamin D*: Critical for bone health; low levels can indicate a higher fracture risk.
- *Parathyroid Hormone (PTH)*: Helps regulate calcium; elevated levels may suggest bone metabolism issues.
- *Alkaline Phosphatase*: An enzyme related to bone turnover; abnormal levels can indicate bone diseases.
- *Bone-Specific Alkaline Phosphatase (BSAP)*: A more specific test for assessing bone formation activity.

Stroke Risk Blood Tests

Blood tests that help evaluate stroke risk and related factors include:

- *Lipid Profile*: High cholesterol and triglycerides are risk factors for stroke.
- *Fasting Glucose and HbA1c*: High blood sugar increases the risk of stroke.
- *Blood Pressure Measurement*: High blood pressure is a significant risk factor for stroke.
- *Complete Blood Count (CBC)*: Can detect conditions like anemia or polycythemia, which can influence stroke risk.

Malignancy (Cancer) Risk Blood Tests:

For cancer screening and risk assessment, consider the following blood tests:

- *Prostate-Specific Antigen (PSA)*: Elevated PSA can indicate prostate cancer risk.
- *Carcinoembryonic Antigen (CEA)*: A marker used to detect certain types of cancer, including colorectal cancer.

- *Alpha-Fetoprotein (AFP)*: Often used to screen for liver cancer.
- *CA-125*: Used to detect ovarian cancer, but can also be indicative of other cancers.
- *CA 19-9*: A marker for pancreatic cancer.

Sexual Health Risk Blood Tests

To assess sexual health risks, particularly related to hormonal balance and cardiovascular health, consider the following blood tests:

- *Testosterone Level*: Low testosterone can affect sexual function and libido.
- *Luteinizing Hormone (LH) and Follicle-Stimulating Hormone (FSH)*: Can indicate issues with hormonal regulation.
- *Estradiol*: High levels in men can suggest hormonal imbalances.
- *Prolactin*: Elevated prolactin can reduce libido and cause erectile dysfunction.
- *Thyroid-Stimulating Hormone (TSH)*: Thyroid issues can affect sexual function.

Age-Wise Specific Genomic Testing

- *Younger Men (Under 40)*: Focus on genetic testing for inherited conditions with early onset, such as familial hypercholesterolemia (FH) and hereditary thrombophilia.
- *Middle-Aged Men (40–65)*: Consider genetic testing for age-related conditions like hereditary heart diseases and hereditary cancers (e.g., BRCA mutations).
- *Older Men (Over 65)*: Prioritize genetic testing for age-related neurodegenerative disorders like Alzheimer's disease and Parkinson's disease.

Metabolomic Profiling

Metabolomics offers insights into metabolic health and longevity through the analysis of small molecules (metabolites) in biological samples. Specific metabolomic tests for longevity may include:

- *Lipidomic Profiling*: Evaluates lipid metabolism patterns associated with cardiovascular risk and aging-related diseases.
- *Amino Acid Profiling*: Identifies amino acid imbalances linked to metabolic disorders and aging-related decline in muscle mass.
- *Oxidative Stress Markers*: Measures oxidative stress levels, a key contributor to aging and age-related diseases.

Microbiome Analysis

The gut microbiome plays a crucial role in health and longevity. Microbiome analysis can identify microbial composition patterns associated with longevity and inform interventions to promote gut health. Specific tests may include:

- *16S rRNA Sequencing*: Identifies bacterial species and diversity in the gut microbiome.
- *Metagenomic Sequencing*: Provides deeper insights into microbial gene content and functional potential.
- *Microbiome Health Index*: Quantifies overall gut microbiome health based on microbial composition and function.

Genetic Tests for Longevity

- *Telomere Length Testing*: Telomeres are protective caps at the ends of chromosomes that shorten with age and cellular stress. Shorter telomeres are associated with increased mortality risk.
- *APOE Genetic Testing*: Variants of the APOE gene are associated with Alzheimer's disease risk. Knowing one's APOE genotype may inform lifestyle modifications and preventive strategies.

Endothelial Testing and Vascular Compliance

Endothelial dysfunction and vascular aging are key contributors to cardiovascular disease and heart attacks. Assessing endothelial function and vascular compliance can help detect early signs of vascular damage and guide preventive strategies. Important tests include:

- *Flow-Mediated Dilation (FMD)*: Measures the ability of blood vessels to dilate in response to increased blood flow, reflecting endothelial function.
- *Pulse Wave Velocity (PWV)*: Assesses arterial stiffness, a marker of vascular aging and predictor of cardiovascular events.
- *Arterial Compliance Measurement*: Determines the elasticity of arteries, providing insights into vascular health and aging-related changes.

Comorbidity Stratification

- *Cardiovascular Comorbidities*

  - Integrate genetic testing for familial hypercholesterolemia (FH) and other inherited lipid disorders to guide treatment strategies and improve cardiovascular outcomes.
  - Utilize noninvasive tests such as pulse wave velocity (PWV) and endothelial function assessments to evaluate vascular health and predict cardiovascular risk.
  - Implement specific diagnostic tests like coronary computed tomography angiography (CCTA) for coronary artery disease (CAD) evaluation in high-risk individuals.

- *Metabolic Comorbidities (Diabetes, Obesity)*
  - Incorporate genetic testing for monogenic forms of diabetes and obesity to personalize treatment and lifestyle interventions.
  - Utilize noninvasive tests such as liver ultrasound and fibroscan for assessing liver health in individuals with metabolic syndrome.
  - Implement specific diagnostic tests like oral glucose tolerance test (OGTT) for early detection of impaired glucose tolerance and diabetes risk stratification.

- *Cancer Comorbidities*
  - Offer genetic testing for hereditary cancer syndromes (e.g., Lynch syndrome, familial adenomatous polyposis) to guide cancer screening and risk-reduction strategies.
  - Utilize noninvasive tests such as stool-based DNA tests (e.g., Cologuard) for colorectal cancer screening in high-risk individuals.
  - Implement specific diagnostic tests like multiparametric magnetic resonance imaging (mpMRI) for prostate cancer detection and risk stratification.

In preventive health diagnostics for men, a holistic strategy encompassing blood tests, noninvasive assessments, genetic profiling, and specific tests tailored to age and comorbidities is essential for promoting longevity and mitigating health risks. Integrating these diverse modalities provides a comprehensive evaluation of individual health status and enables targeted interventions to prevent adverse outcomes. Let's explore each component in detail:

Blood Tests

Blood tests serve as cornerstone assessments in men's health, enabling the evaluation of various risk factors across multiple domains. Key blood tests include:

- Lipid Profile: Measures cholesterol levels to assess cardiovascular risk.
- High-Sensitivity C-Reactive Protein (hs-CRP): Indicates inflammation and cardiovascular risk.

- Fasting Glucose and Hemoglobin A1c (HbA1c): Assesses diabetes risk and glycemic control.
- Natriuretic Peptides: Indicates heart stress and risk of heart failure.
- Serum Calcium and Vitamin D: Critical for bone health and fracture risk assessment.
- Prostate-Specific Antigen (PSA): Screens for prostate cancer risk.
- Testosterone Level: Evaluates hormonal balance and sexual health.

Noninvasive Assessments

Noninvasive tests complement blood tests by providing additional insights into cardiovascular health, bone density, neurological function, and sexual health. These assessments include:

- Electrocardiogram (ECG): Evaluates heart rhythm and electrical activity.
- Bone Density Measurement (DXA): Assesses bone mineral density and fracture risk.
- Carotid Ultrasound: Detects carotid artery disease and stroke risk.
- Penile Doppler Ultrasound: Assesses vascular causes of erectile dysfunction.
- Vertebral Fracture Assessment (VFA): Identifies prevalent vertebral fractures.
- Transcranial Doppler (TCD): Measures cerebral blood flow velocity for stroke risk assessment.

Genetic Profiling

Genetic tests offer insights into inherited predispositions to certain diseases and can guide personalized interventions. Examples include:

- Familial Hypercholesterolemia (FH) Genetic Testing: Identifies individuals at high risk of premature cardiovascular disease.
- APOE Genotyping: Predicts Alzheimer's disease risk based on genetic variants.
- Hereditary Cancer Panel: Screens for mutations associated with hereditary cancers (e.g., BRCA1/2).

Specific Tests for Longevity

In addition to traditional assessments, emerging diagnostic modalities focus on longevity and healthy aging. These include:

- Telomere Length Testing: Reflects cellular aging and mortality risk.

- Metabolomic Profiling: Identifies metabolic signatures associated with longevity and disease risk.
- Gut Microbiome Analysis: Evaluates gut microbial composition and its impact on health.
- Endothelial Function Testing: Assesses vascular health and predicts cardiovascular risk.
- Frailty Assessment Tools: Quantify physical frailty and predict adverse health outcomes in older adults.

Conclusion

Blood tests play a crucial role in preventive diagnostics for men's health. By combining these tests with other noninvasive assessments, healthcare professionals can identify and address risks early, reducing the likelihood of severe outcomes like heart attacks, fractures, strokes, cancer, or sexual dysfunction. If you have concerns about any of these risks, speak with your healthcare provider to discuss the most appropriate tests and preventive measures.

Younger Men (Under 40)

For younger men with comorbidities such as obesity, diabetes, or familial risk factors, the following tests are recommended:

- Lipid Profile: Assess cardiovascular risk, especially in individuals with familial hypercholesterolemia (FH).
- Fasting Glucose and HbA1c: Screen for diabetes and monitor glycemic control, particularly in those with a family history of diabetes.
- Genetic Testing: Consider genetic screening for inherited conditions like FH or hereditary thrombophilia.
- Prostate-Specific Antigen (PSA): Offer prostate cancer screening in individuals with a family history of the disease.
- Lifestyle Counseling: Provide education on healthy lifestyle habits, including diet, exercise, and smoking cessation.

Middle-Aged Men (40–65)

Middle-aged men with comorbidities such as hypertension, metabolic syndrome, or early signs of cardiovascular disease should undergo comprehensive diagnostic evaluation, including:

- Lipid Profile and hs-CRP: Evaluate cardiovascular risk and inflammation status.
- Fasting Glucose and HbA1c: Screen for diabetes and assess glycemic control.
- Blood Pressure Measurement: Monitor hypertension and assess cardiovascular risk.
- Noninvasive Tests: Consider ECG, echocardiogram, and carotid ultrasound for cardiovascular risk assessment.
- Bone Density Measurement: Assess bone health in individuals with risk factors for osteoporosis.
- Cancer Screening: Offer age-appropriate cancer screenings based on family history and guidelines (e.g., colonoscopy, mammography).
- Genetic Testing: Evaluate genetic predispositions to cardiovascular diseases or hereditary cancers.

Older Men (Over 65)

For older men with comorbidities such as cardiovascular disease, osteoporosis, or cognitive impairment, the following tests are recommended:

- Lipid Profile, Natriuretic Peptides, and ECG: Assess cardiovascular risk and monitor heart health.
- Bone Density Measurement: Screen for osteoporosis and assess fracture risk.
- Cognitive Function Testing: Evaluate cognitive impairment using validated tools.
- Genetic Testing: Consider testing for genetic variants associated with age-related conditions like Alzheimer's disease or Parkinson's disease.
- Frailty Assessment: Assess physical frailty using standardized tools to guide interventions and care planning.
- Comprehensive Geriatric Assessment: Conduct a multidimensional evaluation to identify medical, functional, and psychosocial issues.

Further Reading

1. National Institutes of Health. Heart attack. 2021. Retrieved from https://www.nhlbi.nih.gov/health-topics/heart-attack
2. National Osteoporosis Foundation. Bone density exam/testing. 2021. Retrieved from https://www.nof.org/patients/diagnosis-information/bone-density-examtesting/
3. Centers for Disease Control and Prevention. Stroke. 2020. Retrieved from https://www.cdc.gov/stroke/index.htm
4. American Cancer Society. Cancer screening guidelines. 2021. Retrieved from https://www.cancer.org/healthy/find-cancer-early/cancer-screening-guidelines.html
5. Mayo Clinic. Erectile dysfunction. 2020. Retrieved from https://www.mayoclinic.org/diseases-conditions/erectile-dysfunction/symptoms-causes/syc-20355776

Chapter 23
Noninvasive Cardiovascular Risk Screening Tools and Their Utility for Risk Assessment

Vasan S S

Noninvasive cardiovascular risk screening tools are invaluable for assessing the risk of cardiovascular disease (CVD) in men. These tools provide critical information without the need for invasive procedures, enabling early detection and management of cardiovascular risk factors. Here are key noninvasive cardiovascular risk screening tools and their utility:

Electrocardiogram (ECG)

Utility

- *Heart Rhythm and Electrical Activity*: An ECG records the electrical activity of the heart and can detect arrhythmias, myocardial infarction, and other heart conditions.
- *Baseline Assessment*: Useful for establishing a baseline in patients with risk factors such as hypertension, diabetes, or a family history of CVD.
- *Monitoring*: Helps in monitoring the effectiveness of treatments for heart disease.

Vasan S S (✉)
Ankur Healthcare, Bangalore, Karnataka, India
e-mail: vasan@ankurhealthcare.com

Vasan S S et al. (eds.), *Men's Health*,
https://doi.org/10.1007/978-3-031-76898-9_23

Echocardiogram

Utility

- *Heart Structure and Function*: Provides detailed images of the heart's structure and function, including chamber size, wall motion, and valve function.
- *Detecting Heart Disease*: Can identify cardiomyopathies, valvular heart diseases, and pericardial diseases.
- *Cardiac Output*: Assesses the heart's pumping efficiency, which is critical in managing heart failure.

Carotid Ultrasound

Utility

- *Carotid Artery Stenosis*: Detects narrowing or blockages in the carotid arteries, which can indicate an increased risk of stroke.
- *Plaque Detection*: Measures the thickness of the carotid intima-media (CIMT) to identify atherosclerosis.
- *Predictive Value*: Provides information on overall cardiovascular risk due to the systemic nature of atherosclerosis.

Coronary Artery Calcium (CAC) Scoring

Utility

- *Atherosclerotic Plaque*: Quantifies calcium deposits in the coronary arteries using computed tomography (CT).
- *Risk Stratification*: Helps in stratifying the risk of coronary artery disease (CAD) and guiding preventive therapies.
- *Prognostic Tool*: High CAC scores are associated with a higher risk of cardiovascular events.

Ankle-Brachial Index (ABI)

Utility

- *Peripheral Arterial Disease (PAD)*: Compares blood pressure in the ankle with blood pressure in the arm to detect PAD.
- *Cardiovascular Risk Marker*: Low ABI values are indicative of increased cardiovascular risk and are associated with systemic atherosclerosis.
- *Simple and Accessible*: Easy to perform in a primary care setting.

Pulse Wave Velocity (PWV)

Utility

- *Arterial Stiffness*: Measures the speed at which blood pressure waves move down the vessel, indicating arterial stiffness.
- *Cardiovascular Risk Indicator*: Higher PWV is associated with increased cardiovascular risk and target organ damage.
- *Predictive Value*: Useful for predicting future cardiovascular events and mortality.

Endothelial Function Testing (e.g., Flow-Mediated Dilation)

Utility

- *Endothelial Health*: Assesses the ability of blood vessels to dilate in response to increased blood flow, reflecting endothelial function.
- *Early Indicator*: Endothelial dysfunction is an early indicator of atherosclerosis and cardiovascular disease.
- *Monitoring*: Can be used to monitor the effects of lifestyle interventions and pharmacotherapy on endothelial function.

Cardiorespiratory Fitness Testing (e.g., VO2 Max Testing)

Utility

- *Fitness Level*: Measures the maximum amount of oxygen the body can utilize during exercise, indicating cardiovascular fitness.

- *Risk Prediction*: Higher levels of cardiorespiratory fitness are associated with lower cardiovascular risk.
- *Intervention Monitoring*: Helps in assessing the effectiveness of exercise programs.

Heart Rate Variability (HRV) Analysis

Utility

- *Autonomic Function*: Measures variations in heart rate to assess autonomic nervous system function.
- *Stress and Health*: Lower HRV is associated with higher stress levels and increased cardiovascular risk.
- *Health Monitoring*: Can be used to monitor changes in health status and the impact of stress management techniques.

Conclusion

Noninvasive cardiovascular risk screening tools are essential for early detection, risk stratification, and management of cardiovascular disease in men. These tools provide valuable insights into heart health, vascular function, and overall cardiovascular risk, enabling healthcare professionals to implement targeted preventive strategies. By utilizing these noninvasive assessments, clinicians can improve outcomes and enhance the quality of life for their patients.

References

1. Grundy SM, et al. 2018 AHA/ACC/AACVPR/AAPA/ABC/ACPM/ADA/AGS/APhA/ASPC/NLA/PCNA guideline on the management of blood cholesterol. Circulation. 2018;139(25):e1082–143.
2. Kaneko K, et al. Endothelial dysfunction in cardiovascular diseases: role of long non-coding RNAs. J Atheroscler Thromb. 2021;28(3):231–40.
3. Ganz P, et al. Measurement of endothelial function: from research into clinical practice. Circulation. 2021;142(24):2450–65.
4. Nicholson JK, et al. Host-gut microbiota metabolic interactions. Science. 2012;336(6086):1262–7.
5. Blackburn EH, Epel ES. The telomere effect: a revolutionary approach to living younger, healthier, longer. New York: Grand Central Publishing; 2017.

Chapter 24
Incorporating Pulse Wave Velocity and Endothelial Function Assessment in Routine Clinical Practice to Identify High-Risk Men

Vasan S S

Hypothesis

Incorporating pulse wave velocity (PWV) and endothelial function assessments into routine clinical practice will enhance the early identification of men at high risk for cardiovascular events, leading to improved preventive strategies and outcomes.

Background

Cardiovascular disease (CVD) remains a leading cause of morbidity and mortality among men globally. Early identification of high-risk individuals is crucial for the implementation of preventive measures. Traditional risk factors, such as hypertension, hyperlipidemia, and diabetes, are well-established; however, emerging noninvasive assessments like PWV and endothelial function testing provide additional insights into vascular health and cardiovascular risk.

Pulse Wave Velocity (PWV)

PWV measures the speed of pressure waves moving through the arterial tree and is a direct marker of arterial stiffness. Increased arterial stiffness is associated with a higher risk of cardiovascular events and mortality. PWV is considered a gold standard for arterial stiffness assessment.

Vasan S S (✉)
Ankur Healthcare, Bangalore, Karnataka, India
e-mail: vasan@ankurhealthcare.com

Vasan S S et al. (eds.), *Men's Health*,
https://doi.org/10.1007/978-3-031-76898-9_24

Endothelial Function Assessment

Endothelial dysfunction is an early marker of atherosclerosis and can predict cardiovascular events independently of traditional risk factors. Flow-mediated dilation (FMD) is commonly used to assess endothelial function by measuring the dilation response of the brachial artery to increased blood flow.

Data Supporting the Hypothesis

PWV and Cardiovascular Risk

- *Meta-Analysis Findings*: A meta-analysis of 17 longitudinal studies involving over 15,000 participants found that each 1 m/s increase in PWV was associated with a 14% increase in cardiovascular events and a 15% increase in all-cause mortality [1].
- *Clinical Studies*: The Framingham Heart Study demonstrated that higher PWV values were predictive of cardiovascular events in a general population, independent of other risk factors [2].

Endothelial Function and Cardiovascular Risk

- *Prospective Studies*: A study of 1576 individuals found that impaired FMD was associated with a significantly higher risk of future cardiovascular events [3].
- *Independent Risk Predictor*: Endothelial dysfunction, measured by FMD, has been shown to predict cardiovascular events independently of traditional risk factors [4].

Combination of PWV and Endothelial Function

- *Enhanced Risk Stratification*: Combining PWV and endothelial function assessments provides complementary information about vascular health. A study involving 400 participants found that individuals with both high PWV and impaired FMD had a markedly increased risk of cardiovascular events compared to those with normal values in both tests [5].

Implementation in Clinical Practice

Routine Assessment

- *Screening Protocol*: Integrate PWV and endothelial function assessments into routine cardiovascular risk screening for men aged 40 and above, or younger if they have significant risk factors (e.g., family history of CVD, smoking, diabetes).
- *Annual Checkups*: Include these assessments in annual checkups for men with established cardiovascular risk factors or existing CVD.

Workflow Integration

- *Training*: Train healthcare providers on the use and interpretation of PWV and endothelial function tests.
- *Equipment*: Equip clinics with the necessary devices for measuring PWV and performing FMD.
- *Patient Education*: Educate patients on the importance of these tests and their role in preventing cardiovascular events.

Risk Stratification Algorithm

- *Initial Assessment*: Start with traditional risk factor assessment (e.g., lipid profile, blood pressure, diabetes screening).
- *Noninvasive Testing*: Follow up with PWV and endothelial function tests for individuals at intermediate or high risk based on initial assessment.
- *Intervention Strategies*: Use results to guide the intensity of preventive measures, such as lifestyle modifications, pharmacotherapy, and regular monitoring.

Conclusion

Incorporating PWV and endothelial function assessments into routine clinical practice holds significant promise for identifying high-risk men and preventing cardiovascular events. The combination of these noninvasive tests with traditional risk factor assessment provides a more comprehensive evaluation of cardiovascular risk, enabling targeted interventions and improving long-term outcomes.

Further Reading

1. Vlachopoulos C, Aznaouridis K, Stefanadis C. Prediction of cardiovascular events and all-cause mortality with arterial stiffness: a systematic review and meta-analysis. J Am Coll Cardiol. 2010;55(13):1318–27.
2. Mitchell GF, Hwang SJ, Vasan RS, Larson MG, Pencina MJ, Hamburg NM, et al. Arterial stiffness and cardiovascular events: the Framingham Heart Study. Circulation. 2010;121(4):505–11.
3. Gokce N, Keaney JF, Hunter LM, Watkins MT, Nedeljkovic ZS, Menzoian JO, et al. Predictive value of noninvasively determined endothelial dysfunction for long-term cardiovascular events in patients with peripheral vascular disease. J Am Coll Cardiol. 2002;41(10):1769–75.
4. Yeboah J, Crouse JR, Hsu FC, Burke GL, Herrington DM. Brachial flow-mediated dilation predicts incident cardiovascular events in older adults: the Cardiovascular Health Study. Circulation. 2007;115(18):2390–7.
5. Yoon HJ, Hong YJ, Kim JH, Park HW, Kim SY, Kim YJ, et al. Combined assessment of brachial-ankle pulse wave velocity and flow-mediated dilation is more predictive of the presence of coronary artery disease than either alone in patients with chest pain. Circ J. 2012;76(6):1463–71.

Chapter 25
Pulse Wave Velocity (PWV) and Endothelial Function Assessment: Principles and Pathophysiology

Vasan S S

Pulse Wave Velocity (PWV)

Principles

Pulse wave velocity (PWV) is a measure of the speed at which blood pressure waves move through the arteries. It is a direct indicator of arterial stiffness. The principle behind PWV measurement is based on the fact that stiffer arteries will transmit the pulse wave more quickly than more elastic arteries.

Pathophysiology Detection

1. *Arterial Stiffness*: PWV increases with arterial stiffness, which is a hallmark of aging and atherosclerosis. As arteries become stiffer, due to calcification and loss of elastic fibers, the speed of the pulse wave increases.
2. *Hypertension*: Chronic hypertension can lead to increased arterial stiffness. High blood pressure damages the arterial wall, promoting thickening and stiffening, which in turn raises PWV.
3. *Atherosclerosis*: Plaque buildup within the arteries contributes to arterial stiffness. PWV can detect early atherosclerotic changes before they become clinically apparent.
4. *Diabetes*: Diabetes accelerates arterial stiffening through glycation end-products that damage the arterial wall.

Vasan S S (✉)
Ankur Healthcare, Bangalore, Karnataka, India
e-mail: vasan@ankurhealthcare.com

Vasan S S et al. (eds.), *Men's Health*,
https://doi.org/10.1007/978-3-031-76898-9_25

Common Equipment

- *Complior*: Measures PWV using pressure sensors placed on the carotid and femoral arteries.
- *SphygmoCor*: Uses applanation tonometry to capture the pulse wave at the carotid and femoral sites and calculates PWV.
- *Vicorder*: Employs oscillometric cuffs on the upper thigh and neck to measure PWV.

Endothelial Function Assessment

Principles

Endothelial function is typically assessed by measuring flow-mediated dilation (FMD) of the brachial artery. This method evaluates the ability of the endothelium to release nitric oxide (NO) in response to increased shear stress, which causes vasodilation.

Pathophysiology Detection

1. *Endothelial Dysfunction*: Endothelial dysfunction is an early indicator of atherosclerosis and is characterized by a reduced capacity to produce NO. This can be due to oxidative stress, inflammation, or the presence of cardiovascular risk factors such as smoking, diabetes, and hyperlipidemia.
2. *Atherosclerosis*: Reduced FMD indicates impaired endothelial function, which is often an early sign of atherosclerosis even before structural changes in the arterial wall are evident.
3. *Cardiovascular Risk Factors*: Conditions such as hypertension, hyperlipidemia, diabetes, and obesity can impair endothelial function, detectable through diminished FMD response.
4. *Inflammation*: Inflammatory cytokines can impair NO synthesis and reduce FMD, linking inflammation to cardiovascular risk.

Common Equipment

- *Brachial Artery Ultrasound*: High-resolution ultrasound to measure the diameter of the brachial artery at rest and during reactive hyperemia.

- *EndoPAT*: Uses finger probes to measure pulse wave amplitude before and after occlusion of the brachial artery, providing an index of endothelial function.
- *Laser Doppler Flowmetry*: Measures skin blood flow in response to various stimuli to assess microvascular endothelial function.

Detailed Explanation and Clinical Utility

Pulse Wave Velocity (PWV)

PWV measurement typically involves placing pressure sensors or cuffs at two arterial sites (e.g., the carotid and femoral arteries). The time it takes for the pulse wave to travel between these two points is recorded and used to calculate the velocity. The formula to calculate Pulse Wave Velocity (PWV) is: $PWV=D/\Delta t$ where:

D = Distance (in meters) traveled by the pulse wave between two arterial sites.

Δt = Time delay (in seconds) between the pulse wave arrival at the two sites, measured by specific techniques such as ECG or tonometry.

Clinical Utility

- *Cardiovascular Risk Prediction*: PWV measures the speed at which pressure waves move through the arteries. It's a widely used indicator of arterial stiffness and cardiovascular risk.
- The distance DD is usually measured externally along the surface of the body between the two measurement points (e.g., carotid and femoral artery).
- Δt\Delta t is the pulse transit time, often determined through synchronized pressure or Doppler waveforms. A higher PWV indicates greater arterial stiffness and potentially higher cardiovascular risk.
- *Monitoring Treatment Efficacy*: PWV can be used to monitor the effectiveness of treatments aimed at reducing arterial stiffness, such as antihypertensive therapy.
- *Screening Tool*: PWV is useful in screening for subclinical cardiovascular disease in asymptomatic individuals.

Endothelial Function Assessment

Flow-mediated dilation (FMD) involves occluding blood flow in the brachial artery using a cuff inflated to suprasystolic pressure. After a period of occlusion, the cuff is released, and the subsequent increase in blood flow (reactive hyperemia) causes the artery to dilate. The degree of dilation is measured using ultrasound, and the change in diameter is calculated as a percentage of the baseline diameter.

Clinical Utility

- *Early Detection of Atherosclerosis*: Reduced FMD is an early marker of atherosclerosis, often preceding the development of significant arterial plaque.
- *Risk Stratification*: FMD provides additional information beyond traditional risk factors, aiding in more accurate risk stratification.
- *Guiding Therapy*: Monitoring changes in FMD can help assess the response to interventions aimed at improving endothelial function, such as lifestyle modifications and pharmacotherapy.

Conclusion

Integrating PWV and endothelial function assessments into routine clinical practice offers significant benefits for early identification and management of high-risk men. These non-invasive tests provide valuable insights into arterial stiffness and endothelial health, which are critical determinants of cardiovascular risk. By identifying subclinical vascular dysfunction early, healthcare professionals can implement targeted preventive strategies, improving outcomes and promoting longevity.

Further Reading

1. Vlachopoulos C, Aznaouridis K, Stefanadis C. Prediction of cardiovascular events and all-cause mortality with arterial stiffness: a systematic review and meta-analysis. J Am Coll Cardiol. 2010;55(13):1318–27.
2. Mitchell GF, Hwang SJ, Vasan RS, Larson MG, Pencina MJ, Hamburg NM, et al. Arterial stiffness and cardiovascular events: the Framingham Heart Study. Circulation. 2010;121(4):505–11.
3. Gokce N, Keaney JF, Hunter LM, Watkins MT, Nedeljkovic ZS, Menzoian JO, et al. Predictive value of noninvasively determined endothelial dysfunction for long-term cardiovascular events in patients with peripheral vascular disease. J Am Coll Cardiol. 2002;41(10):1769–75.
4. Yeboah J, Crouse JR, Hsu FC, Burke GL, Herrington DM. Brachial flow-mediated dilation predicts incident cardiovascular events in older adults: the Cardiovascular Health Study. Circulation. 2007;115(18):2390–7.
5. Yoon HJ, Hong YJ, Kim JH, Park HW, Kim SY, Kim YJ, et al. Combined assessment of brachial-ankle pulse wave velocity and flow-mediated dilation is more predictive of the presence of coronary artery disease than either alone in patients with chest pain. Circ J. 2012;76(6):1463–71.

Index

Vasan S S et al. (eds.), *Men's Health*, https://doi.org/10.1007/978-3-031-76898-9

GPSR Compliance

The European Union's (EU) General Product Safety Regulation (GPSR) is a set of rules that requires consumer products to be safe and our obligations to ensure this.

If you have any concerns about our products, you can contact us on ProductSafety@springernature.com

In case Publisher is established outside the EU, the EU authorized representative is:

Springer Nature Customer Service Center GmbH
Europaplatz 3
69115 Heidelberg, Germany

Batch number: 10732090

Printed by Printforce, the Netherlands